Community Surveys of Psychiatric Disorders

Series in Psychosocial Epidemiology

Volume 4

Series Editor

ANDREW E. SLABY, M.D., Ph.D., M.P.H.

Series in
Psychosocial
Epidemiology

Volume 4

Community Surveys of Psychiatric Disorders

Edited by
Myrna M. Weissman,
Jerome K. Myers,
Catherine E. Ross

Rutgers University Press
New Brunswick, New Jersey

Library of Congress Cataloging in Publication Data
Main entry under title:

Community surveys of psychiatric disorders.

(Series in Psychosocial Epidemiology; V.4)
Bibliography: p.
1. Mental illness. 2. Epidemiology. 3. Mental health surveys. I. Weissman, Myrna M. II. Myers, Jerome K. (Jerome Keeley), 1921— . III. Ross, Catherine E., 1953— . [DNLM: 1. Mental disorders—Occurrence. 2. Psychiatric status rating scales. W1 PS79E v.4 / WM 100 C7341]
RC455.C618 1986 362.2'0422 83-237045
ISBN 0-8135-1054-6
ISBN 0-8135-1055-4 (pbk.)

Manufactured in the United States of America

Contents

Introduction to Studies in Psychosocial Epidemiology

The rising costs of mental health care and interest in the development of a national health insurance that should include some mental health services have heightened concern both for ways by which health planners may evaluate the extent of behavioral problems and for means to assess the efficacy of various treatment modalities. Questions of paramount importance include: If there are two or more ways to treat an illness, which is the more effective? If two therapeutic modalities are equally effective, which is the more efficient? If two treatments are equally efficient, which is less costly?

Questions regarding the prevalence and incidence rates of specific psychiatric illness in communities are also being raised by those responsible for making policy recommendations for primary prevention and treatment programs. What is the natural history of an untreated behavioral problem, and how is the problem affected by normal growth and development? What does the natural history of a disorder of mood, thought, and behavior tell us about its etiology, and how may it lead to methods of prevention? If an illness is not preventable by currently available knowledge, what interventions may be made in its natural history to arrest and possibly reverse its course? Mental health is now big business and failure to look at specific population needs when planning programs and to build in ways of evaluating cost-efficiency effectiveness results in considerable psychological and economic cost to millions of patients and their families as well as taxpayers in general.

Epidemiology includes a number of technical skills that may be put to use in answering some of the questions facing health planners today. Traditionally, epidemiology has been seen as the study of disease patterns in populations. Epidemiologists have provided data that have led to effective prevention programs for a number of infectious diseases including malaria, smallpox, and poliomyelitis. Epidemiology has, however, played a minor role in psychiatric research until relatively recently. Epidemiologic studies in mental health have tended to be descriptive and focused on the prevalence and incidence of symptoms in broad categories of illness such as "neuroses" or "psychoses." Some infectious and chronic disease epidemiologists, in fact, question whether epidemiology can be used to tackle psychiatric problems. The Society for Epidemiologic Research does not have a section on psychosocial epidemiology, and publication of papers in social and psychiatric epidemiology in the main journal of epidemiology is infrequent. Principal organs of dispersion of knowledge in psychosocial epidemiology have been *Psychological Medicine* and the *Archives of General Psychiatry.* The former journal, published quarterly, has editorial board members who are sophisticated in epidemiology, and it probably publishes the greatest number of articles in this area. However, it is a British journal with limited readership in the United States. On the other hand, the *Archives of General Psychiatry,* a publication of the American Medical Association, is fairly widely read in the United States. It publishes a number of high quality papers in epidemiology, but its broad mandate limits its ability to publish more in the field of mental health.

The *Series in Psychosocial Epidemiology,* of which this is the fourth volume, serves several important functions for epidemiology, psychiatry and related areas in public health. The objectives include: (a) providing a forum for discussion of research strategies in the evaluation of mental health problems in the community and assessing effectiveness of psychiatric treatment interventions; (b) serving as a teaching tool for students in medical schools and schools of public health, hospital administration, social work, and nursing as well as for students in departments of psychology, sociology, and especially epidemiology; (c) keeping prospective researchers alert to problems needing investigation in the area of psychosocial epidemiology; (d) serving as a vehicle to bring together research in the area of psychosocial epidemiology; (e) providing a means of continuing education for epidemiologists working in the field; and (f) providing a means for discussions on how the results of epidemiologic and related behavioral research might be brought to bear on the development of State and Federal health policy decisions.

To achieve these ends, we have chosen a format that gives each monograph a theme of particular interest to investigators in the field of psychosocial epidemiology, such as the study of children, the study of stressful life events, and needs assessment. For each volume of the series we will choose a guest editor with an established reputation in the field to direct the selection of the individual contributors and write the introductory article. In general, the lead article will contain a discussion of methodological considerations in research of a given area (i.e., experimental design, sampling, instruments used, analysis of data, economic considerations, and ethical decisions in planning studies); a critical review of existing studies; information on the current state of the field; and suggested directions for further research.

Volumes in the series to follow this one on community surveys include ones on needs assessment, genetics, aging, alcohol use, ethics of epidemiologic research, drug use, and the methodology of natural experiments. Earlier volumes in the series focused on studies of children, stressful life events, and help-seeking behavior. Barbara Snell and Bruce P. Dohrenwend, Felton Earls, Carl Eisdorfer, Stanislav V. Kasl, David Mechanic, Jerome Myers, Lee N. Robins, Catherine E. Ross, Marc Schuckit, Laurence R. Tancredi, Ming T. Tsuang, George Warheit, and Myrna M. Weissman are the guest editors. In addition to the introductory article and papers selected by investigators in the field, whenever possible, each issue will contain an editorial appearing as the Afterword written by a representative of the World Health Organization (WHO) and an Introduction written by the series editor. The WHO representative, chosen by Dr. Norman Sartorius, Director of the Division of Mental Health, will focus on what is being done internationally in the topic area discussed, what should be done cooperatively and independently to advance the field, what WHO feels are research priorities in the field, and what particular methodologic problems in research in the area exist in pretechnological and Third World nations. I will direct my Foreword to the present state of epidemiological research in the area, the directions the Center for Epidemiological Studies at the National Institute of Mental Health would like to see research take, and the relationship of research in the field to the formulation of health policy.

The mandate of this series is challenging and the task is great. However, with the help of guest editors and other contributors, and with feedback from our readers, the series can fulfill the need for an organ to draw together researchers, students, and health policymakers in an effort to reap conclusions from research in psychosocial epidemiology that will lead to effective and consumer-responsive health policy and programs of preventive psychiatric care.

A.E.S.

Foreword

Case studies, laboratory (experimental) studies, and population studies are the main means used to ascertain associations of phenomena, especially causes and effects in mental disorders. The method essential to epidemiology is the population study, yet this procedure is shared with other sciences that study populations. What epidemiologists have in common with other disciplines are surveys, if the term is used in a broad sense. The degree to which there is convergence and divergence with other disciplines was stated best by Susser (1973): "In saying that elaboration of the 'survey' method is the core of epidemiologic method, we affirm its common ground with the other disciplines involved in the study of society. States of health do not exist in a vacuum apart from people. People form societies, and any study of the attributes of people is also a study of the manifestations of the form, the structure, and the processes of social forces. On the other hand, epidemiology's segregation from other studies of society, in its choice of states of health as dependent variable, gives it common ground with other medical sciences. It differs from other medical sciences in that the unit of study is populations and not individuals" (p.6).

Data obtained from community surveys are important both in obtaining some understanding of the extent of the need for mental health services in a population and in determining factors that may influence use of services when a patient is symptomatic. Severity of symptoms alone, as we have learned in Volume Three of this series *(Symptoms, Illness Behavior and Help-Seeking,* edited by David Mechanic), do not explain all or even the majority of the variance of help-seeking. Prevalence and incidence rates obtained from surveys can be misleading. A health planner unsophisticated in psychosocial epidemiologic strategies may assume naively that presence of illness behavior or symptoms may imply distress or need for services. This is not necessarily so. Many of the elderly depressed members of tightly knit ethnic groups may not seek help despite the presence of symptoms and distress. In addition, individuals with substance use disorders, clearly "mental illness" as defined in the *Diagnostic and Statistical Manual* of the American Psychiatric Association (DSM-III), may not complain of distress nor have significant impairment of functioning on commonly used instruments for measuring psychosocial distress and impairment. Community surveys raise one's consciousness to the fact that health care providers must see the whole person in the whole situation (to use Adolph Meyer's phraseology) to understand who needs, what is needed, and why.

"One use of surveys is descriptive, to set out norms and limits of the distribution of variables in numerical terms. Surveys quantify the attributes of populations, of environments, and of periods of time. They provide an understanding of a selected problem, its size, its nature, among whom and where it is to be found, and, indeed, whether the problem exists. In epidemiology, these are the distributions of states of health referred to in our original definition of epidemiology. A second use of surveys is explanatory or analytical—to compare different populations in relation to environments and trends in time and to account for the variations between them. In epidemiology this is the study of the determinants referred to in our definition." (Susser, 1973, pp. 7-8.)

The purpose of the epidemiologic endeavor is well presented in the charge from the President's Commission on Mental Health to the members of the Task Panel on the Nature and Scope of the Problems:

> Accurate estimates of the burden of illness and appreciation of the realistic potential for prevention have significant bearing on the allocation of resources for research, services and training of appropriate manpower to help ease the illness burden in future years.
> In order to promote mental health effectively and to treat or cure existing mental illness, it is necessary to have knowledge of the full range and magnitude of serious psychological disorder in the population. It will be the task of this group to report figures for the incidence and prevalence of overt mental illness in the total population. It will also be useful to report some comparative figures for socially significant sub-sets of the population, for example, in relation to socioeconomic status, age, sex, etc. (Dohrenwend, et al., 1980, p. 1)

And, indeed, in the *Report to the President from the President's Commission on Mental Health* (1978 Vol. 1, p. 49) it is stated, "Long-term epidemiological and survey research are necessary to understand the incidence and scope of mental disorders in this country. The need for more precise demographic and socioeconomic data is urgent if we are to understand and meet the different needs which exist in our society."

As Kramer (1976) points out,

> However, annual systematic morbidity statistics on the incidence and prevalence of the mental disorders as a group, or of individual disorders within the group, do not exist for the U.S. or any other country. Major impediments to their development continue to be the absence of standard case-finding techniques that can be used in a uniform and consistent fashion in population surveys to detect persons with mental disorder, and reliable differential diagnostic techniques for assigning each case to a specific diagnostic category with a high degree of reliability. As stated by MacMahon (1967): "No problem of definition in medicine is more baffling than that of defining mental illness." (p. 188)

Because these problems are so paramount in psychiatric epidemiology, the editors of this volume devoted five excellent chapters in addition to their introductory chapter to the issue of "Defining a Case." It would be naive to think that the problems besetting mental health epidemiologic survey research would be totally resolved by new instruments such as the Schedule for Affective Disorders and Schizophrenia (SADS), Psychiatric Status Examination (PSE), or the NIMH Diagnostic Interview Schedule (DIS). Nevertheless, as such instruments are used, assessed, and improved they do possess the potential not only of providing the much needed incidence and prevalence data for specific mental disorders but a better insight into the disease process which should improve our ability to define as well as detect a case.

Overall, the selections presented in the Survey section can be summarized as a delight regardless of one's discipline or orientation. To read Lemkau is to be made aware of what used to be called shoe-leather epidemiology. Despite the need for modern techniques in survey research, something is sacrificed when the principal investigators have not absorbed the flavor of the area or gained an intimacy with the people being studied.

To read Dunham is to appreciate how human were the participants in studies we now classify as classics and to realize the ubiquitous presence of serendipity in many of these endeavors. Also, we agree with Dunham that the Chicago study served "as a catalytic agent for initiating what has been a continuing dialogue between psychiatrists and sociologists."

Space does not permit reference to the several other studies now considered classics nor to the few reports representing "the new kids on the block." It is essential, however, to call attention to the Jablensky chapter, for it alone is worth "the price of admission."

Even while we are critical of the methodologies and findings of many of these studies, each survey represents on the part of the principal researchers an enormous expenditure of time, intellectual (and often physical) energies, and challenge to their careers. Such dedication and perseverance warrants respect.

A.E.S.

References

Dohrenwend, B. P., Dohrenwend, B. S., Gould, M. S., Link, B., Neugebauer, R. & Wunsch-Hitzig, R. (1980), *Mental Illness in the United States.* New York: Praeger.

Kramer, M. (1976), Issues in the development of statistical and epidemiological data for mental health services research. *Psychol Med,* 6:185-215.

The President's Commission on Mental Health (1978), Report to the President, Vol. 1. Washington, D.C.: Government Printing Office.

Susser, M. (1973), *Casual Thinking in the Health Sciences: Concepts and Strategies of Epidemiology.* New York: Oxford University Press.

Community Surveys of Psychiatric Disorders

Chapter 1

Community Studies in Psychiatric Epidemiology: An Introduction

MYRNA M. WEISSMAN
JEROME K. MYERS
CATHERINE E. ROSS

Community studies have a long tradition in psychiatric epidemiology. Beginning with the pioneering work of Jarvis in 1855 (Jarvis, 1971), such studies have contributed increasingly to our knowledge of the extent and nature of psychiatric disorder. In the future, community studies should contribute even more toward achieving the goals of psychiatric epidemiology—the identification of the risk factors associated with the development of disorders, the determination of the incidence and prevalence of the disorders, the identification of preventive strategies, and the planning of mental health services.

Identifying the risk factors associated with various disorders is the first step in the search for etiology. Risk factors are those characteristics associated with an increased probability of becoming ill. The characteristics associated with being ill at any one time, recovering slowly, or relapsing can also be identified.

After risk factors are isolated, laboratory experiments are often necessary to determine the specific mechanisms associated with increased risk. Thus a statistical cause may be shown to be a true cause (Robins, 1978). But even if the specific mechanisms associated with developing mental disorders are not isolated in the laboratory, other goals may be met. By determining the incidence and prevalence of mental illness in the community and the groups which are most at risk, preventive measures may be taken to reduce the risk factors, and mental health facilities may be planned to fit the needs of the community.

Parts of this chapter have previously appeared in "Epidemiology of mental disorders: Emerging trends in the United States" by M. M. Weissman and G. L. Klerman (1978), *Arch Gen Psychiatr* 35:705-712. Copyright American Medical Association.

The fit between the actual rates of mental disorder in the community and mental health service utilization has been examined by Regier and his colleagues (Regier et al., 1978). A conservative estimate of the current annual prevalence of mental disorders in community populations is 15%. Yet, in any given year, only 20% of the people with a psychiatric disorder (or 3% of the population) are being treated for mental illness in the professional mental health sector. An additional 3% are in nursing homes or general hospitals, 54% see primary care physicians on an outpatient basis, and 22% receive no medical care (Regier et al., 1978). Because persons with mental disorders have contact with primary care physicians does not mean that they are being adequately or appropriately treated for their disorder. Given the sizable proportion of persons with a mental disorder, most of whom are only seeing primary care physicians, Regier et al. (1978) suggest that more integration of general health and mental health care sectors is needed. They also suggest that primary health care providers be trained in mental health. These suggestions provide an example of the uses of information gathered from community studies. However, the figures reported by Regier et al., (1978) are rough estimates of overall prevalence of psychiatric impairment. Information is needed on both the prevalence and the incidence of specific psychiatric disorders including both treated and untreated cases. Such information is currently being collected in several ongoing large-scale community epidemiologic studies (see chapter by Eaton et al., this Monograph).

Community Studies Versus Treated Rates

Arriving at actual incidence and prevalence rates of specific mental disorders is a difficult task, dependent primarily on case definition and case location (Manis et al., 1964). Two ways to locate cases are the patient census (that is, counting persons in treatment) and the community survey. The patient census often takes case definition as given: anyone in psychiatric treatment is a case. The procedure of counting persons in treatment as cases has many problems. First, different psychiatrists often use different diagnostic concepts, and this means the diagnoses may not be reliable. Next, the persons in treatment are not a random sample of all persons with mental disorders. Many persons with psychiatric problems never reach the mental health treatment sector (Regier et al. 1978), and those who do reach treatment may be different from those who do not. Treated rates are contaminated by social characteristics that determine utilization of psychiatric services, self-referral versus referral by others (including police or courts), recognition of symptoms, or the length of time the disorder is present before treatment is administered. In addition, both the length of stay in a hospital or readmissions to a hospital influence treated prevalence rates. In terms of outpatient treatment, persons may be in treatment for a longer or shorter time depending not only on their illness but also on the psychiatric orientation of the therapist. Thus, simply counting treated cases provides biased, unreliable information on the actual rates of disorders.

The community sample provides information on the actual rates in the community, but it makes case definition problematic. No longer is a case defined as anyone who seeks treatment and receives a diagnosis from a psychiatrist. Instead, impairment or symptom scales measuring specific psychiatric diagnoses are used. Impairment or symptom scales are objective, reliable, and economical, and they avoid the problem of differences in psychiatric judgment (see chapter by Langner, this Monograph). Moreover, they do not distinguish between different diagnoses, and in fact may not capture many categories of severe mental illness (Weissman and Klerman, 1978). The newer, more diagnostic specific instruments now being used in clinical settings can be used by nonpsychiatrists to determine rates of psychiatric diagnoses in the community. These rates, in conjunction with rates of persons being treated in institutions, provide the best estimates of actual prevalence and incidence. The rates of persons in institutions such as mental hospitals, nursing homes, or prisons must be added to the community rates so the most serious cases are not missed. These rates of persons in institutions should be determined by the same diagnostic specific instruments that are used in the community. If the same objective diagnostic schedule is administered to persons in various communities and institutions over time, comparisons of rates of mental disorders over time and among different cultures can be obtained. As will be shown, the range of such information is not yet available, but substantial progress is being made (see Chapters 2-6).

The History of Community Studies in Psychiatric Epidemiology in the United States: Pre-World War II

In 1855 Edward Jarvis conducted the first study of the prevalence of psychopathology (Jarvis, 1971). By surveying key informants, including general practitioners, clergymen, and community leaders, and examining hospital and other official records, Jarvis attempted to determine the frequency of idiocy and insanity, the two major nosological distinctions of the time. In so doing, Jarvis hoped to determine the etiology of mental disorders. The key-informant methodology was used by Lemkau et al. (1942) in the Eastern Health District of Baltimore in 1933 and 1936, and by Roth and Luton (1943) in Williamson County, Tennessee in 1935. Lemkau et al. (1942) supplemented the information from the key informants with direct interview data on the frequency of "nervousness" (Weissman and Klerman, 1978) (see chapter by Lemkau).

Although it was not a community study, in the 1930s Farris and Dunham (1939) examined the ecological distribution of first admissions to mental hospitals in Chicago. They found that the highest rates of first admissions for schizophrenia were concentrated in the central city; in the areas that were deteriorated, lower class, and characterized by social disorganization and social isolation (see chapter by Dunham).

These pre-World War II methodologies—key informants and hospital records—had a number of limitations. Case ascertainment was incomplete and probably biased. Behavior that was obvious and disturbing to the community, such as personality disorders or schizophrenia, was likely to be reported, while depression or anxiety was probably less noticeable and less troublesome and therefore less likely to be reported. In addition, little attention was given to the reliability or validity of diagnosis in these studies (Weissman and Klerman, 1978).

World War II and After

World War II had a major impact on the development of psychiatric epidemiology. The Selective Service System rejected large numbers of men for psychiatric reasons, and this focused public attention on the magnitude of mental problems in the community. Also, rates of psychoneuroses in soldiers who had previously been screened and declared psychiatrically well fluctuated in relation to the amount of combat stress present. Because these psychiatric reactions occurred in men who had already been screened for mental disorders, it was concluded that stress can precipitate mental illness. The emphasis on the role of stress in the etiology of mental illness remained strong in the post-World War II epidemiologic studies. In addition, the military put considerable effort into developing neuropsychiatric screening and impairment scales. Results on these standardized scales could be statistically related to the amount of combat stress. Modifications of these impairment scales were used in community studies after the war.

After World War II, community surveys employed face-to-face interviews with large random samples of subjects. Such direct procedures ensured that all study subjects would be evaluated, and made possible more thorough and unbiased counts of total prevalence. These studies concentrated on social and cultural influences on mental health. Srole et al. (1962), for example, were interested in the stressful impact of urban life on mental health. They interviewed more than 1,000 adults selected by probability sampling in midtown Manhattan (see chapter by Srole and Fischer). Leighton et al. (1963) sampled 1,600 residents of Stirling County in rural Canada to evaluate the stressful impact of social change on mental health (see chapter by Murphy). Both studies found high rates of mental impairment, as did Gurin et al. (1960) in their nationwide survey of mental health. Such community surveys assumed an underlying unidimensional concept of mental health and did not differentiate between various categories of mental disorder. All of them based impairment ratings on symptoms derived from sources such as the Neuropsychiatric Screening Adjunct developed during World War II, the Cornell Medical Index, and the MMPI. Most such studies utilized short symptom scales that were easy to administer, standardized, objective, and reliable.

Both the Midtown and the Stirling County studies, however, employed more lengthy procedures to judge psychiatric impairment. Although nonpsychiatrically trained interviewers administered standardized interview schedules, psychiatrists later reviewed and evaluated the protocols, judging the degree of impairment, severity of symptoms, and the likelihood that a respondent would be a "case" if given a full diagnostic evaluation. As with symptom scales, specific diagnostic categories were not used, and cases were identified by the degree of nonspecific impairment. Moreover, while the symptom questions were standardized, the evaluations made by the psychiatrists were not. Thus, there was uncertainty as to the reliability of the psychiatrists' judgments.

The importance of these post-World War II studies should not be underestimated for a number of reasons. First, attention was given to the social and cultural influences on mental health. These influences included stress, social change, anomia, and social class. Previously the impact of the social environment on mental health had been de-emphasized. With the new attention given these social variables, more sophisticated approaches to their measurement were developed. Second, it was recognized that there is no single cause of mental disorder. Third, the survey methods produced complete probability samples. Finally, the use of impairment scales produced standardized, reliable information that could avoid problems of diagnostic unreliability, expensive and time-consuming use of psychiatric interviews of all subjects, or reliance on variable records of treated patients.

At the same time pioneering work was being done in community studies, Hollingshead and Redlich (1958) were conducting research that established the importance of social class as a determinant of treated mental illness (see chapter by Hollingshead). A 10-year follow-up of their study by Myers and Bean (1968) reaffirmed the Hollingshead and Redlich findings. These studies had limitations because they examined only treated mental illness. On the other hand, community studies faced the limitations associated with using impairment scales that assumed an underlying unitary dimension of mental illness rather than examining distinct diagnostic categories. The respective limitations of the two types of studies indicated the need for an objective and reliable diagnostic schedule that could be used in the community. The importance placed on social factors as the primary cause of mental illness had two implications. First of all, it reinforced the concept of the dependent variables as unitary (coded from low to high impairment), thus obscuring the heterogeneity of psychiatric disorders. The underlying theory was that the more stress present in the social environment, the greater the impairment. Next, it meant that other possible causes such as genetics, birth defects, infections, nutrition, early childhood experiences, or biological variations were de-emphasized. Thus, although one strength of the post-World War II studies was the introduction of social causation, this was also a weakness in that genetic and biological factors were ignored.

After the initial postwar studies, many community studies were done in which objective impairment scales were administered to a random community sample (Myers et al., 1971; Warheit et al., 1973; Dohrenwend and Dohrenwend, 1969) (see also chapters by Warheit et al. and Dohrenwend et al.). These studies did not have psychiatrists judging the impairment scales for their caseness. Instead, the impairment scales were used either as interval variables with no case designation, or an objective cutoff point was used above which a subject was designated as a case. While this method eliminated the problem of unreliability, the problem of validity remained. What, if any, portion of the spectrum of mental illnesses did these scales capture? Let us examine the characteristics of the impairment scales used in these community studies in more detail.

Impairment Scales

Impairment scales (also called symptom scales) are checklists of symptoms. The symptoms are added together and the resulting score indicates the degree of impairment. Some of these scales, such as those developed by Langner, MacMillan, and Gurin, measure overall impairment (see chapter by Langner). Others, such as the Center for Epidemiologic Studies-Depression scale (CES-D), measure specific symptoms.

Development and Validity

During World War II, the Army was faced with the problem of how to screen out recruits who would break down under the stress of combat. They needed to develop procedures for identifying psychological disorder among individuals who had never been treated (Dohrenwend et al., 1977). A questionnaire was developed which contained over 100 questions in 15 scales, yet one of these scales provided as good a discrimination between active soldiers and soldiers hospitalized for neurosis as did all 15. This was the psychosomatic scale, which later became the core of the Neuropsychiatric Screening Adjunct (Dohrenwend et al., 1977). This psychosomatic scale differentiated between inductees who were rejected on the basis of psychiatric interviews and those who were accepted. This method of seeing whether the impairment scale differentiates between a "known-ill" and a "known-well" group became the basic procedure for validating psychiatric impairment scales.

After World War II considerable work was done on the development of short screening scales that could be used in community studies. Two of the best known are the MacMillan index and the Langner index. Most work has been done on validating the Langner 22-item screening scale (see chapter by Langner). This scale is a shortened version of the list of 120 symptoms of emotional disorder used in the Midtown Manhattan Study (Srole et al., 1962). These 120 items, in turn, were chosen from the Neuropsychiatric Screening Adjunct and the MMPI. The 120-symptom checklist was administered to a "known-well" and a "known-ill" group. The "known-well" group was selected on the basis of interviews with psychiatrists, and the "known-ill" group was composed of psychiatric patients.

The 22 items that comprise the Langner scale distinguished between the patient and the normal group at $p < 0.01$ (Langner, 1962; Shader, 1971). In addition to discriminating between patients and normals, the 22-item index demonstrated a fairly high correlation (0.41-0.79) with the overall judgments of impairment made by the psychiatrists in the Midtown Manhattan study (Langner, 1962). This suggests that the psychiatrists considered these symptoms to be somewhat important in their ratings of impairment. Langner also found that 28% of the nonpatient group, 50% of the ex-patients, and 60% of the current outpatients in the Midtown Manhattan study reported four or more of the 22 symptoms (Langner, 1962). Langner chose the cutoff point of four or more symptoms because it captures only 1% of the respondents categorized as well by the psychiatrists, and 84.4% of the respondents categorized as incapacitated. The incapacitated group showed serious symptoms and high impairment in social functioning.

Manis and his associates (1963) have also validated the Langner index. They found that persons in the receiving ward of a psychiatric hospital had much higher scores (6.1) than predischarge ward patients (2.8), college students (3.6), and community respondents (2.8). The predischarge ward patients had scores that were equal to the community group and lower than the college students. This indicates that the scale probably captures acute rather than enduring traits. This conclusion is reinforced by the findings that the Langner scores fluctuate with life events (Dohrenwend, 1967; Myers et al., 1972). Manis et al. (1963) conclude that persons who score above 10 on the Langner index have a very high probability of being mentally ill, but it does not necessarily follow that all mentally ill persons receive high scores and all well persons receive low scores. It is also not clear that a high Langner score means the same things for psychiatric patients as it does for persons in the community (Seiler, 1973).

The fact that impairment scales differentiate *between* patient and nonpatient populations has been the basis for the claim that the scales are valid. But what exactly do they measure? Do they capture psychiatric disorder in untreated populations? Langner states that his index does not capture organic brain-damaged persons or sociopaths, but implies that it will screen other mental disorders. Other researchers modify this claim. Dohrenwend et al. (1977) state that although impairment scales may distinguish between patients and nonpatients, they do not make finer distinctions *among* groups of patients. Within a group of patients or within a group of nonpatients, impairment scales will not indicate the relative amounts of the full spectrum of psychopathology. In addition, the scales are not diagnostic; they do not identify subtypes of psychiatric disorder.

According to Dohrenwend and Crandell (1970) and Seiler (1973) the symptoms in the Langner index indicate mild forms of psychological disorder. Thus many mild symptoms summing to a high score are not necessarily indicative of serious mental illness. The index only differentiates between mild forms of mental illness, and in fact may not capture serious disorders at all. Dohrenwend and Crandell (1970) find evidence for this in the findings that outpatients scored higher than inpatients. Muller (1971) found that neurotics scored higher than psychotics. In addition to capturing only mild forms of psychological disorder, the scale may also pick up persons who are physically but not psychologically ill since the scale contains many psychophysiological and physiological symptoms. (The impairment scales were developed in large part from the psychosomatic sub-scale of the Neuropsychiatric Screening Adjunct.) It may best screen those persons who express their psychological distress in somatic terms. It may not capture those persons who express psychological distress in terms of aggression or hostility.

Therefore, it may be able to capture distress as women traditionally express it, but be less sensitive to the masculine expression of psychological disorder (Philips and Segal, 1969). In addition, there are two dimensions of mental illness: symptomatology and role functioning. The impairment scales do not measure the latter aspect of disorder at all.

Response Bias

Extraneous factors may also influence the number of symptoms reported. Respondents may consciously over or under-report symptoms in order to influence the readers of the symptom scale (the Army, a work organization, etc.) one way or the other. In addition, some groups may find the symptoms less undesirable and therefore be more likely to report them. Dohrenwend and Dohrenwend (1969), for example, attribute the findings of high Langner scores among Puerto Ricans to the fact that they do not think the symptoms are as undesirable as others do. Similarly, Philips and Segal (1969) attribute the high scores of women to response bias, although Clancy and Gove (1974) find no evidence for this assertion.

The Symptom Checklist-90 Items (SCL-90) and the Center for Epidemiologic Studies Depression Scale (CES-D)

Other symptom scales include the SCL-90 and the CES-D. The SCL-90 includes constructs measuring somatization, obsessive-compulsive behavior, interpersonal sensitivity, depression, anxiety, hostility, phobic anxiety, paranoid ideation, and psychoticism. This checklist has been validated by finding a high degree of convergence between its nine dimensions and those of the MMPI (Derogatis et al., 1976).

The CES-D is a 20-item, self-report symptom rating scale designed to measure depressive mood in the community. The scale was used in household surveys in Missouri and Maryland, sponsored by the Center for Epidemiologic Studies (Comstock et al., 1976; Radloff, 1977). In terms of validating the scale, it was found that acutely depressed patients (as determined by clinical judgment) scored the highest on this scale, followed by recovered depressives, alcoholics and drug addicts, and schizophrenics. The normal community sample scored the lowest (Weissman et al., 1977). Since this symptom scale differentiates between the depressed and other psychiatric populations, it is not simply measuring overall psychiatric impairment.

Strengths and Weaknesses of Impairment Scales

In summary, Langner (1962) originally developed the 22-item index as a screening instrument measuring psychiatric impairment. This scale can be used to screen candidates for further examination of mental illness or to assess gross symptomatology of various subgroups in order to get clues as to the etiology of mental disorder (Langner, 1962). According to Langner, the index provides a "rough indication of where people lie on a continuum of impairment in life functioning due to very common types of psychiatric symptoms" (Langner, 1962, p. 269). It does not screen persons with organic brain damage, the mentally retarded, or sociopaths. Over the years other researchers have examined and modified the original claims. Less critical attention has been paid to the Health Opinion Survey developed by MacMillan (1957) for the Stirling County Study and later modified by Gurin et al. (1960), although Seiler (1973) states that the criticisms of the Langner index also apply to the MacMillan and Gurin indices.

Impairment scales have limitations. They do not differentiate between categories of psychiatric disorder, and, in fact, may be better at capturing the milder forms of disorder than the serious forms. They may also pick up persons with physical problems unrelated to psychiatric disorder. Furthermore, they do not measure role functioning and may be weak in capturing masculine forms of psychological disorder. Also, different racial or ethnic groups may express their distress in different forms. Thus high scores on the impairment scales may mean different things in different cultures. This is one form of response bias. Social desirability, differential desirability of the symptoms, and yea-saying are others. These extraneous factors might affect scores on the impairment scales. If a cutoff point is used to differentiate cases from noncases, it is not clear which is the best cutoff. It depends on whether the researcher would rather err on the side of calling well persons impaired or impaired persons well. In addition, although the scales differentiate between "known-well" and "known-ill" groups, scale scores cannot be used to rank order the degree of mental illness among respondents (Seiler, 1973).

The limitations of the impairment scales do not mean they are not useful. The limitations simply alert researchers to the appropriate use of the scales. Although symptom scales do not differentiate specific psychiatric disorders, they are good measures of reactions to stress, including chronic social stressors such as low social class and social isolation, and acute social stressors such as life events (Myers et al., 1971, 1972, 1974). This response has been called reaction to psychological stress (Seiler 1973), demoralization (Dohrenwend et al., 1977), or psychological distress, and it is best measured as an interval level variable.

Researchers may also use the scale as a screening device in which respondents who score over a certain level are more extensively interviewed. In this case a cutoff point is established, and the scale is made dichotomous.

Researchers are beginning to solve some of the problems associated with impairment scales, such as the presence of physical symptoms and response bias. Symptom scales may be broken down into subindices that isolate physiological symptoms, psychological symptoms, or psychophysiological symptoms (Crandell and Dohrenwend, 1967). This allows researchers to separate the purely psychological symptoms from those that include physical problems. Other researchers have begun to examine the problems of response bias in the impairment scales (Philips and Segal, 1969; Clancy and Gove, 1974). Gove and his associates (1976) have found that response styles, including the belief that symptoms are undesirable, the tendency to give socially desirable answers, and the tendency to yea-say or nay-say, do not account for the effects of race, sex, income, education, or marital status on psychological distress. Furthermore, the estimated effects of these variables are not seriously biased when the three response styles are left out of the equation (Clancy and Gove, 1974; Gove et al., 1976).

Case Definition: Diagnostic Instruments

While impairment scales are reliable and easy to administer, they do not differentiate between specific psychiatric disorders. In the 1960s, advances in the fields of psychopharmacology, genetics, psychopathology, and neurobiology indicated that mental illness is not a unitary phenomenon and that diagnostic categories needed to be differentiated (Weissman and Klerman, 1978).

Research in genetics strengthened evidence for the biological as well as the psychosocial factors in the causation of mental illness. The studies by Heston (1966) and those done in Scandinavia by Mednick et al. (1974) and Rosenthal and Kety (1968), using the cross-rearing adoptive technique, established the high likelihood that genetic factors are involved in schizophrenia. In the 1960s, independent research groups in the United States, Europe, and Scandinavia studied primary affective disorders and found that by dividing their population into unipolar and bipolar groups based on the presence of a history of manic episodes, strong familial associations could be found that supported a genetic transmission for the primary affective disorders, especially the bipolar forms (Perris, 1966; Winokur et al., 1969; Angst, 1966; Leonhard et al., 1962).

Studies in psychopharmacology demonstrated that the new psychotropic drugs, which had been shown to have varying neuropharmacologic modes of action, had different patterns of clinical efficacy, explainable partially by diagnostic types. For example, schizophrenic patients responded to phenothiazines whereas depressed patients responded to tricyclic antidepressants, and the bipolar subtype of affected patients showed response to lithium carbonate. These findings supported the concept that psychiatric disorders were discrete and heterogeneous and prompted reevaluation of diagnosis (Weissman and Klerman, 1978).

By the mid-1960s, there was growing awareness among clinicians and researchers that the absence of an objective and reliable system for description of psychopathology and for psychiatric diagnosis was limiting research. Since psychiatrists were using different criteria in their classifications, this led to unreliability and noncomparability across diagnoses made by different psychiatrists. In addition, it was time-consuming and expensive to have psychiatrists give clinical interviews in the community. Reliable diagnoses of community respondents were needed. Spitzer and Endicott and their associates, in an attempt to develop reliable psychiatric diagnoses, identified five sources of unreliability in diagnoses (Spitzer et al., 1975; Spitzer and Fleiss, 1974): *(a)* the patient actually has different conditions at different times; *(b)* the patient is in different stages of the same conditions at different times; *(c)* the clinicians have different sources of information; *(d)* the clinicians, presented with the same stimuli, differ in what they observe; *(e)* the formal inclusion and exclusion criteria the clinicians use to summarize patient data into psychiatric diagnosis differ. Standardized, specified diagnostic schedules were developed to reduce these sources of variance. A structured clinical interview was developed to elicit the patient's signs and symptoms in a systematic fashion in order to reduce variance due to differing interview styles and coverage. Operational definitions with specific inclusion and exclusion criteria were developed to reduce criterion variance, the largest source of error (Endicott and Spitzer, 1978; Spitzer et al., 1978; Feighner et al., 1972). And two schedules were developed, one for current episodes and one for lifetime disorders, in order to reduce the error due to changes in the patient's condition over time (see chapter by Williams et al.).

Historically, before the publication of the first Diagnostic and Statistical Manual of Mental Disorders (DSM-I) in 1952, clinicians seeking guidance on the criteria for diagnosis relied on textbooks and articles that described typical cases (Spitzer et al., 1975). The DSM-I and DSM-II reduced unreliability due to varying diagnostic criteria but did not eliminate it. There are a number of reasons why unreliability remained a problem. There were no formal definitions of the diagnostic categories. It was not clear which features were usually, but not necessarily, present and which needed to be present for a diagnosis. Nor was it clear which features distinguished one condition from similar conditions, or which conditions were mutually exclusive. And even when concepts were clear, there were no operational definitions of the concepts (Spitzer et al., 1975).

Research Diagnostic Criteria (RDC)

Because of these inadequacies, efforts were made to develop explicit criteria and classification schemes. Work begun at the Washington University School of Medicine by Feighner, Robins, and their colleagues (1972) was later modified and elaborated by Spitzer, Endicott, and their colleagues into the Research Diagnostic Criteria (RDC) (Endicott and Spitzer, 1978; Spitzer and Fleiss, 1974; Spitzer et al., 1975; Spitzer et al., 1978).

The RDC, developed in conjunction with the latest Diagnostic and Statistical Manual (DSM-III), has 25 major diagnostic categories, many of which are divided into subtypes. The RDC explicitly specifies inclusion and exclusion criteria, which refer either to symptoms, signs, course of illness, or levels or severity of impairment. Terms are defined. Criteria are based on their ability to predict outcome, response to treatment, or familial association. This information comes from past research. Other criteria are based on clinical experience. Special attention was given to reliability, to the extent that a clinical feature traditionally used in making a diagnosis would not be included in the criteria if reliable judgments of it could not be made. For example, blunted affect, which is traditionally a criterion of schizophrenia, was not included. In addition to an emphasis on reliability, the Research Diagnostic Criteria decrease the probability of false positives. All diagnoses are judged as either not present, probable, or definite. Thus researchers may choose different degrees of certainty. There is also a category for "other psychiatric disorder" in which patients with obvious psychiatric disturbance who do not meet the criteria for any of the specific diagnoses can be placed. (Approximately 5% of an inpatient group are in this category.) This increases the likelihood that a patient will be incorrectly placed in the "other" category, although he has a specific disorder. This is in contrast to traditional approaches in which patients are often placed in specific categories although they do not belong there. Spitzer et al. (1975) feel the consequences associated with false positive diagnosis are worse than those associated with a false negative, since a false positive will lead to incorrect treatment that may be expensive or potentially toxic. On the other hand, a false negative only delays treatment, which they consider a minor cost.

The Schedule for Affective Disorders and Schizophrenia (SADS) is used to directly interview patients or community respondents in order to make an RDC diagnosis. With the SADS both a current diagnosis and lifetime diagnosis can be made. Each diagnostic category contains three components: symptoms, course (duration of episode), and impaired social functioning. The respondent must meet the criteria in all three components for a diagnosis to be present.

The reliability of the RDC categories has been most extensively tested with inpatients. Both interrater reliability and test-retest reliability were found to be high within the major diagnostic categories (Spitzer et al., 1975). Most reliability coefficients were higher than those reported in other research studies (Spitzer and Fleiss, 1974). Reliability was lower within the category subtypes but still satisfactory for research use. Although reliability has been tested less extensively with outpatients and community respondents, such testing is ongoing.

Preliminary Findings: RDC Diagnoses in the Community

Weissman, Myers, and their colleagues were the first to use the Research Diagnostic Criteria in a community study in order to obtain rates of specific psychiatric disorders (Weissman et al., 1978; Weissman and Myers, 1978) (see also chapter by Myers and Weissman). Weissman et al. (1978) found that 15.1% of the population had a probable current psychiatric disorder. Major depression was the most frequent disorder (the current rate of both definite and probable depression was 4.3%), followed by anxiety, minor depression, and alcoholism. The current rate of definite schizophrenia was 0.4%. No current cases of schizoaffective, manic hypomanic, or obsessive-compulsive disorders were found (Weissman et al., 1978). The lifetime rates of both probable and definite major depression were 20%, and those for minor depression were 9.2% (Weissman and Myers, 1978). There was also a high rate of multiple diagnoses: 46% of the subjects with a current major depression had one or more other current diagnoses, and 53% had one or more other past diagnoses. The most common additional diagnosis was alcoholism. Weissman and Myers (1978) also found that only about 25% of persons with a diagnosis had sought professional medical or psychiatric treatment in the past year.

Weissman and Myers (1978) also examined the risk factors associated with various RDC diagnoses. They found, for example, that rates of current major depression were higher in the lower social classes, but not significantly so. On the other hand, lifetime rates of major depression were higher in the upper social classes. Current minor depression was highest in the lower social class. Bipolar disorders were highest in the upper social class. Rates of all affective disorders were higher for women than for men. Although inconclusive, these risk factors may begin to give researchers clues to the etiology of specific disorders, and can help in the planning of mental health services.

Present State Exam (PSE)

In addition to the Research Diagnostic Criteria, another objective diagnostic schedule, the Present State Exam, was developed in England by Wing and his associates (Wing, 1976; Wing et al., 1974, 1978) (see also chapter by Wing). The Present State Exam (PSE) defines eight levels of psychiatric symptomatology. Level 1 is the absence of PSE symptoms. Levels 2 and 3 contain nonspecific neurotic symptoms. In level 4 specific symptoms are present, but there is insufficient information to justify an attempt at a clinical classification. Level 5 is the threshold level, at which a classification can be made. Levels 6, 7, and 8 are definite disorders which provide increasing degrees of certainty that the symptoms can be classified into a diagnostic category (Wing et al., 1978). These diagnoses correspond to those in the International Classification of Disease (ICD). At the threshold level and above, CATEGO, a computer program that classifies each case into a specific diagnosis, can be used. This program classifies cases in a purely standardized and objective manner. Both the PSE and CATEGO have been validated. Case identification based on the type, number, and severity of PSE symptoms correlated highly with independent global clinical judgment. Above the threshold level, CATEGO can, within limits, match broad clinical diagnoses such as schizophrenia, mania, or depression (Wing et al., 1978). The PSE has been used in community studies in the United Kingdom and in Africa.

Unlike the SADS (the interview schedule that gathers information to make an RDC diagnosis), which includes both a current mental status examination and lifetime diagnoses, the PSE primarily uses the current mental status examination. Both the SADS and the PSE depend primarily on direct observation and questioning of the respondent, although, unlike the PSE, the SADS also gathers information from multiple informants, increasing the likelihood of cross-validating information (Luria and Guziec).

Diagnostic Interview Schedule (DIS)

A third diagnostic instrument, the NIMH Diagnostic Interview Schedule (DIS), has recently been developed (see chapter by Robins). When the Division of Biometry and Epidemiology of the National Institute of Mental Health decided to launch a major program to assess the treated and untreated prevalence and incidence of specific psychiatric disorders in the general population, the need for a diagnostic instrument that could be taught quickly to a large number of lay interviewers became acute. At this junction, a group at Washington University had completed testing the Renard Diagnostic Interview (RDI), an instrument usable by nonpsychiatrists that allows computer scoring of lifetime diagnoses according to the explicit criteria described in Feighner et al. (1972). NIMH implemented a collaboration of Spitzer, Endicott, and Robins to produce an instrument based on the format of the Renard Diagnostic Interview, which would allow the application of criteria from the new Diagnostic and Statistic Manual (DSM-III), the RDC, and Feighner and would assess current as well as lifetime prevalence (Robins 1979).

According to its developers (Robins, Helzer, Croughan, and Spitzer), the DIS provides a more systematic and replicable format than prior diagnostic instruments. Its fully structured format means that lay interviewers can become proficient in its administration in a short time. Clinical judgment is minimal. Validity testing of the DIS is ongoing.

In addition to making both current and lifetime diagnoses, the DIS provides a flexible definition of current diagnosis, depending on whether the symptoms of each syndrome occurred within four time periods ranging from the last two weeks to the last year (and also the last three years for syndromes such as alcoholism, drug dependence, and antisocial personality, which are known to have a fluctuating or sporadic course).

Diagnoses are made by asking respondents whether they have had each of the criterion symptoms in their lifetime, and whether those symptoms met specified levels of severity. The criteria for severity include taking medication for the symptom, seeing a physician about the symptom, and having a symptom significantly interfere with one's life. In addition, the interview ascertains whether the symptom was explained entirely by physical illness or as a complication of the use of medication, illicit drugs, or alcohol. A number of additional factors can be determined from the DIS including the first-appearing diagnosis, number of nonoverlapping diagnoses, level of current functioning, history of treatment for psychiatric disorder and physical illness, and demographic characteristics.

This information will be useful both descriptively and analytically. Descriptively, the current and lifetime prevalence of specific diagnoses in the population can be ascertained. Analytically, the number of correlations can be examined. Do certain diagnoses tend to occur together? In what sequence do multiple diagnoses typically appear? What is the association between severity of the disorder and the likelihood of seeking treatment? What is the relationship between demographic factors and diagnosis and functioning? Do persons in remission from specific disorders continue to have impaired functioning? The DIS is being used in a multisite NIMH-sponsored epidemiologic catchment area study of the rates of psychiatric disorders in the community (see chapter by Eaton et al).

Work to be Done

These diagnostic interview schedules represent a significant advance for psychiatric epidemiology. They can be used in community studies and in clinical settings, and they can help integrate clinical and epidemiological studies. They reduce the unreliability of psychiatric diagnoses by providing explicit inclusion and exclusion criteria for making a diagnosis. Although most of the reliability studies have been done on inpatients, information on interrater and test-retest reliability is now being conducted in the community. Much work remains to be done on validity.

Although the validity of a classification is limited by its reliability, reliability *per se* does not establish validity. The usual approach to validity testing in psychiatry is to correlate the diagnostic classification with clinical judgment. Robins and Guze (1970, 1972) put forth additional methods for establishing diagnostic validity on a scientific basis. The methods identified were careful clinical description, delimitation from other disorders, laboratory studies, follow-up studies, family and genetic studies, response to treatment, and correlation with independent psychological or social variables. Studies such as these can help establish validity of diagnostic criteria through the correlation of these criteria with variables such as long-term outcome, response to treatment, and familial association.

Work is also progressing on sampling procedures, delimitation of independent variables, longitudinal studies, and the development of diagnostic schedules for children. Respondents should include random samples of the community, stratified community samples of persons especially at risk, and samples of institutionalized persons. Independent variables should be included to identify persons at risk. These variables, which should include social, genetic, biological, birth defect, nutritional, and psychological factors, may provide clues to etiology. In addition to a concern with sampling and the independent variables, researchers should continue work on longitudinal studies, such as those undertaken by Srole (1974) and Myers, Weissman, and their colleagues (Myers et al., 1971, 1972, 1974; Weissman et al., 1978; Weissman and Myers, 1978). These studies, which examine psychiatric disorder over time, can begin to establish under what conditions psychiatric disorders develop and how they change over time. Soon researchers will also be able to examine psychiatric disorders of children in the community since an epidemiologic version of the SADS is being developed for children (Orvaschel et al., 1982).

Summary

Future research in psychiatric epidemiology should be concerned with three factors: *(a)* the dependent variables, *(b)* the independent variables, and *(c)* the samples. Beginning with the dependent variables, emerging evidence from psychopharmacology, genetics, and psychopathology demonstrates the heterogeneity of psychiatric disorders. This heterogeneity should be reflected in the dependent variable. Since objective interview schedules such as the RDC, the PSE, and the DIS provide the most reliable rates of disorders in the community, diagnoses should be based on these instruments. Impairment scales may also be included as dependent variables in order to screen respondents for more intensive diagnostic evaluation. Although they do not measure discrete diagnostic categories of psychiatric disorder, impairment scales may be used to measure psychological distress or demoralization, especially in response to social stressors.

Turning to independent variables, there is no single cause of mental illness, and it is possible that factors from various realms may interact with one another. For example, genetic factors probably interact with the environment. Thus the independent variables should include social variables such as life stress, social class, social mobility, alienation, and childhood experiences as well as genetic and biological variables such as nutritional, hormonal, developmental, and prenatal.

Finally, samples must be taken from which actual incidence and prevalence rates can be extracted and risk factors identified. Thus random community samples are needed, in conjunction with institutional samples, in order to capture all persons with both mild and severe mental disorders. When these studies are longitudinal and the same persons are measured at certain time intervals, information on changes in disorders can be gathered. In addition, longitudinal studies bring the researcher closer to determining the causes of psychiatric disorders.

References

Angst, J. (1966), Etiological and nosological considerations in endogenous depressive psychosis. In: *Monographien aus dem Gesamtgebiete der Neurologie und Psychiatrie*, Berlin: Springer-Verlag, p. 112.

Baldessarini, R. J. (1975), An overview of the basis for amine hypotheses in affective illness. In: *The Psychobiology of Depression*, ed. J. Mendels. New York: Spectrum Publications, pp. 69-84.

Clancy, K. & Gove, W. (1974), Sex differences in mental illness: An analysis of response bias in selfreports. *Am J Sociol* 80:205-216.

Comstock, G. W. & Helsing, K. J. (1976), Symptoms of depression in two communities. *Psychol Med* 6:551-564.

Crandell, D. L. & Dohrenwend, B. P. (1967), Some relations among psychiatric symptoms, organic illness, and social class. *Am J Psychiatr* 123:1527-1538.

Derogatis, L. R., Rickels, K. & Rock, A. F. (1976), The SCL-90 and the MMPI: A step in the validation of a new self-report scale. *Br J Psychiatr* 128:280-289.

Dohrenwend, B. P. (1967), Social status, stress, and psychological symptoms. *Am J Public Health* 57:625-632.

Dohrenwend, B. P. & Crandall, D. L. (1970), Psychiatric symptoms in community, clinic and mental hospital groups. *Am J Psychiatr* 126:1611-1621.

Dohrenwend, B. P. & Dohrenwend, B. S. (1969), *Social Status and Psychological Disorder: A Causal Inquiry*. New York: Wiley.

Dohrenwend, B. P., Oksenberg, L., Dohrenwend, B. S. & Cook, D. (1977), What psychiatric screening scales measure in the general population. Unpublished manuscript, p. 10.

Endicott, J. & Spitzer, R. L. (1978), A diagnostic interview. *Arch Gen Psychiatr* 35:837-844.

Faris, R. E. L. & Dunham, H. W. (1939), *Mental Disorders in Urban-Areas: An Ecological Study of Schizophrenia and Other Psychoses*. Chicago: University of Chicago Press.

Feighner, J. P., Robins, E., Guze, S. B., et al. (1972), Diagnostic criteria for use in psychiatric research. *Arch Gen Psychiatr* 26:57-63.

Gove, W. R., McCorkel, J., Fain, T. & Hughes, M. (1976), Response bias in community surveys of mental health: Systematic bias or random noise? *Soc Sci Med* 10:497-502.

Gurin, G. J., Veroff, J. & Feld, S. (1960), *Americans View Their Mental Health*. New York: Basic Books.

Heston, L. L. (1966), Psychiatric disorders in foster home reared children of schizophrenic mothers. *Br J Psychiatr* 112:819-825.

Hollingshead, A. B. & Redlich, F. L. (1958), *Social Class and Mental Illness*. New York: Wiley.

Jarvis, E. (1971), *Insanity and Idiocy in Massachusetts: Report of the Commission on Lunacy, 1855*. Cambridge, MA: Harvard University Press.

Langner, T. S. (1962), A twenty-two item screening score of psychiatric symptoms indicating impairment. *J Health Hum Behav* 3:269-276.

Leighton, D. C., Harding, J. S., Macklin, D. B., MacMillan, A. M. & Leighton, A. H. (1963), *The Character of Danger: Stirling County Study*. Vol. 3. New York: Basic Books.

Lemkau, P., Tietze, C. & Cooper, H. (1942), Complaint of nervousness and the psychoneuroses. *Am J Orthopsychiat* 12:214-223.

Leonhard, K., Korff, I. & Shulz, H. (1962), Die temperamente in den familien der monopolaren und bipolaren phasischin psychosen. *Psychiatr Neurol Med Psychol* 143:416-434.

Luria, R. E. & Guziec, R. J., Comparative description of the SADS and PSE. Unpublished manuscript.

MacMillan, A. M. (1957), The Health opinion survey: Technique for estimating the prevalence of psychoneurotic and related types of disorders in communities. *Psychol Rep 3:325-339.*

Manis, J. G., Brawer, M. J., Hunt, C. L. & Kercher, L. C. (1963), Validating a mental health scale. *Am Sociol Rev* 28:108-116.

Manis, J. G., Brawer, M. J., Hunt, C. L. & Kercher, L. C. (1964), Estimating the prevalence of mental illness. *Am Sociol Rev* 29:84-89.

Mednick, S. A., Shulsinger, F., Higgins, J., et al., eds. (1974), *Genetics, Environment and Psychopathology*. New York: North Holland Publishing Co.

Muller, J. D. (1971), Discussion of Langner's psychiatric impairment scale: A short screening device. *Am J Psychiatr* 128:601.

Myers, J. K. & Bean, L. L. (1968), *A Decade Later: A Follow-up of Social Class and Mental Illness*. New York: Wiley.

Myers, J. K., Lindenthal, J. J. & Pepper, M. P. (1971), Life events and psychiatric impairment. *J Nerv Ment Dis* 152:149-157.

Myers, J. K., Lindenthal, J. J. & Pepper, M. P. (1974), Social class, life events, and psychiatric symptoms: A longitudinal study. In: *Stressful Life Events.*, ed. B. P. Dohrenwend & B. S. Dohrenwend. New York: Wiley.

Myers, J. K., Lindenthal, J. J., Pepper, M. P. & Ostrander, D. R. (1972), Life events and mental status: A longitudinal study. *J Health Soc Behav* 16:421-427.

Orvaschel, H., Puig-Antich, J., Chambers, Tabrizi, M. A. & Johnson, R. (1982), Retrospective assessment of prepubertal major depression with the Kiddie-SADS-E. *J Am Acad Child Psychiatr* 4:392-397.

Perris, C. (1966), A study of bipolar (manic depressive) and unipolar recurrent depressive psychoses. *Acta Psychiatr Scand* (Suppl) 194:1-189.

Philips, D. L. & Segal, B. F. (1969), Sexual status and psychiatric symptoms. *Am Soc Rev* 34:58-72.

Radloff, L. S. (1977), The CES-D Scale: A self-report depression scale for research in the general population. *Appl Psychol Measurement* 1:385-401.

Regier, D. A., Goldberg, I. D. & Taube, C. A. (1978), The de facto U.S. mental health services system. *Arch Gen Psychiatr* 35:685-693.

Robins, L. (1979), *Diagnostic Interview Schedule.* Developed under contract from the Center for Epidemiologic Studies, National Institute of Mental Health (ADAMHA), Rockville, MD.

Robins, L. (1978), Psychiatric epidemiology. *Arch Gen Psychiatr* 36:697-702.

Robins, E. & Guze, S. B. (1972), Classification of affective disorders: The primary-secondary, the endogenous-reactive, and the neurotic-psychotic concepts. In: *Recent Advances in the Psychobiology of the Depressive Illness,* ed. T. A. Williams, M. M. Katz & J. A. Schield. Washington, D.C.: U.S. Government Printing Office, pp. 283-293.

Robins, E. & Guze, S. B. (1970), Establishment of diagnostic validity in psychiatric illness: Its application to schizophrenia. *Am J Psychiatr* 126:107-111.

Rosenthal, D. & Kety, S. S. (1968), *The Transmission of Schizophrenia.* New York: Pergamon Press.

Roth, W. F. & Luton, F. H. (1943), The mental health program in Tennessee. *Am J Psychiatr* 99:662-675.

Seiler, L. H. (1973), The 12-item scale used in field studies of mental illness. A question of method, a question of substance, and a question of theory. *J Health Soc Behav* 14:252-264.

Shader, R. I., Ebert, M. H. & Harmatz, J. S. (1971), Langner's psychiatric impairment scale: A short screening device. *Am J Psychiatr* 128:88-93.

Spitzer, R. L., Endicott, J. & Robins, E. (1975), Clinical criteria for psychiatric diagnosis and the DSM-III. *Am J Psychiatr* 132:1187-1192.

Spitzer, R. L., Endicott, J. & Robins, E. (1978), Research diagnostic criteria: Rationale and reliability. *Arch Gen Psychiatr* 35:773-782.

Spitzer, R. L. & Fleiss, J. L. (1974), A re-analysis of the reliability of psychiatric diagnosis. *Br J Psychiatr* 125:341-347.

Srole, L. (1974), Measurement and classification in socio psychiatric epidemiology: Midtown Manhattan study (1954) and Midtown Manhattan re-study (1974). *J Health Soc Behav* 16:349-364.

Srole, L., Langner, T. S., Michael, S. T., Opler, M. D. & Rennie, T. C. (1962), *Mental Health in the Metropolis: The Midtown Manhattan Study,* Vol. 1. New York: McGraw-Hill.

Warheit, G., Holzer, C. & Schwab, J. (1973), An analysis of social class and racial differences in depressive symptomatology: A community study. *J Health Soc Behav* 4:291-199.

Weissman, M. M. & Klerman, G. L. (1978), Epidemiology of mental disorders: Emerging trends in the United States. *Arch Gen Psychiatr* 35:705-712.

Weissman, M. M. & Myers, J. K. (1978), Affective disorders in a U.S. urban community. *Arch Gen Psychiatr* 35:1304-1311.

Weissman, M. M., Myers, J. K. & Harding, P. S. (1978), Psychiatric disorders in a U.S. urban community: 1975-1976. *Am J Psychiatr* 134:459-462.

Weissman, M. M., Scholomskas, D., Pottenger, M., Prusoff, B. & Locke, B. (1977), Assessing depressive symptoms in five psychiatric populations: A validation study. *Am J Epidemiol* 106:203-214.

Wing, J. K. (1976), A technique for studying psychiatric morbidity in inpatient and outpatient services and in general population samples. *Psychol Med* 6:665-671.

Wing, J. K., Cooper, J. E. & Sartorius, N. (1974), *The Measurement and Classification of Psychiatric Symptoms.* London: Cambridge University Press.

Wing, J. K., Mann, S. A., Leff, J. P. & Nixon, J. M. (1978), The concept of a case in psychiatric population surveys. *Psychol Med* 8:203-217.

Winokur, G., Clayton, P. & Reich, T. (1969), *Manic Depressive Illness.* St. Louis: C.V. Mosby Co.

Part One

The Surveys

Chapter 2

The 1933 and 1936 Studies on the Prevalence of Mental Illnesses and Symptoms in the Eastern Health District of Baltimore, Maryland

PAUL V. LEMKAU

The interpretation of surveys of the prevalence of mental illnesses done in 1933 and 1936 requires an appreciation of the state of the art of psychiatric epidemiology at that time and of the setting in which the surveys were carried out.

Studies of the epidemiology of the mental illnesses before and during the early 1930s were based almost entirely on changes in hospitalized populations; very few data on patients outside hospitals had been collected. Tietze, Lemkau and Cooper (1943) summarized the few community based studies then available. These surveys were of relatively small European populations except for the Eastern Health District (EHD) studies reviewed here, and a sister study of a rural area, Franklin county, Tennessee (Roth et al., 1943). The EHD and the Tennessee studies were designed independently.

A number of events contributed to beginning work in the Eastern Health District of Baltimore. William H. Welch, the founder of the Johns Hopkins School of Hygiene and Public Health, had had military experience on the Mexican border and in World War I, which convinced him of the importance of mental ill health in the congeries of issues public health must grapple with. When Welch and Wickliffe Rose composed the Prospectus for the new school in 1917, mental hygiene was one of the subjects listed in which health officers were to be educated. Efforts were made to find a person to lead a mental hygiene group in the School's faculty from 1918, when it opened, and parttime faculty was employed to teach an elective course as early as 1921 (Lemkau, 1961). No scheme for establishing a research effort in the field could be found, however, until 1934.

Studies on the distribution of disease in the EHD had begun as a part of the National Health Survey. Adolf Meyer, then Professor of Psychiatry in the Medical School, insisted that mental ill health should be included in any such survey. He originated a study, carried out by Katherine Brown, of cases seen at the Henry Phipps Psychiatric Clinic of the Johns Hopkins Hospital, which demonstrated the clinical burden of mental disorders in the population of the District (Fairbank, 1937). Wade Hampton Frost, Professor of Epidemiology, and Allen W. Freeman, Professor of Public Health Administration, collaborated with Meyer in establishing an epidemiologic research group. Dr. Meyer released one of his senior staff, Ruth E. Fairbank, to head the group and Bernard E. Cohen, an experienced statistician, was recruited as the technically trained epidemiologist. Later, Elizabeth Greene joined the group as social worker to ease collaboration with agencies in which the cases were expected to be found. This team was replaced after a few years by Lemkau, Tietze, and Cooper, who were mainly responsible for the analysis and publication of the second (1936) survey. They also collaborated in the analysis of the data of the study established in Tennessee and based on the Medical School of Vanderbilt University.

The Setting of the Studies

The Eastern Health District of Baltimore was a service area of the Baltimore City Health Department developed cooperatively with the School as a service and field research population. The Department of Biostatistics of the School, chaired by Lowell J. Reed, was in charge of the repeated censuses of the area to establish the epidemiologic parameters of the population of the District. It also trained the public health nurse enumerators who investigated the presence of disease in the population. The availability of this basic data made the addition of studies on the prevalence of mental illnesses relatively easy. It also made it possible in most instances to relate discovered cases of mental disorders directly to families and individuals identified in the censuses (Downs and Simons, 1954).

The 1933 survey may be considered a pilot study in which case-finding and analytic methods were worked out for use in the more definitive second survey. For the most part, this review will present data from the 1936 survey. The following is a short-ended paraphrase of a description of the District made at the time of the 1936 survey:

The Eastern Health District is an area of about one square mile located in the northeastern quadrant of the city of Baltimore. The western part of the district touches one of the oldest areas of the city, Old Town. The homes in this section are the oldest and have the fewest modern conveniences. The eastern part is newer, showing the difference in its architecture, in the greater width of the streets, and in the larger number of trees that line them. The homes throughout the district are of the Baltimore row-house type; there are almost no detached dwellings in the area. At the western end, the homes are almost uniformly built of painted red brick; at the eastern end, there is more variation in material, and the rows are frequently set back and have small grass plots and front porches of various types.

The southern boundary street of the district is lined with small stores, cafes, saloons, and so forth, the buildings usually also serving as residences for one or more families. A similar situation prevails in the northwestern corner of the district. There is a rapidly growing business section close to the geographic center of the district along one of the important east-west streets. In this section the stores are newer and larger. There is some manufacturing, largely in the more open areas at the eastern end of the district.

The Johns Hopkins Hospital, Medical School and School of Hygiene and Public Health, and Sinai Hospital dominate the high ground in the central section of the district. These institutions draw many of their less skilled employees from people living in the district. The neighborhood immediately surrounding the hospital differs from the rest of the District in that medical students, physicians, and technical workers connected with the hospitals make up a significant part of the population (Lemkau, Tietze, and Cooper, 1941).

The population of the District was 55,129, 77% white and 23% black. The age distribution agreed closely with that for the urban population of the United States. There was an excess of blacks between the ages of 25 and 45, probably related to recent immigration. The District population was economically less well off than that of the U. S. urban population and blacks were considerably poorer than whites. The District consisted of Wards 6 and 7 of the City, with Ward 7 being north of Ward 6. It was also possible to divide the wards into census tracts and group these into four east-west divisions. Blacks made up a larger proportion of the population in Ward 7 than in Ward 6 (15.9 and 29.5%) and were concentrated in the western end of the District, the older area. The District also included areas of concentration of people of Jewish and of Czech extraction.

Sources of Cases

The questionnaire of the National Health Survey of 1936 contained a question asking whether anyone in the household was "nervous." Cases so reported were used in some analyses to be discussed later. Other cases were found by searching medical, social service, educational and police records for individuals with diagnoses or symptoms of mental disorder. The files of 43 different agencies were searched for cases, and 4,500 useful entries were identified. The number was reduced to 3,337 individuals by excluding duplications. Whenever medical diagnoses were included in case records they were accepted, the ones of latest date being used if there were more than one. Where no psychiatric diagnosis was included in the record and appeared justified the staff concluded on a diagnosis in conference, consciously tending toward understatement rather than overstatement in the translation from recorded symptoms to diagnosis. Multiple illnesses diagnosed (at the same time) in the same individual were retained.

Classification of Cases

In 1936, no less than at present, the classification of the mental disorders was unsatisfactory. The standard used for the 1936 survey was the Statistical

Manual for the use of Hospitals for Mental Disease of the American Psychiatric Association (A.P.A., 1934) so far as possible. It was, of course, not useful for the classification of much of the data originating with social, police, and to some extent, educational agencies, so certain new groupings were made.

Furthermore, the classifications used had to be arranged in a certain order so cases with more than one diagnosis could be dealt with. This was accomplished by setting up a hierarchy of diagnoses with more "serious" disorders being at the top of the hierarchy and those considered less serious at the end. The order was as follows:

Psychosis
Psychoneurosis
Psychopathic personality
Personality disorder (in adults)
Behavior disorder (in children)
Minor or possible disorder
Epilepsy
Mental deficiency
School progress problem
Adult delinquency

This method of classification allowed for the counting of individuals with one or more diagnosis for the calculation of overall rates of disorder, but also allowed the calculation of rates for each type of disorder. If a case were diagnosed, for example, as psychosis with mental deficiency, a not unusual diagnosis in Maryland Psychiatric hospitals in 1933 and 1936, it would be counted for overall rates as psychotic, but it could also be counted in calculating the rate of mental deficiency in the population.

The groups of illnesses included in each rubric of the hierarchy could be further broken down into more discrete diagnostic groups. Psychoses, for example, included 10 diagnoses from "schizophrenia and paranoid states" to "other" and "undiagnosed psychosis." This procedure allowed statistical analysis of the larger diagnostic groups while making it obvious that smaller ones were not suitable for such treatment.

The continuing problem of relating diagnoses in children to those in adults was apparent in 1936. It was resolved by making separate analyses (for some purposes) of the juvenile population. Since very few children were diagnosed before the age of 7 and the 17th birthday marked the end of the jurisdiction of the Juvenile Court in Baltimore at that time, and because the court had a psychiatric service furnishing useful data on some of its cases, the base population upon which rates of disorder for children was calculated was that of the ages 7 through 16 (Lemkau et al., 1943).

Results

The 3,337 persons included as mentally disordered in the 1936 survey of the EHD were distributed over the classification scheme as shown in table 1.

TABLE 1
Cases of Mental Disorders Active in 1936, by Leading Classification.[a]

Disorder	*Subtotals*	*Totals*	
Psychosis		367	
Psychoneurosis		171	
Psychopathic personality		30	
Personality disorder — in adults			
Psychotic traits	26		
Neurotic traits	60		
Psychopathic traits	13		
Behavior deviation	119	218	
Behavior disorder — in children			
Neurotic traits	162		
Conduct problems	287	449	
Minor or possible disorder			
"Nervous in census"	294		
"Police only"	17[illegible]		
All others	279	651	
Epilepsy	75		
Mental deficiency	375		
School progress problem	434		
Adult delinquency	567	1,451	
Total			3,337
All epileptics			126
All mental deficients			694

[a]*From* Lemkau et al., 1941.

It indicates that roughly 6% of the population of the EHD was identified as showing at least one deviation from a mentally healthy status as defined by the Study. Since earlier studies in the United States had been confined to the analysis of hospitalized cases only, this study may be seen as the beginning of the trend toward finding a significant proportion of the general population to be mentally disordered, a trend which perhaps culminated in the Stirling County and Manhattan studies where much larger proportions were reported (Leighton et al., 1962, and Srole et al., 1962).

Psychoses

The cases of psychosis discovered in the Survey of 1936 were distributed as shown in table 2. The prevalence rate of psychosis increased with increasing age from 0.2 per 1,000 in the age group 10 to 14 (one case) to 21.6

TABLE 2
Distribution of Psychotic Cases
by Type of Psychosis, Sex, and Race, 1936 Survey.[a]

	Distribution among				
Type of psychosis	*Males*	*Females*	*Whites*	*Blacks*	*Total*
Schizophrenia	79	799	140	18	158
Manicdepressive	13	28	36	5	41
Involutional	4	3	7	-	7
Senile and arterio-sclerotic	20	18	34	4	38
Alcoholic	10	5	9	6	15
Syphilitic	26	3	20	9	29
With epilepsy	9	-	9	-	9
With mental deficiency	10	18	18	10	28
Other	7	4	8	3	11
Undiagnosed	11	20	28	3	31

[a]*From* Lemkau et al., 1942.

at age 65 and over (58 cases). The rates for whites (blacks were too small in number to allow this analysis) were highest in the lowest and highest economic groups, with the mid-income group showing the lowest rate. Twenty-five percent of all psychotic cases were not in hospital; these were older than those in hospital and there was an excess of females in this group.

This study is believed to be the first in the United States to investigate the proportion of psychotic persons living in the community; thus it may have been one of the sources of concern which has reached a high level as hospital populations have been so markedly reduced since 1950.

The data also showed that blacks tended to be hospitalized for psychosis more often than whites, but that their stay was likely to be shorter. It was suggested that one factor in this situation might be a higher death rate for hospitalized blacks.

An incidence for all psychoses was calculated. For all cases it was 1.0 case per 1000 per year, with somewhat higher rates for males and blacks than for females and whites in this population.

The Neurotics

Four groups of cases had to be considered in addressing the issue of the prevalence and distribution of neurotic illnesses in the population. These were:

1. Psychoneuroses—cases seen and diagnosed by physicians (171 cases)
2. Adults with neurotic traits—Adults for whom individual symptoms or incomplete syndromes of the psychoneuroses were recorded (60 cases)
3. The "nervous in census"—cases who were reported or reported themselves as "nervous" and on whom no further information was available (191 cases)
4. Children with neurotic traits—as defined in the 1934 APA Statistical Manual (162 cases)

Group 4 was so obviously different in its distribution in the population (not only by age) that it was analyzed and discussed separately. The first three were found to have very similar demographic traits and were, for some purposes, treated as a single group (tables 11-14 in Lemkau et al., 1942).

The basis for this treatment is the epidemiologic principle that groups of patients with similar sex, age, economic and/or other demographic parameters may be assumed to have the same or similar diagnoses. So far as is known, this study represents the first time the principle was applied in the epidemiology of mental illnesses (Lemkau et al., 1942B).

Unlike the psychotics where the male/female ratio was not statistically different from 1/1, the adult neurotics showed higher rates for females and relatively low rates for blacks, as shown in table 3.

The white exceeds the black rate significantly. The rate for females is so much higher than that for males that there is only the remotest possibility that the difference could be accounted for by a sampling error ($p < 0.00001$).

In economic status white adult neurotics and psychotics were similarly distributed with an excess of cases at both ends of the economic scale, though the number of cases of higher income is too few to establish firm rates. This is, so far as is known, the first demonstration that the neurotic type of illness follows the trend of illness in general, namely, greater prevalence in economically deprived groups.

The Epileptics

All cases in which the records used the word "epilepsy" were counted under that classification. Where only the words "convulsions" or "fits" were entered on the records, the cases were not included. The latter were rare and were known in some cases to refer to hyperpyrectic convulsions in children.

A total of 126 cases of epilepsy was found. In 51 of these (40%), the records showed other personality problems in addition to the epilepsy. In 70 cases

TABLE 3
Distribution by Age and Sex of "Adult Neurotics" Discovered in 1936 Survey.

		Rate per 1,000 of the population		
	No. of Cases	*Crude*	*Adjusted*	*Standard*
White males	99	4.73	4.63	.47
White females	261	12.09	11.56	.73
Black males	19	3.11	3.44	.76
Black females	46	7.05	8.12	1.11
All whites	360	8.47	8.20	.43
All blacks	65	5.15	5.80	.68
All males	118	4.37	4.38	.40
All females	307	10.92	10.87	.62
TOTAL	425	7.71	7.71	.37

in which the intellectual status was known, 50 were mentally defective. Prevalence of epilepsy in 1936 was 2.3 cases per 1000 of the population. The illness was present somewhat more often in males than females.

The Mental Deficients

A total of 694 persons was found to be mentally deficient (IQ < 70). Of these, 326 or 47% had other personality disorders as well. Fifty-nine were psychotic, 8 showed psychotic traits, 50 were epileptic, 46 were in the "adult neurotic" group and the rest were scattered among other classes of cases.

Cases were classified by the then usual terms for severity of retardation: idiots, IQ < 25; imbeciles, IQ 25-50; morons, IQ 50-70. Idiots, so named in the records or classified by recorded IQ, numbered 25, imbeciles 111, four times as many, and morons 470, again about four times as many as the next more profoundly retarded group. Of the 694 cases of mental retardation recorded, only 88 were without a record of an IQ test indicating to some degree the intensity of psychological and psychiatric care available to the EHD population at the time of the surveys.

The age distribution of the mentally deficient cases showed high rates during the school period with markedly lower ones for adults. The highest rate, 43.6 per 1000, was found in the 10 through 14 age group. Table 4 presents this data. Differential death rates did not explain the "disappearance" of retardates in the adult years.

TABLE 4
Distribution by Race, Sex and Age
of Mental Deficients Discovered in 1936 Survey.[a]

	Distribution among					*Rate per 1000 of the general population*
Age Group	*Whites*	*Blacks*	*Males*	*Females*	*Total*	
0-4	3	-	3	-	3	0.7
5-9	33	23	37	19	56	11.8
10-14	108	131	137	102	239	43.6
15-19	75	84	96	63	159	30.2
20-24	29	9	14	24	38	7.2
25-34	61	16	32	45	77	8.1
35-44	47	22	28	41	69	8.3
45-54	30	9	20	19	39	6.4
50-64	8	1	1	8	9	2.6
65 and over	3	2	4	1	5	1.9
TOTAL GROUP	397	297	372	322	694	12.2

[a]*From* Lemkau et al., 1942.

The definition of retardation was for the most part on the basis of IQ tests, which were generally available only for children in school or recently in school. Thus low IQ scores brought a larger proportion of child cases to the attention of the agencies surveyed than did the ability to live in the community, which was test applied for adults.

Mental retardation is a condition usually regarded as present at birth, of relatively low incidence thereafter, and not subject to any marked changes in severity over the life span. Other surveys had noted the marked variation in prevalence rates by age and this one called renewed attention to the fact and eventually led to improved survey design to "flatten the curve" (Imre, 1967).

Mental Disorder in Children

As already noted, children (persons aged 7 through 16) could not be analyzed by the same scheme as the adults. To a considerable extent, this was because the diagnostic classification for children, then as now, was quite different from that of adults. Also, the public school system was the source of almost half of the child cases but not, of course, of any adult ones.

The population of the EHD between the ages 7 and 17 was 10,636, 19.3 percent of the total population. Records indicating mental health problems were found for 1,242 individual children (1,862 contacts). The APA Statistical Manual was used as the basis for classification of cases and resulted in table 5. Eighty-four percent of the 1,242 cases had IQ scores included in their records. Only four cases of psychosis, two males and two females, were recorded in children. All were above 15 years of age except a 12-year-old diagnosed as psychotic with mental deficiency.

TABLE 5
Distribution by Diagnoses of Active Cases
Seven through Sixteen Years.

Diagnosis	*Total cases with diagnosis*	*Cases with diagnosis as leading classification*
Psychosis	4	4
Neurotic traits	140	140
Conduct problems	371	311
Minor personality traits	62	56
Epilepsy	40	18
Mental deficiency	403	282
School progress problems without mental deficiency	592	431
TOTALS	1612	1242

Tables 6 and 7 present the data available on the children with neurotic traits and those with conduct problems, as the terms were defined in 1936 and used in the Survey. Neurotic traits were found to be more prevalent in white than black children. Unlike adults, however, neurotic traits (as defined in 1936) were not higher in females than in males. Speech and reading defects, however, showed almost five times as many cases among males as females, though the numbers were small.

The conduct disorders show a markedly different distribution. Blacks present significantly more cases than whites and males many more than females. The mean age of children with conduct problems is higher than for those showing neurotic traits. The prevalence of neurotic traits, conduct disorders, and mental deficiency in children 7-17 are all linked to family income: the greater the income, the fewer disorders in each case.

TABLE 6
Problems Presented by 140 Children (7-16) with Neurotic Traits, by Sex and Race.[a]

	Distribution among				
Problem	*Males*	*Females*	*Whites*	*Blacks*	*Total*
Temper tantrums	15	19	29	5	34
Eneuresis	16	15	23	8	31
Fears	11	15	18	8	26
Speech and reading defect	19	4	19	4	23
Nailbiting	11	9	17	3	20
Overactivity	7	8	15	-	15
Sleep disturbance	7	7	12	2	14
Feeding problems	3	5	8	-	8
Masturbation	6	1	7	-	7
Tics and habit spasms	2	4	6	-	6
Vomiting	2	4	5	1	6
"Nervousness"	15	21	32	4	36
Other	8	11	16	3	19
TOTAL PROBLEMS	122	123	207	38	245
Total cases	70	70	116	24	140

[a]*From* Lemkau et al., 1943.

Technical Note: The Index of Case Finding

Early in the 1933 and 1936 survey analyses it became apparent that prevalence for most disorders was higher in Ward 7, the more northerly section of the EHD, than in Ward 6. The finding was so consistent and arresting that it generated no end of hypotheses to explain it. While the puzzle was never completely cleared up it led to very close scrutiny of sources of bias. It was realized, of course, that families requiring economic assistance were subject to greater chances of having personality deviations recorded than were other families. Since more black than white families were poor, their rates for disorder were likely to be inflated. It was also possible to segregate the Jewish families using name indicators, and the Jewish population was found consistently to have higher rates of disorder than other groups. The suspicion arose that the social workers of the Jewish agencies

TABLE 7
Conduct Problems Presented by 371 Children (6-17) by Sex and Race.[a]

	Distribution among				
Problem	*Males*	*Females*	*Whites*	*Blacks*	*Total*
Violence against persons	14	1	9	6	15
Stealing	105	8	58	55	113
Miscellaneous delinquency	111	25	68	68	136
Truancy	62	27	52	37	89
Other school misbehavior	64	20	66	18	84
"Other problems"	29	35	44	20	64
TOTAL PROBLEMS	385	116	297	204	501
TOTAL CASES	279	92	221	150	371

[a]*From* Lemkau et al., 1943.

were more likely to record personality disorders than were the workers of the other agencies. The availability of the National Health Survey data offered an approach to these problems. Lemkau et al. (1942B) explained the approach as follows:

> We make the assumption that the number of cases reported in the National Health Survey by their relatives or by themselves as insane, nervous, epileptic, or in similar terms, represents a constant proportion of the "true" number of psychotics, adult neurotics, and epileptics in the district. These groups were chosen because in the aggregate they most nearly correspond to the layman's conception of mental and nervous diseases. To be sure, not all cases whose illness was active in 1936 were reported in the survey. The failure to report might be due to a variety of causes. The condition may not yet have been apparent; it may have been unknown to the informant, or the informant may have been unwilling to reveal it; or may have reported it under the name of some somatic disease. It is obvious that level of intelligence and of education might influence the extent and the correctness of reporting. Nevertheless, every informant had the same opportunity to report, and we make the assumption that the proportion reported is the same for all groups. We hasten to add that, while this assumption is plausible, there is no way of verifying it.
>
> The assumption made, the total number of cases found by all sources in any section of the population and identified in the household rosters of the National Health Survey is divided by the number of cases reported as insane, nervous, and so on, for the section in question.

> We thus arrive at a figure we have called the "index of case finding." Perhaps a fictitious example will make the procedure clearer: Suppose our 43 sources found 50 cases in Block No. 14. The National Health Survey enumerator received 25 reports indicating mental illness in that identical area. The index of case finding, then, is computed 50/25 = 2.00, which index would show that the coverage of our sources was exceptionally good in that area. In using the index, Block No. 14 of this example may be replaced by any other grouping, whether on the basis of geography, race, income, family size, and so forth, so long as the required comparable figures can be obtained (pp. 11-12).

This procedure, applied to the various subgroups of the population available, produced the data from which an Index of Case Finding was derived. Table 8 gives the data and indices.

It will be noted that the index rises with lowered socioeconomic status, indicating that more cases were recorded for the poor than for the better off. The high index for the Jewish ("Hebrew") population is very clear. Had the intensity of case-finding for Hebrews (index 2.47) been applied to the total population of the District, the number of cases discovered would have been 1035 rather than 658. A small subgroup of the Jews in the District were on relief; this group had an index of case-finding of 3.57. Such an intensity of case reporting would have resulted in 1496 cases, more than twice the number actually recorded.

A Note on the Prevalence of "Psychopathic Personality" in 1933 and 1936

The concept of a constitutionally determined tendency to anti- or asocial personality was strong in the 1930s. Such cases were considered to be unmodifiable by any treatment then known. The general concept appears to have derived from the notion of "degeneracy" and constitutionalism, which was then waning but still strongly represented in European and some American psychiatry. The diagnosis of psychopathic personality was usually based on the history of poor work record, frequent changes of life goals, repetitive delinquency, and relative absence of anxiety and guilt feelings. Drug addictions, alcoholism, and homosexual and other sex deviations were also considered symptomatic of psychopathic personality. The data on psychopathic personalities in the EHD in 1933 and 1936 are presented in table 9.

The rubric, Personality Disorder in Adults, Psychopathic Traits, was not used in 1933—the group so diagnosed in 1936 is added to the group diagnosed psychopathic personality for the purposes of this discussion. It will be noted that about one-third more such cases were diagnosed in 1933 as compared to 1936. The rates were 1.21 per thousand in 1933 and 0.78 per thousand in 1936.

TABLE 8
Psychotics, Adult Neurotics and Epileptics Found in all Sources and Identified in the National Health Survey;
Cases Reported in the National Health Survey as Insane, Nervous and Epileptic; and Index of Case Findings by Race, Ethnicity, Social-Economic Status of Household, Relief and Income.[a]

Group	*Cases found in all sources and identified in National Health Survey*	*Cases reported in National Health Survey*	*Index of case finding*
Total group	658	418	1.57
Whites	539	356	1.51
Blacks	119	62	1.92
Hebrew	89	36	2.47
Non-Hebrew whites	450	320	1.41
Socioeconomic status	56	38	1.47
Unskilled labor	155	98	1.58
Skilled labor	168	114	1.47
Clerical	74	49	1.51
Professional and business	62	41	1.51
Unclassified	24	16	-
Relief and income Relief	101	53	1.91
Non-relief under $1000	189	130	1.45
$1000-$1500	150	101	1.49
$1500-$2000	51	41	1.24
$2000-and over	38	25	1.52
Unknown	10	6	-

[a]*From* Lemkau et al., 1942B.

Whites only.

[b]Whites only.

TABLE 9
"Psychopathic Personality" in the Eastern Health District in 1933 and 1936.[a]

Cases active	*1933*	*1936*
Psychopathic personality	68[a]	30[b]
Psychopathic traits	-	13
TOTAL	68	43
Population	56,048	55,129
Rate/1000 population	1.21	0.78

[a]Cohen and Fairbank, 1933, p. 1160.
[b]Lemkau et al., 1941.

The explanation for the marked reduction of rate over a period of only three years is undoubtedly complicated. However, it will be recalled that inability to hold a job was one of the cardinal elements of the congeries of factors entering the making of the diagnosis of psychopathic personality during this period. It would appear that in 1933, still early in the Great Depression, it was not yet generally realized that the loss of a job was likely due to general economic conditions rather than individual pathology, while by 1936 a greater appreciation of the displacing effect of the Depression was clearly grasped. This appears to be one of the first pieces of evidence in the modern literature supporting the notion that social conditions strongly influence the prevalence of at least some psychiatric disorders.

Comment

This review of work done 40 years ago makes one feel he is engaged in a sort of intellectual archeology. The nomenclature is dated as are some attitudes underlying it. "Hebrews," for example, very rarely appears in the scientific literature of the 1980s. "Psychopathic personality," much used in Baltimore psychiatry in the 1930s, is now heard extremely rarely.

Methodology is also much different. So far as I can remember, it occurred to none of our group to test the reliability of the diagnoses made. By the end of the studies (dictated to a considerable extent by World War II, which broke up the research group) the conviction had been reached that dependence upon secondary sources such as psychiatric case records and social agency files would not suffice again, but systems for evaluation of the mental status of individuals in a population still lay in the future. The development of psychiatric case registers, indeed registers of any group of diseases, had hardly begun.

These studies did make certain contributions to the field of psychiatric epidemiology. The most important ones appear to me, in 1983, to have been these:

1. Attention was called to the relatively large proportion of psychotic persons living in the community.
2. The idea was generated that a group of psychiatric cases having the same demographic distribution as that of a diagnosed group of cases would have the same diagnosis.
3. The idea was generated that in surveys of psychiatric disorder in populations, the economically poor and certain other particularly intensively served groups will produce more cases than the general population and that methods can be devised under certain conditions to estimate the extent of bias this factor introduces.
4. The idea was generated that diagnoses that depend on social criteria may vary widely with general social conditions, in this case probably the realization by the diagnosticians of the effect of the Great Depression on the ability to hold a job.
5. Finally, the study demonstrated the advantages of having a relatively exact census of the population surveyed, and of its demography for use as the denominator in the calculation of prevalence for the various conditions diagnosed.

Acknowledgements

Dr. Christopher Tietze, presently with the Population Council, and the statistician with the group that did the 1936 survey, has read and commented helpfully on this review. These studies were supported by grants from the Rockefeller Foundation.

References

American Psychiatric Association, Committee on Statistics (1934), *Statistical Manual for the Use of Hospitals for Mental Disease.* Utica, N. Y.: State Hospital Press.

Downs, E. & Simons, K. (1954), Characteristics of psychoneurotic patients and their families as revealed in a general morbidity study. *Milbank Quarterly,* Jan. 1954.

Fairbank, R. E. (1937), Mental hygiene component of a city health district. *A J Publ Health* 27:247-252.

Imre, P. D. (1967), Mental Retardation in a Maryland County. American *Psychiatric Assn., Psychiatric Research Report 33.*

Leighton, D., Harding, J. S., Macklin, D. B., Macmillan, A. M., & Leighton, A. H. (1962), *The Character of Danger.* New York: Basic Books.

Lemkau, P. V. (1961), Notes on the development of mental hygiene in the Johns Hopkins School of Hygiene and Public Health. *Bull Hist Med* 35:169-174.

Lemkau, P. V., Tietze, C., & Cooper, M. (1942), Complaint of nervousness and the psychoneuroses. *Am J Orthopsychiatry* 12:214-223.

Lemkau, P. V., Tietze, C. & Cooper M. (1941), Mental Hygiene Problems in an Urban District. *Ment Hyg,* 25:624-646.

Lemkau, P. V., Tietze, C., & Cooper, M. (1942), Mental hygiene problems in an urban district. Second paper. *Ment Hyg* 26:100-119.

Lemkau, P. V., Tietze, C., & Cooper, M. (1942B), Mental hygiene problems in an urban district. Third paper. *Ment Hyg* 26:275-288.

Lemkau, P. V., Tietze, C., & Cooper, M. (1943), Mental hygiene problems in an urban district. Fourth paper. *Ment Hyg* 27:279-295.

Lemkau, P. V. (1956), Epidemiological aspects of mental deficiency. In: *Evaluation and Treatment of the Mentally Retarded Child in Clinics* New York: National Association for Retarded Children, Inc.

Roth, W. F. & Luton, F. H. (1943), The mental health program in Tennessee. *Am J Psychiatr* 99:662-675.

Srole, L., Langner, T. S., Michael, S. T., Opler, M. K. & Rennie, T.A.C. (1962), *Mental Health in the Metropolis.* New York: McGraw-Hill.

Tietze, C., Lemkau, P. & Cooper, M. (1943), A survey of statistical studies on the prevalence and incidence of mental disorder in sample populations. *Public Health Reports* 58:1909-1927.

Chapter 3

The Geographic Distribution of Functional Psychoses in Croatia, Yugoslavia: A Collaborative International Study

PAUL V. LEMKAU

In 1951, I was requested by the Yugoslav Government through the World Health Organization (WHO), to survey and report upon the mental health services of the country. After six weeks of intensive study and travel and three days of discussion with Yugoslav colleagues of a draft, a final report was published in English (Lemkau and Pavković, 1952). In the course of the survey, several areas inviting epidemiological research were noted, including the northern littoral of the Adriatic Sea and the islands of that region, which allegedly produced a relatively larger number of schizophrenics than did the rest of Croatia. In a preliminary opinion survey of 34 psychiatrists in Croatia, 32 believed this area produced an excess of cases (Lemkau et al., 1971).

In 1959, Branko Kesić, then director of the Andrija Štampar School of Public Health in Zagreb, suggested that research on the problem begin. There followed almost two decades of collaborative effort by the Andrija Štampar School, the Institute of Public Health of Croatia (personnel often holding appointments in both institutions), and the School of Hygiene and Public Health of The Johns Hopkins University, Baltimore.

The work falls into four segments. The first was a "quick and dirty" test to see whether hospital statistics supported the hypothesis that an excess of cases existed in what became the Study Area (fig. 1).

This study led to the question: "Are there sufficient psychotic persons living outside mental hospitals to account for different prevalence rates in the Study and Control areas?" To answer this question, two pilot studies were made. First, 100% samples of four communes (counties) were subjected to household interviews. Second, 22 cluster samples of households in Rijeka, a city in the Study Area, and of Zagreb, in the Control Area, were surveyed.

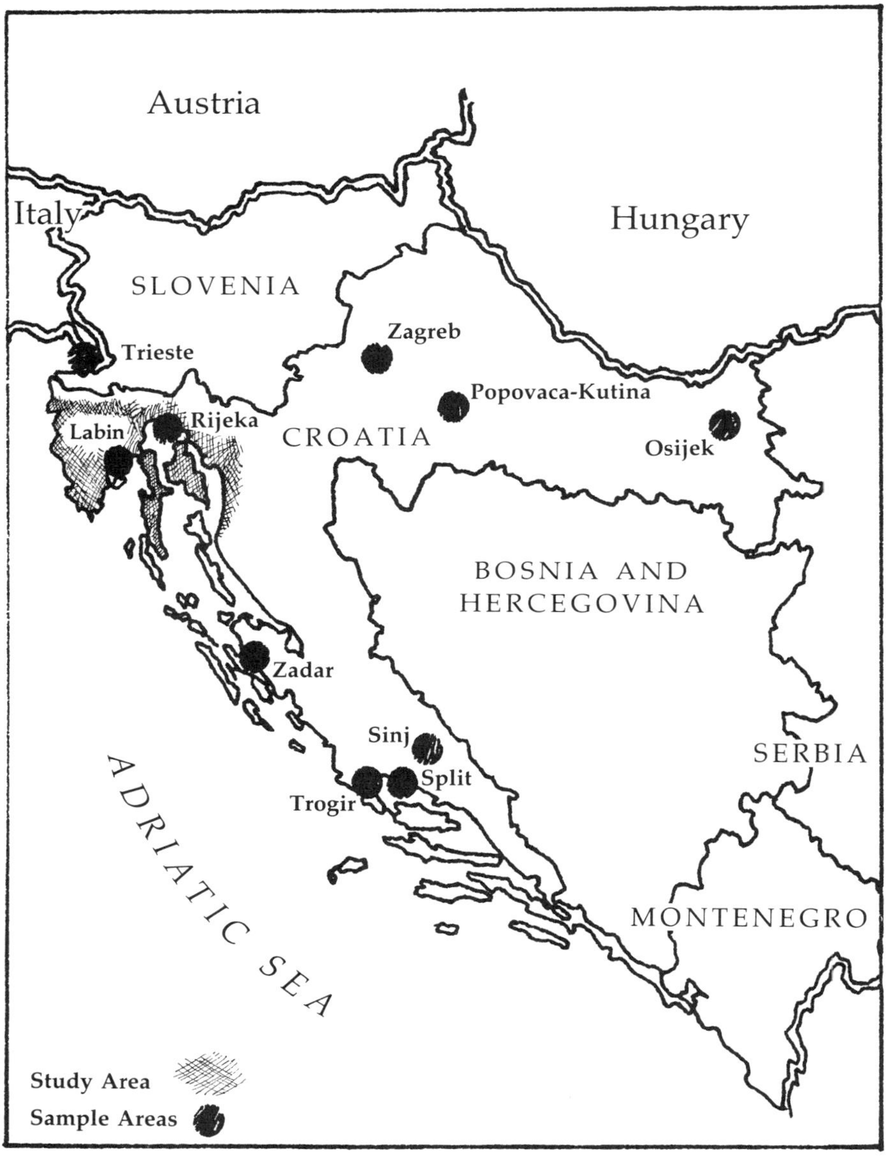

FIGURE 1
Geographic location of Croatia, showing bordering countries and Republics of Yugoslavia, Study and Control Areas and Areas involved in particular sub-studies.

Both these studies showed higher rates of functional psychoses in the Study Area, but neither could be said to be representative of the area in which they were situated.

Finally, a representative sample was constructed for the Study and Control Areas in the hope of reaching a conclusive answer to the question, "Is there an area of Croatia (Study Area) which has a higher prevalence rate for functional psychotic cases than the rest of Croatia (Control Area)?"

The Setting

Yugoslavia as a whole and Croatia in particular has a long and distinguished history in public health. The influence of Andrija Štampar, over many years a world leader in public health, led to the establishment of local and regional public health services combining curative and preventive medicine in a single authority. The view of public health was broad, including housing, nutritional, and agricultural policies as health issues (Štampar, 1966). The country developed a social security and health insurance program after World War II.

What is today Yugoslavia straddled the great trade routes between the Occident and Orient and its ancient history is marked by waves of conquest from the North, West, and East. The South Slavs gave the area its name.

Both Rome and Venice controlled ports on the eastern shore of the Adriatic and most of the area was part of the Roman Empire for a period. Split provided Rome with an Emperor, Diocletian, who returned home after his retirement and built the walled town that remains the core of that modern coastal city.

The Turks conquered the Serbian kings and ruled most of the eastern Yugoslav territory for 500 years. Napoleon controlled Western Yugoslavia (and most of the Study Area of this research) for a period. Croatia and other parts of Yugoslavia were part of the Austro-Hungarian empire from about the middle of the 19th Century to World War I. The Empire administered the various sections of the area under more or less separate administrative structures, as an attempt to control the political movement toward the unification of the South Slavs, a nationalistic ideal held ambivalently by many. After World War II, the union was accomplished, incorporating Slovenia, Croatia, Bosnia-Herzegovina, Serbia, Macedonia, and Montenegro (plus certain other provinces) into the Union of Socialist Republics. Zadar and Fiume became Yugoslavian, and Trieste was annexed to Italy after a plebiscite. The people were allowed individually to decide whether they wished to remain in Yugoslav territory and become Yugoslav citizens or to move to Italian territory.

The coastal areas have always supported a fishing and seafaring industry, while the great valleys of the Sava, Drava, and Danube are a part of the "breadbasket of Europe," with fertile alluvial valleys producing mostly small grains. The littoral is a karst formation geologically, with the typical sinkholes and caves. The topsoil is thin and, compared with the northern river valleys, infertile. Corn is the principle crop. There are mountains in the north of the country, the Dinaric Alps, and along the Adriatic limestone mountains rise dramatically from the sea. The Adriatic Islands, of which there are hundreds, are the tops of mountains that were not fully exposed as the Coast rose.

A land so often invaded has many population isolates. Geography dictated this on the Islands until petroleum made boat transport easy. In the south, there are Italian speaking towns; Italian speaking interviewers had to be trained to work in some communes in the Istrian Peninsula. There are also populations of Rumanians and Hungarians in the Republic, mainly in the north. There are dialects within the range of the Croatian language; at times accents were so different that students from Zagreb had difficulty being understood when pronouncing names in Istria (Lemkau and Kulčar, 1971).

Many of the items just listed militate against the suitability of the population for epidemiological studies. The population is not homogeneous. The geography and geology of Croatia are varied. Such items presaged difficulty in segregating factors responsible for differences in prevalence rates for functional psychoses even if they were to be discovered. Furthermore, at the time the studies were begun in the early 1960s, myths of marked differences in prevalence rates for mental illness were being exploded. Eaton and Weil had demonstrated that schizophrenia had about the same prevalence rate among the Hutterites as it did in surrounding populations (Eaton and Weil, 1955). A WHO study had exploded the notion that depression did not occur among Africans (Carothers, 1953). These reports led us to expect that initial findings would be negative and would preclude further research.

These factors were offset, however, by others that made the opportunity inviting. Public health services were highly organized, had strong leadership and welcomed collaborative research. Local health services proved willing to supply space for keeping records, provide field training of personnel, and arrange housing and board for interviewers. In addition, they frequently helped in transportation of interviewers and in finding households included in the sample. The local Red Cross health educational facilities were also helpful, particularly in the 100% sample studies, encouraging the local population to receive the interviewers and to furnish the needed information.

Croatia also offered a sophisticated medical record system that could be employed in the proposed studies. All hospital discharges were reported to the Institute of Health of Croatia. This made it possible to segregate psychiatric diagnoses and, after a special census of the population of psychiatric hospitals and the psychiatric wards of general hospitals, to construct a register of psychiatric cases who were or had been hospitalized because of psychiatric illnesses.

Finally, the political situation was favorable for epidemiologic studies. In general, the health officers enjoyed excellent relations with the political authorities so census data and, particularly, voters lists were made available for use in sample selection. The health officers, like the psychiatrists, had been trained for the most part in Zagreb so they had common traditions. This meant so far as health officers were concerned, receptivity toward field research and, for psychiatrists, relatively uniform systems of examination and diagnosis.

Although the situation was not ideal, the advantages appeared to more than offset the disadvantages and the decision was made that the research should be attempted.

Study of Hospitalized Patients

It will be recalled that according to the legend, it was schizophrenia that was supposed to be in excess in the Study Area. The study of hospitalized patients was nevertheless designed to consider all cases discharged from or resident in psychiatric hospitals as of the time of the survey.

Tables 1 and 2 show the results of the study of hospital discharges and of the census of patients in hospital, respectively. The tables indicate that the Study Area does have significantly higher prevalence rates for hospitalized psychoses than the control area. As already noted, this was an unexpected finding.

TABLE 1
Discharged Patients from Mental Hospitals and Psychiatric Wards of General Hospitals in Croatia by Residence in Study and Control Areas and by Age, 1965.

	No. of patients			*Rate per 10,000 population*		
Diagnosis and age (years)	***Study area***	***Control area***	***Total***	***Study area***	***Control area***	***Total***
Schizophrenia	330	1,706	2,036	7.92[a]	4.41[a]	4.76
< 15	-	6	6	-	0.06	0.05
15-19	12	56	68	3.58	1.71	1.88
20-39	152	912	1,064	11.72	7.67	8.06
≥ 40	166	732	898	11.13	5.40	5.97
All other psychoses	610	1,422	2,032	14.64[a]	3.68[a]	4.76
< 15	-	12	12	-	0.12	0.10
15-19	6	28	34	1.79	0.85	0.94
20-39	198	326	524	15.26	2.74	4.00
≥ 40	406	1,056	1,462	27.22	7.79	9.72
Total psychoses	940	3,128	4,068	22.56[a]	8.09	9.50

[a] $p < 0.001$

TABLE 2
Patients with Psychotic Illnesses in Mental Hospitals and Psychiatric Wards of General Hospitals in Croatia on August 15, 1962, by Residence in Study and Control Areas.

	No. of patients from Croatia		*Rates per 10,000 population*	
Diagnosis	***Study area***	***Control area***	***Study area***	***Control area***
Schizophrenia	321	1,763	8.1[a]	4.6[a]
All other psychoses	91	366	2.3[a]	1.0[a]
Total psychoses	412	2,129	10.4[a]	5.6[a]

[a] $P < 0.001$

A number of possible explanations for the finding were tested. The age-sex distribution of the Study and Control populations was not significantly different. Urban vs. rural living was not markedly different. Distances from psychiatric hospital or ward were not controlling. As already noted, most psychiatrists have been trained in a single center; differences in diagnostic practice did not appear very influential. The ratio of available beds to population was not remarkably different in the two areas. In summary, there appeared no sufficient reason to discount the finding of a significant difference in the prevalence rates for psychoses in the Study and Control areas.

It was disappointing, however, that the difference in rates between the Study and Control Areas was not confined to schizophrenia alone but extended to all psychoses as shown in table 2. Had the excess been confined to schizophrenia alone, the finding might have contributed to the detection of possible specific factors in the etiology of that disease complex. The finding, however, indicated that whatever was responsible for the difference in prevalence rates, it must apply to some general vulnerability to psychosis. Had the finding been otherwise, it could have led at once to the search for factors specific to schizophrenia.

The finding immediately raised the question of whether hospitalization practices in the two areas might be different, with the Control Area retaining more psychotic persons in the community and the Study Area tending to hospitalize more readily. Further studies were directed to answering this question.

Studies Identifying All Psychotic Patients

Development of Methods for Household Surveys

An initial attempt to find cases in the community through the use of key informants proved unpromising and was soon dropped in favor of direct interviewing in households. Because of the particular interest of local health officers, four communes were selected as pilot areas, Sinj, Trogir, and Popovača-Kutina in the Control Area and Labin in the Study Area (fig. 1).

A two-step case finding procedure was developed. Medical students (and a few advanced students in psychology) who were members of the Public Health Club of the Medical School of the University of Zagreb were recruited as interviewers. This club was established by Stampar to encourage field public health researches by students during vacation periods. It was well organized and had strong leadership. The Club agreed to supply interviewers who would attend training sessions during the school year and do field work in the project during the summer (Lemkau and Kulčar, 1980). Training consisted of familiarization with the symptoms of psychoses through the examination of hospitalized cases under the supervision of psychiatrists in conveniently placed mental hospitals, and instruction in the art of interviewing (Novosel, 1981). Local health officers taught the peculiarities of the dialect of their localities and the names used for mental symptoms and syndromes in the communes concerned.

Forms for the interviews were developed to allow uniform recording of findings for statistical analysis. Household interviewing in the closely knit families of Yugoslavia was found difficult because the interviews became the center of family conclaves with many distractions intruding upon the gathering of data. Training of the interviewers included experience in overcoming this difficulty.

The form employed for the household interviews was the result of numerous conferences by the study staff, in consultations with psychiatrists, social psychologists, sociologists, and public health personnel. It began with general questions concerning the health of family members and proceeded through questions concerning physiological symptoms (sleep, appetite, weight variations, headache, palpitation, etc.) to more specific psychiatric symptoms (Kovačić, Kulčar and Persić, 1981).

A census of the household preceded the household interview. In this wave, the adult considered most likely to be informed was selected as the informant. At the end of the interview, persons in the household suspected of being psychotic were noted. Instructions included urging inclusion of all possible suspects; usually two to three times as many suspects were identified as were later diagnosed psychotic by the psychiatrists. All suspects were interviewed by psychiatrists, either at the local health center or, if the patient would or could not come for the interview, at his home or elsewhere. The form the psychiatrist used to record findings was more detailed and specific as to psychiatric symptoms.

As the series of studies matured, the field team included statistical clerks who reviewed the forms of both household interviewers and psychiatrists daily and saw to it that errors and omissions were corrected. These statisticians also compiled records, checked that all households were covered, and kept the financial records. Responsible supervisors were recruited from more experienced interviewers. They assigned households to the interviewers and were available to work with refusals and other difficult cases.

Public health nurses, usually borrowed from the local health department, visited suspects and arranged the psychiatric examinations. In this process, they also collected information on the work history of the patient as well as other social and self-care information.

In the opinion of the staff, the use of medical students as interviewers implied their being collaborators in the research rather than merely data collectors and that they could not be denied knowledge of the hypothesis being tested. Having made this decision, this material was incorporated in their training. Thus the interviewers were not "blind" as to the object of the research. On the other hand, they did not know how rates were running from day to day, and the interviewing of the Control and Study Areas was done in two different years (in the final wave) so that bias introduced by knowing the object of the research was hoped to be minimal. In the initial wave of the field work, some effort was made to exchange interviewers between Study and Control Areas, but the transportation expense was too great for this precaution to be used in later waves.

The Communes Surveyed

Labin, a commune in the Study Area, contains the only large coal deposit in Yugoslavia. It lies on the east coast of the Istrian Peninsula (fig. 1) and, in addition to its mines, includes large agricultural areas. The population is predominantly Slavic and the rural population fairly stable. Miners, however, are recruited from many areas of Yugoslavia and make up a more transient population. A feature of Labin is that the main town is situated high on a hill which has begun to sink because of the removal of the coal that underlies it. It was still the administrative center of the Commune when this survey was done, but has since been abandoned, its suburbs having been extensively built up. It has a desirable coast and includes many tourist hotels and other services.

Trogir, a commune in the Control Area, lies on the Dalmatian Coast, about 20 kilometers northwest of the large city of Split. It is primarily an agricultural area but has considerable tourist trade. It is an ancient town with interesting Roman buildings and ruins juxtaposed to modern apartment houses and business structures.

Sinj lies about 30 kilometers east of Trogir behind the first range of coastal mountains. Although it has a river flowing through it from mountains in the north, irrigation is not used. It, too, is the site of an ancient Roman town; one can see stones carved by Romans built into the structure of much later homes. At the time of this study it had the lowest per capita income of the communes of Croatia.

Popovača-Kutina lies about 20 km east of Zagreb in the Sava valley. At the time of this survey it was largely agricultural, growing small grains, but has since become fairly heavily industrialized as a result of the discovery of oil and gas in the area.

Trogir was surveyed in 1964 and provided the first test of the instruments. Experience there led to their revision as well as development of the administrative structure needed to make the operation of field teams effective. Sinj and Labin were surveyed in 1965, and Popovača-Kutina in 1965 and 1966.

Results

To avoid the diagnostic problems inherent in dealing with psychotic adolescents and the aged, the studies were limited to cases occurring in the 20-64 age group. Table 3 gives the population concerned, the number of functional psychotic cases found, and the prevalence rates for the areas studied. It will be noted that the prevalence rate for Labin, in the Study Area, is much higher than for the three Control Area populations and that the probability of this being due to chance is < 0.001. Two to three times as many individuals were classified as suspects as received diagnoses of psychosis. The excluded individuals were usually diagnosed as alcoholic or neurotic by the psychiatrists. The prevalence rate for Labin is one of the highest recorded in the literature (Kulčar et al., 1971).

Of 132 psychotics identified in Trogir, 25 were without discoverable previous diagnoses; that is, they were newly discovered cases. Of 55 schizophrenics, only three were in this group, while 22 of 77 individuals with other psychotic diagnoses were previously unknown.

The data of table 3 include all known psychotic cases, whether active at the time of the survey or not. Table 4 presents data on cases active within the three-month period immediately preceding the survey date. These rates approach a point or period prevalence for these usually chronic conditions. Such data could not be prepared for the Popovača-Kutina area; this area is excluded from table 4 for this reason. Trogir and Sinj are geographically close to each other and both are in the Control Area. The data for them are combined in table 4.

There is a highly significant difference in the prevalence rates for the areas. The difference in rates for the functional psychoses, defined as the schizophrenic and manic depressive cases, is also highly significant. The category "all other psychoses" (other than functional as defined) shows prevalence rates for the Study and Control areas that are not significantly different.

This table also shows that age does not appear to be a factor in the prevalence of schizophrenia and paranoid states between the ages of 20 and 64. Manic-depressive and involutional disorders, on the other hand, are considerably more prevalent in the older age group.

There is no evidence whatever that Labin is typical of the Study Area or Sinj, Trogir and Popovača-Kutina of the Control Area. The surveys of these 100% samples, however, served to standardize and field test instruments for collecting data through home interviews and to develop an administrative structure to control the quality of the data collected.

TABLE 3
Suspected Psychotics, Verified Psychotics and Rates
Per 10,000 Population 20-64 years old only:
Total Accumulated Prevalence in Four Communities.

Community (survey year)	*Population surveyed: 20-64 years old only*	*Suspected psychotics*[a]	*Verified psychotics*[b]	*% of suspects diagnosed psychotic*	*Rate/10,000 20-64 years old only*
Labin (1965)[c]	15,756	627	253	40.8	160.6
Trogir (1694)[d,e]	9,592	262	92	35.1	95.9
Sinj (1965)[e]	26,734	531	215	40.4	80.4
Popovača-Kutina (1965-66)[d]	18,933	391	83	21.2	43.84

[a] Includes cases later determined to be outside predetermined age range and residence requirements for the study.
[b] Only cases within the definition of the research, that is, excludes those outside age range and residence requirements.
[c] Labin is in study area, Sinj, Trogir and Popovača in control area.
[d] Rate of psychosis, study area vs. control area: $\chi^2=31.169$, n=1, p 0.001
[e] Rate of psychosis, Trogir vs. Sinj: $\chi^2=1.7$, n=1, $p < 0.25$

TABLE 4
Number of Cases, Prevalence Rates[a] per 10,000 Population 20-64 Years of Age by Age Group: Statistical Significance of Differences by Age and Diagnostic Groups, Labin and Sinj-Trogir.

	Age group 20-39					*Age group 40-64*					*Age group 20-64*				
	Labin		***Sinj-Trogir***			***Labin***		***Sinj-Trogir***			***Labin***		***Sinj-Trogir***		
Diagnostic Group	*Cases*	*Rate*	*Cases*	*Rate*	*P*	*Cases*	*Rate*	*Cases*	*Rate*	*P*	*Cases*	*Rate*	*Cases*	*Rate*	*P*
300, 303 Schizo-phrenic & paranoid	56	64.4	53	26.6	0.001	60	84.6	52	31.7	0.001	116	73.6	105	28.9	0.001
301,302 Manic-depressive and involutional	8	9.2	7	3.5	0.10	30	42.3	16	9.8	0.001	38	25.1	23	6.3	0.25
304-309 All other psychoses	9	10.4	15	7.5	0.50	21	29.6	34	20.7	0.25	30	19.0	49	13.5	0.25
300-309 All psychoses	73	84.2	75	37.6	0.001	111	156.5	102	62.2	0.001	184	116.7	177	48.7	0.001
300, 301, 302, 303 "Functional psychoses"	64	73.9	60	30.1	—	90	126.9	68	41.5	—	154	97.7	128	35.2	0.001

[a] "Point prevalence" or "period prevalence" (see text for definition).

The test of the hypothesis that the Study Area really does have higher prevalence rates for functional psychoses, however, must rest on data collected from a representative sample population of the two areas.

The Cluster Sample and the Results of the Pilot Survey

The next survey wave was to have accomplished this for the whole of Croatia but the attempt had to be aborted. It served, however, for a further field test of the instruments and as a pilot project in sample construction as well as for developing techniques for entering households that were much less prepared than in the earlier waves. In the previous study, the total population was involved so the question "why me" did not have to be faced. Furthermore, complete coverage of the commune allowed use of the cooperating health department and its health officer, the political authorities, and the Red Cross. These assets could not be available when the sample population was scattered over the whole of Croatia and where, of two neighbors, one might be in the representative sample while the other was not.

It was decided that a cluster sample of households in Control and Study Areas could be drawn so that every person aged 20-64 in the population had an equal chance of being included. About 200 households appeared to be a convenient cluster size. The households were to be as nearly contiguous as possible in order to keep travel expense to a minimum. The total households of the two areas were, therefore, divided by two hundred, thus reaching the number of clusters available. Clusters were now drawn from each commune in proportion to the number of households in it. The clusters were numbered and those to be surveyed selected from a table of random numbers. Eighty-six clusters were selected containing about 11,200 households. This number would supply a sufficient number of people and cases to test any differences found for statistical significance.

At this point it became clear that there was insufficient money to complete a survey of all the 86 clusters selected. In order not to lose the interviewers trained in the earlier wave and because prospects for renewed funding appeared bright, 22 or about one-fourth of the clusters were selected as the base for another pilot study. To economize on automobile transportation, the clusters in Rijeka and Zagreb made up the sample, again sacrificing the goal of a representative sample.

Zagreb is the capital of Croatia and at the time of the survey had about 610,000 population. It is an inland city on the Sava River near the western end of its broad and fertile valley. Zagreb is in many ways a typical administrative, industrial and agricultural trade center. It is in the Control Area. Rijeka (Fiume), a smaller city of about 200,000 population, is a seaport. The port and its supporting industries make up its economic core.

Table 5 shows the number of the population 20-64 years of age surveyed, the number of cases found, and the rates per 10,000 population. The prevalence rates for all psychoses and for functional psychoses are reliably higher in Rijeka than in Zagreb. The subgroups within the classification,

TABLE 5
Population, Number of Cases, and Prevalence per 10,000 Population Aged 20-64, by Diagnostic Group and Residence.

	Rijeka (pop. 4,919)		*Zagreb (pop. 4,282)*		*Total pop. 9,201*	
Diagnostic group[a]	*No. of cases*	*Rate*	*No. of cases*	*Rate*	*No. of cases*	*Rate*
300,303 Schizophrenic and paranoid	36	73.2	18	42.0	54	58.7
301,302 Manic-depressive and involutional	26	52.9	13	30.4	39	42.4
304-309, All other psychoses	12	24.4	88	18.7	20	21.7
300-309, All psychoses	74	150.4[b]	39	91.1[b]	113	122.8
300-303, "Functional psychoses"	62	126.0[c]	31	72.4	93	101.1

[a] International Classification of Diseases, VIIth Rev., 1955
[b] $p < 0.02$
[c] $p < 0.025$

functional psychoses, are not significantly different between the two areas, probably because the number of cases is too small. The Rijeka population was significantly older than that of Zagreb, but rates were significantly different only for the 35-49 age group ($P < 0.01$) for both sexes and, for females, in the 50-64 age group.

This wave included designs to test certain features of the method of case finding. First was the question of the efficacy of household interviewing as compared to the psychiatric register and other records as ways of discovering cases. Of the total of 113 cases found in the Rijeka and Zagreb surveys, 44 (39%) were not identified in any available medical records. Furthermore, persons suspected of being psychotic by the household interviewer were asked by the psychiatrists about prior hospitalizations. Twenty-four records included statements of previous hospitalization for psychosis, and nine said the patient had received outpatient treatment for an illness diagnosed as psychotic. Assuming that the patients' reports of previous treatment were correct and that records could have been found, the number of cases newly discovered only by the survey is reduced to 11, or 9% of the total. This corresponds to a rate of about 1 case per 10,000 of the population.

It will be recalled that in the first survey wave the household respondent was selected as the available person judged best able to report on the health of family members. It was found that respondents made up 45.1% of the population aged 20-64 but that this segment produced 60.2% of all verified psychotics, a statistically significant difference ($P < 0.001$). A review of the survey methods led to the realization that respondents and nonrespondents had different risks of being labelled "suspect"; respondents were available for direct observation, and their being at home at the time of the interview could depend on their being in poor health. If the Rijeka population surveyed contained more respondents than a similar population in Zagreb, this would explain the excess cases in Rijeka. On test, however, there was no significant difference between Rijeka and Zagreb on this parameter.

Next, the issue arose as to whether cases among persons who were not respondents were differentially missed in the two areas. If it is assumed that this happened, its effect can be tested by proportionally raising the rate for nonrespondents to that for respondents and observing whether the difference remains significant. This computation results in a case number of 149 as compared to the 113 actually found, and differences in rates became more marked. In spite of this demonstration that differential rates for respondents and nonrespondents did not affect the conclusions of the study, the method of respondent selection was changed for the final wave of the study to one of pre-selection by a rotation system among the adult family members available (Kulčar et al., 1971).

In summary, the survey of 22 urban clusters in Rijeka and Zagreb showed that the Study Area city (Rijeka) had a significantly higher rate for functional psychoses than did Zagreb, a city in the Control Area. Furthermore, this pilot wave indicated that the controlling cases lay in the 35-49 age group for both sexes and in the 50-64 age group for females. Differences in age distribution of the population of Rijeka and Zagreb did not explain the difference in rates, nor did differences in the proportion of respondents as compared to nonrespondents in the two areas. Thus, this pilot study showed an excess prevalence in a Study Area city compared to a Control Area one. The wave did demonstrate the feasibility of interviewing to find persons suspect of being psychotic in households unprepared by public education and independent of the influence of the local health department. It also showed that the cluster sampling method worked in the field. It allowed further stabilization of instruments, training methods, field supervision, and administrative organization.

The Survey of The Representative Sample of Croatia

The final test of the hypothesis that the Study Area has higher prevalence rates for functional psychoses than the Control Area rests on a survey designed so that every person 20-64 years of age in the Study and Control Areas had an equal chance of being included in the sample.

A new cluster sample of Croatia was drawn because of the passage of time between the last pilot and this final wave, adjusting for changes in the number of households in the areas, for differences in household size in rural as compared to urban areas, and to make use of contemporary voters lists of the population over 18 years of age. Fifty clusters of 160 households each were drawn for the Study Area, using a table of random numbers to determine the first cluster and the interval number. A similar procedure was followed for drawing the 50 clusters of the Control Area.

It would have been desirable for the Control and Study Areas to have been surveyed in the same year, alternating interviewing teams between the two areas, but this was financially impossible. The Study Area was surveyed in 1969, the Control Area in 1970. As already noted, the interviewing teams were not "blind" as to the purpose of the surveys; the time between the two surveys, it is hoped, lessened the possibility of bias due to this factor. Field personnel were made up of statisticians and supervisors with experience in the earlier waves, and these and new and experienced interviewers were trained for this final wave.

The "false negative," a case missed at the household interview level, was of particular concern, since such cases could not be recovered unless they had medical records, and at least one case per 10,000 population aged 20-64 had been shown to be without discoverable records. In addition, every 30th person included in the survey was tagged for psychiatric examination as a means of determining the number of cases being missed at the suspect level. Eight hundred and three such examinations were carried out; two persons were found to be psychotic, a rate of less than two per 10,000 of the population aged 20-64.

Two studies were done to test the reliability of the psychiatrists' examinations. In the first, 62 cases were examined by three psychiatrists, each interviewing a patient in rotation with all three recording the examination and reaching a diagnosis independently. Hospital diagnoses on these patients were also available. Of the 35 cases diagnosed as schizophrenic by the hospital, 33 were identically diagnosed by all three psychiatrists as either schizophrenic or questionably so, while all agreed that one case diagnosed as schizophrenic by the hospital was actually a manic-depressive case. One case was considered primarily epileptic by two of the psychiatrists. Ten manic-depressives by hospital diagnosis all received that diagnosis by the three psychiatrists, though two of them designated one case with a question mark. Of 10 cases diagnosed as psychoneurotic by the hospital diagnosis, one was diagnosed as schizophrenic by all three field psychiatrists, two were diagnosed as manic-depressive or questionably so by one field psychiatrist, and two cases were considered as questionable psychoneurotics by the other two field psychiatrists. All agreed with the hospital that four cases were alcoholic and two primarily epileptic. The field psychiatrists agreed better among themselves than with the hospital diagnoses, a not unexpected result considering the conditions of the experiment.

In the second study, a group of 107 individuals was set up, of which 33 had earlier diagnoses of functional psychoses. These were subjected to the household interview by four teams of two interviewers, each of whom alternated in questioning the subjects and recording the interview. All cases were also examined by field psychiatrists. Two cases were missed at the "suspect" level. In one of these, the case was missed by both interviewers of the team, but the other case was unusual in that one interviewer discovered a psychotic in the group interviewed who had not been "salted" into it. This basic group had been used for interviewer training and was previously not known to contain any psychotic persons. The data, so difficult to present verbally, are shown in table 6 (Lemkau et al., 1971).

TABLE 6
Agreement Between Interviewers Evaluating 107 Subjects For "Suspect" Status by Psychiatrists' Diagnosis: "Salted" Sample (n = 107) Including 33 Known Psychotics.

			Interviewer A		*Interviewer B*	
	No. Interviewed	*Psychiatrist's diagnosis*	*Susp.+*	*Susp.−*	*Susp.+*	*Susp.−*
Group I	26	Psychotic, 5	4	1	4	1
		Nonpsychotic, 21	3	18	5	16
Group II	27	Psychotic, 5	5	0	5	0
		Nonpsychotic, 22	5	17	6	16
Group III	26	Psychotic, 11	12	0	12	0
		Nonpsychotic, 15	4	10	2	12
Group IV	28	Psychotic, 11	10	1	11	0
		Nonpsychotic, 17	3	14	4	13

TABLE 7
Number of Households and Household Members, Age 20-64, by Study and Control Areas in Representative Cluster Sample: Number Interviewed and Response Rate.

	Sex	*Study area*	*Control area*	*Total*
Number of households interviewed		5,376	5,598	10,974
Number of persons in the sample	Male	5,500	6,810	11,558
	Female	5,880	6,810	12,690
	TOTAL	11,380	12,868	24,248
Number of individuals covered in interview	Male	5,386	5,929	11,315
	Female	5,786	6,653	12,439
	TOTAL	11,172	12,582	23,574
Response percent	Male	97.9	97.9	97.9
	Female	98.4	97.7	98.0
	TOTAL	98.2	97.8	98.0

Table 7 shows the size of the samples and the extraordinarily high rates of response achieved. We believe that two factors account for the high rates: first, the long experience in health education of the Croatian population plus the respect that local health services receive; second, the compliance of the population in a venture that had the support of the government. Of the two factors, the first appears the more significant.

Results

The prevalence rate per 1000 persons between the ages 20 and 65 was 7.3 for the Study Area and 3.8 for the Control Area, the rates being based on 82 and 48 cases respectively. The ratio of the rates is 1.9 to 1, indicating that the two areas differed in the prevalence of functional psychosis at greater than the 0.05 level of confidence. The basic hypothesis of the research was therefore supported.

Further analysis showed that although cases among males occur more frequently in the Study Area than in the Control Area, the difference did not reach the usual level of statistical significance. For females, however, the rate for the Study Area is 8.6 per 1000, for the Control Area, 4.2 per 1000, indicating a significant excess of cases in the Study Area females. Table 8 presents the figures and indicates further that there is a significant excess in rates for functional psychoses over the age of 40 and that the difference in rates is greater in the older the population. From these data it is concluded that the Study Area has higher prevalence rates than the Control Area for functional psychosis, and that the excess cases lie in the female population and the older groups of both sexes. Further analysis indicates that elderly females with the diagnosis manic-depressive psychosis have high rates for the Study Area as compared to the Control Area.

Test of Secondary Hypotheses

The demonstration that there is a difference in the rate of functional psychoses in the Study and Control Areas indicates a need for further studies to determine whether any features of the two populations can throw light on the differences and perhaps explain them. The features available for testing, in addition to age and sex already discussed, were marital status, insurance status, educational level, cigarette smoking, migration history, coastal or inland location, and other illnesses showing similar distribution.

All except the last of these involved the use of a fictitious population in which all features were adjusted for except the one under consideration at the moment. For example, when marital status differences were being looked at in the Study and Control areas, any difference in the other features such as family size, or place of residence were automatically adjusted by the computer program. The data on smoking collected for this study are unique for Yugoslavia.

The findings can be rather quickly summarized. Single females are overrepresented in the functional psychotic group. As is found in most such

TABLE 8
Number of Cases of Functional Psychoses and Rate per 1000 Covered by Interview, Study and Control Areas, by Age Group and Sex.

	Male					Female									
	Study area		*Control area*			*Study area*		*Control area*			*Total Study*		*Total control*		
Age group	*No.*	*Rate*	*No.*	*Rate*	*Ratio of rates*	*No.*	*Rate*	*No.*	*Rate*	*Ratio of rates*	*No.*	*Rate*	*No.*	*Rate*	*Ratio of rates*
20-29	3	2.4	3	2.1	1.14	3	2.4	2	1.4	1.7	6	2.4	5	1.8	1.3
30-39	4	2.7	8	4.8	0.6	0	5.9	7	4.0	1.5	13	4.3	15	4.4	0.1
40-49	10	7.8	5	2.3	32.3	19	13.2	13	7.7	1.7	29	10.6	18	4.7	1.9
50-64	14	11.0	4	2.9	3.8	19	12.2	6	3.4	3.59	34	11.7	10	3.1	3.8
Total	31	5.9	20	3.4	1.74	50	8.6	28	4.2	2.05	82	7.3	48	3.8	1.9

studies, the married show lower rates than the divorced, widowed, or single. There is no significant difference for the factor of marital status between the Study and Control Areas.

Health insurance in Yugoslavia is universal, but coverage varies with the type of employment. The total population is covered for emergency conditions, infectious diseases, and psychiatric illnesses requiring hospitalization. Coverage for other conditions varies, however, between farmers, industrial workers, the unemployed, pensioners, and other occupations. The Control Area shows a smaller proportion of the population employed in industry (active workers) than the Study Area. This is probably related to the greater fertility of the land in the Control Area, which allows farmers to support themselves from agriculture alone, while the poorer soil of the Study Area makes holding a job necessary in addition to farming. None of the differences, however, are sufficiently large to account for the difference in rate of functional psychosis in the two populations.

The educational level of the two areas is not conspicuously different. The Control Area population contains a larger proportion who did not complete elementary education as well as more who have completed 13 or more years of schooling. The differences, none of which reach statistical significance, are mostly confined to the older age groups.

Cigarette smoking was of interest because of its association with ill health generally and because the habit is alleged to be symptomatic of nervousness. As the first study of the epidemiology of cigarette smoking in Yugoslavia, the data are valuable in their own right. Table 9 presents the results. A higher proportion of cases smoke as compared to the general population. Significantly, ($P < 0.03$) more of the population of the Study Area smoke than of the Control Area. As is commonly found, males smoke more than females.

Data available to estimate the effect of migration on rates of functional psychosis consisted in whether an individual was born in the area in which he was interviewed, elsewhere in Croatia or Yugoslavia, or in another country. A significantly larger proportion of people in the Study Area live in places other than where they were born. It is found that the native rather than the migrant population provides the excess of cases. The difference is significant at the 0.003 level. This finding may be related to the fact that rates are highest in the elderly. Adult migrants are generally younger than native populations.

Because the Adriatic Sea is a much more dominant factor in the life of the Study Area than of the Control Area, coastal or inland residence was examined. Furthermore, the Study Area is geologically a karst region while the Control Area is predominantly alluvial plain. Corn is the main crop in the Study Area, small grains in the Control Area. Eleven percent of the Control Area population lives near the coast, while 65% of the Study population is so located. In both areas, rates for functional psychoses are higher in coastal than in inland regions, but the difference is not significant. The Study Area's higher rates hold up for both coastal and inland locations.

The geologic and agricultural differences between the Study and Control Areas are so striking that they invite hypotheses relating them to the dif-

TABLE 9

Population Sample and Cases of Functional Psychoses,[a] Study and Control Areas, by Cigarette Smoking and Sex—Percentages.

	Percent smoking in study area (Pop. n = 11,172; Case n = 82)						*Percent smoking in control area (Pop. n = 12,528; Case n = 48)*					
	Males		***Females***		***Total***		***Males***		***Females***		***Total***	
Amount smoked	*Pop.*	*Case*	*Pop.*	*Case*	*Pop.*	*Case*	*Pop.*	*Case*	*Pop.*	*Case*	*Pop.*	*Case*
Non-smokers	41.2	18.8	88.0	82.0	65.4	57.3	43.2	40.0	90.0	82.0	67.9	64.6
1-10 cigarettes/day	11.1	21.9	4.9	4.0	7.9	11.0	10.4	15.0	4.3	0.0	7.2	6.3
10+ cigarettes/day	47.6	50.0	7.1	—	26.6	28.0	46.3	40.0	5.6	17.9	24.8	27.1
Unknown	0.2	9.4	0.1	0.0	0.1	3.7	0.1	5.0	0.1	0.0	0.1	2.1
Total	100	100	100	100	100	100	100	100	100	100	100	100

[a] International Classification of Diseases, WHO, 295, 296, 297, VIIIth Ed.

ferences in rates of functional psychoses found. Two present themselves at once, one that nutritional differences may be controlling, the second that the excess of psychosis in the Study Area may simply be a part of a picture of general ill health in this more impoverished population. Nutritional disorders (as indicated by hospital discharge diagnoses) were not, however, different in the two areas. This does not dispose of the hypothesis since nutritional disorders are almost as difficult to diagnose as psychiatric ones, and hospital discharge data would be concerned only with the more severe cases. The hypothesis is still a haunting one.

Diseases of the bones (I.C.D. 740-759) were marginally higher in the Study Area, but this category includes conditions ranging from infectious to degenerative and will certainly require further definition before any even tentative conclusions can be reached.

Diabetes mellitus is considerably more common in the Study Area than in the Control Area and is concentrated in older females. Psoriasis also shows this feature and is of special interest since an association between psoriasis and mental illness has been suggested in the literature. Urticaria is also more common in the Study Area, a matter of interest since this skin disease involves mesodermal rather than ectodermal tissue. The findings on cardiovascular disease are confusing and impossible to interpret, probably because of diagnostic problems in this area. Alcoholism is more often reported for the Study Area but it was not, as tentatively predicted, associated with an excess of pellagra. Tuberculosis, often treated as an indicator of lowered general health, was found to be lower in the Study Area than in the Control Area.

Summary

A study of the prevalence of functional psychoses in Croatia extending over about 15 years and involving different field methods and data bases is presented. The study began as an attempt to test a long-standing belief on the part of Yugoslav psychiatrists that an area around the northern end of the Adriatic Sea showed higher prevalence rates for schizophrenia than the rest of Croatia. The first method used, a study of hospitalized patients, indicated that there was an excess of schizophrenia in the Study Area, but that the excess was present for all functional psychoses and not confined to schizophrenia.

To be certain that the differences observed were not artifacts related to practices of hospitalization of the mentally ill, methods were developed for identifying cases in households. The method finally used consisted of a two-step identification and diagnostic procedure. In the first step, a member of the household was interrogated by a specially trained interviewer who identified household members suspected of being psychotic. These suspects and certain control individuals were examined by psychiatrists who determined whether a psychosis was present and made a diagnosis. The method was subjected to tests for reliability and, to some extent, validity. In the final wave of the study, a representative sample of households in the Study and Control Areas was interviewed. The results were as follows:

1. There exists in Croatia, Yugoslavia, an area with a population, aged 20-64, with a higher prevalence rate for functional psychoses than the rest of Croatia (Control Area).
2. The excess of cases in the Study Area is unevenly distributed over the population by age and sex. The differences are greatest in the group over 40 and are most marked in older women who show high rates for affective disorders.
3. The difference in prevalence rates for functional psychoses in the Study as compared to the Control Area is not related to educational level, inland or coastal home site, or occupational group.
4. The excess of cases in the Study Area appears to arise from native-born population rather than from immigrants.
5. Cigarette smoking is slightly more common in the Study than in the Control Area, and cases are found to smoke more than the general population.
6. Although diabetes mellitus, psoriasis, urticaria, and alcoholism are more prevalent in the Study Area than in the Control Area, tuberculosis is less so. Nutritional disorders are not significantly different in the two areas. In any case, the hypothesis that the excess prevalence of psychoses in the Study Area might be related to stresses of general ill health in that area as compared to the Control Area, could not be supported.
7. The research has tested only a very few of the hypotheses that can be put forward in relation to its findings. It is hoped that at least some of these will be tested in the future.
8. The research made necessary the establishment of a computerized register of hospitalized psychiatric patients. The register has made it possible to determine that the prevalence rates for hospitalized cases have not markedly changed from 1969 to 1975.
9. The existence of two contiguous areas, one of which has significantly higher rates for functional psychoses than the other, is considered to have been demonstrated by this series of investigations. While nothing has been shown which explains the difference, the existence of the areas offers the opportunity to test both genetic and ecological theories concerning the etiology of the functional psychoses.

Acknowledgments

The initial grant to test the feasibility of these studies was made by the Milbank Foundation. The studies themselves were supported by the National Institute of Mental Health, to some extent through the use of counterpart funds in Yugoslavia. Local Health Departments in Croatia provided many useful services. Branko Kesić, Živko Kulčar, Luca Kovačić, and the late Guido Crocetti were principal investigators for the studies reported here, and many others, particularly in Yugoslavia were involved in their execution.

References

Carothers, J. D. (1953), *The African Mind in Health and Disease.* Geneva: World Health Organization.

Eaton, J. W. & Weil, R. J. (1955), *Culture and Mental Disorders.* Glencoe, Ill.: Free Press.

Kovačić, L., Kulčar, Ž. & Persic, VII (1981), Development of field instruments and methods. In: *Epidemiology of Psychoses in Croatia,* eds. Kesić, B., Kulčar, Ž. and Lemkau, P. V. Zagreb: Yugoslav National Academy of Science, pp. 77-93.

Kulčar, Ž., Crocetti, G. M., Lemkau, P. V. & Kesic, B. (1971), Selected aspects of the epidemiology of psychoses in Croatia, Yugoslavia. II. Pilot studies of communities. *Am J Epidemiol* 94:118-125.

Kulčar, Ž., Rogina V. & Gorwitz, K. (1976), Long-term followup of schizophrenics in Croatia. *J Croatian Med Soc* 4:3-18.

Lemkau, P. V. & Pavković, A. (1952), Report on a survey of mental health facilities in Yugoslavia. In: Lemkau, P. V. and Pavković, A.: *Problemi i zadaci mentalne higijene,* Zagreb. *Medicinska Knjiga.*

Lemkau, P. V., Kulčar, Ž., Crocetti, G. M. & Kesić, B. (1971), Selected aspects of the epidemiology of psychoses in Croatia, Yugoslavia. I. Background and use of psychiatric hospital statistics. *Am J Epidemiol* 94:112-117.

Lemkau, P. V., Kulčar, Ž., Kesić, B. & Kovačić, L. (1980), Selected aspects of the epidemiology of psychoses in Croatia, Yugoslavia. IV. Representative sample of Croatia and results of the survey. *Am J Epidemiol* 112:661-674.

Novosel, M. (1981), The training of personnel. In: *Epidemiology of Psychoses in Croatia,* ed. Kesić, B., Kulčar, Ž., and Lemkau, P. V., Zagreb: Yugoslav National Academy of Science, pp. 94-102.

Štampar, A. (1966), *Serving the Cause of Public Health: Selected Papers of Andrija Štampar,* ed. M. D. Grmek. Andrija Štampar School of Public Health, Medical Faculty, Univ. of Zagreb. Monograph Series No. 3.

Chapter 4

Mental Disorders in Urban Areas: A Retrospective View

H. WARREN DUNHAM

To look back 50 years and come up with a substantive summation of the Faris-Dunham study, while it produces much nostalgia, is not an easy task. It is not easy for two reasons. First, the perspective of a half century of accumulated epidemiologic studies of mental disorders makes one critical of this study on several counts. Second, in any attempt to make an analysis of this early epidemiologic study, one must strive for complete honesty so that the students who read the account will recognize that significant research does not always follow the formula of assumptions, hypotheses, methods, data, and findings but may emerge by serendipity. The memories associated with this research bring me closer to Watson's account (Watson, 1968) of those very human experiences that accompanied the discovery of the structure of DNA rather than the formal structure posed by the editors of this volume.

To begin at the very beginning, one must note that this work was conceived and executed during my graduate years in the 1930s at the University of Chicago. This was a period when most empirical efforts in the social sciences were conducted on infinitesimal budgets. The affluent period of social science research was still two decades away. These low budgets accounted for two characteristics of sociological research at that time. First, as the collection of data was mostly in the hands of students, it was marked by keen interest and high motivation as the students were concerned with getting their dissertations out of it. Second, much of it was an example of crude empiricism—raw data in search of a hypothesis. Then later, after the findings were clear, an attempt was usually made to fit them into some larger theoretical framework. Deductive sociology at that time was a rarity. While a professor who suggested an area of work for the student usually harbored some theoretical concern, the student began to learn about the state of the problem in the library while collecting data in the field.

So it was with the Faris-Dunham research. I had completed a year of graduate study in 1931. By September of that year I found myself without funds to continue formal graduate study. The Depression was in full swing, but I was lucky enough to secure a position as a social worker. The work consisted of sorting and processing the unemployed men who were drifting into the "hobohemia" areas at the city's center. My task along with that of the other social workers—this was before the Federal government assumed responsibility for the unemployed—was to secure face-sheet information on each man, pass him on to a doctor for a physical and psychiatric examination, and then provide him with a bed and a meal ticket until he secured a job. However, this rarely happened in those Depression days. I found out later that some of these men would get themselves committed to a state hospital. The meals were better and so were the beds. They also often provided a leadership role among the patients, being of sounder mind than even those patients with the more benign symptoms.

In December of that year, after I had been on my new job for three months, I received a phone call from Professor Burgess. He asked me to stop by his office at some time soon when I was not working. At the appointed time I was there, and after some ritualistic conversation that may take place between teacher and student, he asked me if I would be interested in a research assistantship at a state hospital collecting case data on first admissions. In discussing the procedure I was to follow, Professor Burgess mentioned that I would receive a stipend of $50.00 a month plus board and room at the hospital. This magnificent stipend was about one-third of my social work salary, but I jumped at the chance. It seemed to be just the opportunity I very much wanted. It would reestablish my University connection, which I so desired, and would enable me to collect data that I could use for my Master's dissertation. By early January of 1932 I was ensconced at the Elgin State Hospital collecting data, reading psychiatry, sharing a room with a psychiatric intern, getting acquainted with state hospital life, and playing monthly poker with the young doctors.

With the Elgin State Hospital as background, my psychiatric education was about to begin. Since the hospital was footing the bill for my research, the hospital superintendent required that I pass out the mail to the employees for a couple of hours in the afternoon. All my other time was devoted to the collection of data. From the post provided by the mail room, I was able to make numerous observations about the hospital world. I came to know all the employees—from attendants to the doctors—to discover the hospital grapevine, to note the class divisions in the hospital, and to become acquainted with selected patients with ground privileges who would stop at the mail room to talk. I saw all the patients as they marched to their meals, served cafeteria style, from their respective wards. It was during this early state hospital experience that the ideas behind my sociocultural study of the state mental hospital began to take shape (Dunham and Weinberg, 1960).

My observations of state hospital life went hand in hand with my initial excursions into the psychiatric literature. My ignorance of psychiatry was colossal. My only academic experience with the "abnormal" was through a course with Franz Alexander during the third quarter of that first graduate year. Alexander had been invited to spend a year at the University, but as the medical school would have nothing to do with such a "nonscientific" body of lore as psychoanalysis, he found himself assigned to the law school. His first course, "Introduction to Psychoanalysis," was given before seven students—four budding sociologists, two maidenly public school teachers, and one professional student who made a life for himself by collecting various university degrees. Alexander, utilizing the clinical case method, presented a clear picture of the structure of psychoanalytic theory illustrated with reference to the treatment of individual patients in which repressed experiences were supposedly the cause of the development of both physical and mental symptoms. But that was all. At this very beginning of my education in psychiatry, I felt very keenly that if I was ever able to make any significant contribution about mental disorders from a sociological perspective, I should at least know as much and more about psychiatry than medical school graduates.

First, I started to read psychiatric textbooks. At least I thought I would learn what the doctors had found out about psychiatry in the medical school. I turned first to A. Rosnoff's *Manual of Psychiatry*, 1927; next I turned to D. K. Henderson and R. P. Gillespie, *A Textbook of Psychiatry*, 1927; and finally, I consulted A. B. Noyes, *Textbook of Psychiatry*, 1928. Then with the discovery of E. E. Southard's and M. Jarrett's *The Kingdom of Evils*, 1922, and later the works of Abraham Myerson (1925 and 1927), I was on my way.

This initial reading was only a start. When I finally returned to formal graduate training in 1938-39 (just prior to the publication of *Mental Disorders in Urban Areas)*, I was permitted, along with three other graduate students in sociology, to offer psychiatry as an outside field for the doctoral examinations. To prepare for this examination we were required to take two seminars in psychiatry designed for medical school seniors, to make morning bed rounds with a psychiatrist for the observation of the current psychiatric patients who were hospitalized, and to work for a couple of quarters in the outpatient clinic preparing the clinical case histories of the persons referred to us by the other hospital departments. In those days if a person presented himself to the hospital with a physical complaint and if on a physical examination all tests were negative, he was automatically referred to the psychiatric department. As young graduate students in sociology, we received the same training as senior medical students who took this clinical experience as an elective in the outpatient department. The teachers from whom I received my formal psychiatric education were Jules Masserman, Henry Brosin, and Hugh Carmichael. I am in debt to all of them.

When the editors of this volume requested an account of this 50-year-old study from me and suggested that I include its objectives, methodology, methods, sample size, findings, and significance, they demonstrated that their social science education was of a time when social research had developed a more self-conscious theoretical character than was true at the time of our study. In fact, if such had been the case, the logic of our study might have been presented in the following propositions with the organized data serving as a test of the theory.

1. Symbolic communication is essential for normal development and a lack of such communication leads to mental breakdown.
2. In an urban community certain areas have a greater degree of social disorganization than other areas.

3. Social disorganization is characterized by excessive mobility, ethnic conflict, breaks in communication and lack of consensus.
4. Seclusiveness is a key trait in schizophrenia.
5. Persons who develop seclusive traits do so as a result of social isolation or breaks in communication.
6. These conditions are found in certain urban areas identified as being disorganized.
7. Therefore, these areas will have the highest rates of schizophrenia.

Now, while these propositions depict the logical deductive structure of our study, this structure was developed after the data were collected and the findings had emerged. This was exactly the reasoning on which Leighton inaugurated his Sterling County study in 1951. Leighton asked, will those communities we can show are disorganized have the highest rates of mental illness as compared to communities not characterized by disorganization? In other words, will high incidence rates be found where theory suggests they will be found? (Leighton, 1950.)

Data comprising patient's case number, address at commitment, date of first admission, age, sex, marital status, occupation, nativity, race, and diagnosis were collected from the clinical records of state and private mental hospitals receiving patients from Chicago. These data, taken from 34,864 clinical records, were transferred to Hollerith cards and then distributed by coded address on local community maps of Chicago. As is well known, maps were constructed that showed the distribution of rates for total mental disease, for several separate diagnostic categories, and in the case of schizophrenia and manic-depressive psychosis, for their respective subtypes. For these functional psychoses certain rate distributions were constructed on the basis of both sex and age. Our next step was to compute a number of ecological correlations that purported to measure the correspondence between the local community rates of the several diagnostic categories and selected demographic indexes—percentage of foreign-born, percentage of hotel and lodging house residents, sex ratio, median rental, percentage of home ownership, percentage of single homes, and median school grade. It was assumed that such indexes provided measurements for social disorganization in the subcommunities of Chicago.

Finally, when these data were collected and analyzed by maps, tables, and correlation coefficients, the isolation hypothesis was advanced as an explanation for the schizophrenic distributions. Faris had already explored the behavior of persons who had experienced extreme social isolation and inferred that this isolation might be an antecedent condition to the emergence of the trait of seclusiveness so characteristic of the beginning of schizophrenic symptoms.

However, it should be at once apparent that for social isolation to provide an explanation for schizophrenia certain facts must be established. First, it must be shown that where schizophrenic rates are high, the patients making up the rates were born there and/or spent most of their formative years in one of those high rate communities. Second, it must be shown that the high rate communities are characterized by social disorganization. Third, it must be shown that the persons who became schizophrenic experienced periods of extreme social isolation in growing up. Finally, it must be shown that persons who developed schizophrenia and were found in lowrate communities experienced extreme social isolation even though these communities could not be regarded as socially disorganized. It is clear that we were not able in this study to establish these facts and so what we have is a suggestion—a tentative hypothesis—to account for the distribution of schizophrenic cases in a large city.

These data, necessary to validate the isolation hypothesis, point to the dual theoretical concerns of this study. Here, attention should be focused on the subtitle, *An Ecological Study of Schizophrenia and other Psychoses.* The human ecology model developed by R. E. Park (1926 and 1931) was one of the two theoretical positions that dominated the "Chicago School" in my graduate days. The other model was represented by symbolic interactional theory found in social psychology. Park developed the human ecology model by applying certain concepts developed by the plant ecologists to human communities. Thus the model provided an explanation for the settling, growth, and decline of human communities. Park saw the same continuous struggle and competition of the plant and animal communities taking place in the human communities but with a difference. This difference was provided by the cultural order in human society, which did not permit this Darwinian "struggle for existence" and "survival of the fittest" to work itself out to its logical conclusion of extinction but rather helped to soften the struggle, making for various kinds of survival.

The human ecologist is interested in all types of data that reveal the working of the social process by which individuals and institutions find their "ecological position" in the community, the interdependence of the institutional structures, and the various situations that encourage different modes of survival. Thus the human ecologist who collects data on every type of social problem is not so much interested in isolating etiological factors as in showing how the location of problems in the urban environment contributes to the emergence of a social organization to which humans make various responses. For the physician, human ecology becomes medical ecology. Thus the central concern is to show how the precarious balance among disease agents, persons, and their sociocultural environment can be maintained to encourage a healthy and not an illness response (Dunham, 1966).

The investigator who desires to study mental disorders within the theoretical framework of human ecology should ask the following questions: *(a)* What are the pressures and factors at work in the urban community that can account for the distribution patterns of all types of detected mental disorders? *(b)* What are the consequences of such distribution patterns on the organization of the urban community? *(c)* If such patterns vary by type of mental disorder, what will be the consequences on urban social organization? *(d)* What social and demographic indicators show high positive or high negative associations with the various rate distribution patterns?

The findings of research guided by human ecological theory reveal little about the cause of specific mental disorders but tell us something about the different urban environments and subcultures that attract or repel those persons who have developed or are developing a mental disorder. Such research might also reveal selected high risk social factors that are associated with the development of mental disorder.

However, if the investigator conducts his research using the epidemiologic method, he is working in the field of medicine. Thus, he examines the distribution of a disease in a given population for clues as to the etiologic factors that may be relevant to a better knowledge of the disease process. Such etiologic clues may point to factors of a genetic, physiologic, psychologic, or sociologic character. The epidemiologist asks these questions: *(a)* Why does the incidence of a given disease show a significant variation between two populations of risk? *(b)* What does the distribution pattern of a given disease suggest as to the factors that might have an etiologic significance? *(c)* What hypothetical risk factors, associated with the disease, has the sick person had contact with before developing the disease? *(d)* What do the epidemiologic findings suggest with respect to the control and/or prevention of a specific disease? Thus, after examining the various distribution patterns of a disease, the epidemiologist asks questions about factors associated with it. In contrast, the ecologist inquires about factors that disrupt the social structure to the extent that unhealthy responses are produced by persons that compose the community.

Now, it is just this double perspective that one can find tucked away in our study. We started out by examining the ecologic structure of the city and how mental disorder distributions appeared to reveal new knowledge about the urban structure. We ended up, however, as epidemiologists attempting to suggest the factor—for us a sociological one—that might account for the development of schizophrenia. We failed to call attention to other theoretical orientations that might be relevant to the etiology of schizophrenia as suggested by our epidemiologic findings. Thus we began with ecological theory but ended with social psychological theory.

But with the airing of these theoretical concerns, I want to return to the main story. It was late in 1933 that Professor Burgess suggested to Faris and me that we collaborate on a joint effort to present our data, findings, and theory in a book-length manuscript. Faris and I had known each other during our undergraduate days—we first became acquainted on a job painting the seats of the Stagg Stadium—and so the suggested collaboration was an easy adjustment for both of us. At the time we both had completed manuscripts analyzing our respective data—my Master's dissertation and Faris' Doctoral dissertation. Then, following Burgess' suggestion, Faris and I met on several occasions to decide on the division of labor. It was agreed that I would handle the empirical data—rate distributions, correlations, tables, populations used—while Faris would devote several chapters to developing the theory of social isolation he had used in his dissertation. We worked hard and fast and so, by the end of 1935, we had produced a manuscript which we turned over to Professor Burgess. He was to see that it was reviewed by several critical readers.

I do not have any idea as to who these critical readers were, though I heard many rumors. I am sure that Professor Burgess read our manuscript, and also that a couple of psychiatrists read it. Anyway, after four months the criticisms were in and did not prove very supporting. Much of the criticism centered on the theoretical section in the manuscript. It was not that Faris had not done a commendable job, but when all was said there just was not any hard evidence to support the elaborate theoretical structure that Faris had developed. The psychiatric readers were particularly critical about that and objected heatedly to the idea that schizophrenia might result from social isolation, especially in the absence of any solid evidence. We took these criticisms in stride, and because our findings were interesting and suggestive, we were urged to report them in a revised manuscript.

If my memory serves me, it was in the late fall of 1936 that Faris and I met in New York to lay out the division of labor for a revised manuscript. (Faris was then teaching at Brown University and I was collecting some new data for my doctoral dissertation.) At this meeting we decided to include some distribution data for Providence, Rhode Island, which Faris had been collecting with some colleagues, and he was also to write a brief theoretical chapter on "Mind and Society" and Chapters I and II. I was to be responsible for the chapters dealing with the distribution of the different psychoses in the city and both of us would take a joint responsibility for the concluding chapter. Each was to examine and raise any questions about what the other had written and differences were to be resolved in a face-to-face discussion. And so it went.

The revised manuscript was presented to Professor Burgess some time late in 1937. This time it apparently was accepted by the review committee. Dr. Burgess responded to our request to write an Introduction and I asked Dr. Singer, who had read the manuscript, to write a Foreword. He was willing. The volume was accepted for publication in the University of Chicago Sociological Series and came off the press in 1939 at about the same time that the German Army marched into Poland signalling the start of World War II.

The central findings of this study include the following:

1. All types of mental disorders are distributed in the city in such a manner that the highest rates are concentrated in and around the central business district, with rates declining in every direction toward the city's periphery.
2. The distribution patterns for schizophrenic rates by sex and type except the catatonic are very similar to those for all types of mental disorders.
3. The distribution patterns for the types of schizophrenia showed sharp contrasts. The pattern distribution of catatonic rates differed significantly from the rate patterns for the paranoid and hebephrenic types. The catatonic rates were highest in the impoverished foreign-born communities, while the paranoid and hebephrenic rates were highest in those communities having high percentages of hotel and rooming house populations.
4. By contrast the distribution pattern for manic-depressive rates by sex and type for every series show a scatter within the city that can be described as random.

5. The highest rates of schizophrenics for native-born and foreign-born are highest in areas populated primarily by blacks, while rates for blacks are highest in areas primarily populated by whites.
6. The distribution pattern for alcoholic psychosis showed the highest rates in the impoverished rooming house areas in the city.
7. The distribution pattern for general paresis also showed a high concentration of rates in the rooming house areas.
8. The distribution pattern for senile psychoses showed the highest rates in the most economically deprived areas of the city and the pattern of rates for psychoses with arteriosclerosis followed this pattern closely.

These propositions constitute the basic findings as reported in *Mental Disorders in Urban Areas.* They were based on all first admissions for the years 1922-34 to the four state hospitals and eight private hospitals that admitted patients with a residence in Chicago.

The ink was hardly dry on this first edition before the debate began. The ensuing discussion centered around two questions: *(a)* What was the nature of the evidence that supported the interpretation of the distributions suggested by the authors? *(b)* What were the significant methodologic issues that, because they are still unresolved, made it difficult to accept the findings at face value?

With respect to the first question, which incidentally involved a major methodologic issue, I would have to admit that there is hardly a shred of hard evidence in the book that supports the hypothesis that a person is more likely to develop schizophrenia because he experiences a higher degree of social isolation in a slum community of a large city than he would in a more socially organized community. If this were a valid proposition, the argument would be that a person might experience isolation in any urban community but the risk of isolation would be many times greater in a slum community. Therefore, one expects these communities to have the highest rates, which indeed they do. A series of case studies that could show that persons who developed schizophrenia experienced a marked social isolation in their formative years would constitute additional supporting evidence (Clausen and Kohn, 1955). But we had suggested a hypothesis that was, as Professor Burgess stated at the time, "congenial to the sociological student" but had no hard evidence to support it.

The isolation hypothesis as presented in our work also points to a grave methodologic error. Data comprising rates of schizophrenia are presented on one level of observation, that is, the social system level, and then inferences and hypotheses are suggested involving data on another level of observation—the level of interpersonal relations (Robinson, 1950).

The critics quickly moved in for blood. There were two statistical criticisms that we were able to answer satisfactorily. The first was the charge that the distribution pattern of rates as found represented a statistical illusion. In other words, a computation of the standard errors of the rates showed that there often were not any significant differences between the rates in the local communities. However, by combining contiguous areas, significant differences did appear and the rate pattern held up. Another criticism was that the population base for certain communities was not valid as the population turned over about three times a year. Such a consideration reduced the rates in these communities by two thirds. Again, when we did increase the population for these chief offending communities, the rates were still very high. A final criticism still with us is the issue of coverage. It was argued that we only based our rates on first admissions to state and private hospitals, while every psychiatrist knows that this only represents about 50% or 60% of all mental patients. The other 40% or 50% are supposedly never detected or are not counted in the year that the first symptoms of their mental illness appear.

Another major criticism emerged as the "drift" hypothesis. This was the argument that Abraham Myerson (1940) made in one of the early reviews of the book. He argued that the authors ignored the generally recognized fact that the handicapped, the homeless, and the failures drifted down to these slum communities where they could lead an anonymous existence. Thus he set the stage for several empirical attempts to resolve the issue.

In addition to this methodologic issue, relating to the interpretation of our distribution pattern, there were two other methodologic problems that began to emerge in the progress of our research. These problems had a bearing on the question as to whether the distribution pattern of rates for the several psychoses could be taken at face value. One issue centered around the reliability and validity of the diagnosis. This particularly applied to the functional psychoses. For example, what assurance does one have that all cases given a schizophrenic diagnosis are suffering from the same disease? Or, for that matter, is schizophrenia a true disease in the sense that some embedded pathology of the neurologic system accounts for the mental symptoms? Without the assurance that the schizophrenic rate structure is made up of the same type of cases, it is pointless to search for a meaningful explanation of the pattern.

The second methodologic issue that gradually took shape as we examined our distribution patterns centered on the extent of the mobility of the individual cases. What social route had each case traveled to get to the community in which he was picked up and sent to a mental hospital? To what extent were the individual cases indigenous to the community in which they were picked up? What percentage of cases found in any community had been born and raised in that community? These questions, where answers were needed, were crucial for interpreting the various distribution patterns. The drift hypothesis was beginning to take shape. However, instead of facing the question directly, we proceeded to amass what evidence we had to support the validity of the distributions as found. The facts that we did produce to support our distribution findings were suggestive but not definitive.

There are two other methodologic issues that have been recognized as a result of further epidemiologic study of mental disorders. One issue has to do with the changing character of the ecology of urban social structure over time. I became aware of this issue when I began to focus my attention on the epidemiology of schizophrenia. Here it is not without point to note that Levy and Rowitz (1973), in replicating the Faris-Dunham study a generation later, wrote about "hospital utilization rates." They did not take the rate patterns at face value as we tended to do.

There is one final problem that I attempted to face in my recent epidemiologic study of schizophrenia (Dunham, 1965). It is the "gap" problem. The "gap" refers to the length of time between the recognition that a disease exists and the entry into a treatment situation. Let me illustrate this issue for schizophrenia with respect to two hypothetical cases. A person from a lower class family is observed by other family members to act strangely by sitting in the same corner for two hours, for speaking nonsense, and accusing his mother of serving him poisoned food. Within the week, the family has had him taken to the city's psychopathic hospital. On the same day a person in an upper middle class family shows the same symptoms. His family, however, does not act immediately. The members wait and observe the sick member and talk the matter over with friends, their minister, and their family doctor. This all takes time. But the person does not improve, and so, two years after the first appearance of his symptoms, is admitted to a psychiatric facility. Now, the point is that the first case enters into the incidence rate for the community immediately, where the second case does not enter into the incidence rate for the community until two years later. This suggests that the case detection rate and the incidence rate would be the same for one community, while cases making up the detection rate in another community might be staggered over a period of years. This situation, when carried to its logical conclusion, would suggest that all rate distribution patterns of schizophrenia have a spurious quality.

Finally, we confront the important question, as posed by the editors: What has been the significance of this study? How significant was its contribution? I do not think that it should be up to me to formulate answers to these questions. Its significance at the beginning was attested by both favorable and critical reviews. It has been called a "classical" study; it has been reissued twice, the first time in hard cover by the Hafner Press in 1960 and the second time in paperback by the University of Chicago Press in 1965. It has served as a stimulus for numerous studies by both social scientists and psychiatrists in order to test or support our findings. Numerous studies have also centered around the theoretical model we developed to explain rate distribution patterns for schizophrenia. All of these efforts have served to enrich our knowledge and understanding, both positively and negatively, of how the physical, social and cultural environments act upon a malleable human organism to move it in a direction where its mental and behavioral responses will not be understood by family, friends, or employers.

There is one very important contribution of this study that has received little public attention. Here I am referring to the role of the study as a catalytic agent for initiating what has been a continuing dialogue between psychiatrists and sociologists. True, the interchange had begun earlier in 1927 with the appointment of a committee of sociologists and a committee of psychiatrists to explore their mutual interests, but these efforts had died down after two colloquiums on the human personality had been held (Proceedings: First and Second Colloquiums, 1930). However, the dialogue stimulated by our study has continued to this day. At the Ninth World Congress of Sociologists held in Uppsala, Sweden, in August 1978, there were six sessions of the committee on Sociology of Mental Health in which psychiatrists participated along side the more numerous sociologists.

In this continuing dialogue, sociologists seemed to be on the constant search for evidence that might tighten the influence of social factors in the development of mental disorders. The psychiatrists who reacted to our study seemed to fall into two groups: those who took a highly critical position, tending to downgrade our findings as they continued with their own research interests, exploring possible genetic and bio-chemical factors; and a second group of psychiatrists who in general had a favorable reaction to our findings due to the particular theoretical position which they held. It seemed to me that these were the psychiatrists who would have preferred to have been trained as social scientists.

Thus, despite methodologic problems that have persisted and have remained largely unresolved to this day, the study has held up, continues to be widely quoted, and requests to reprint chapters and maps continue until this day. The research has been a stimulus for numerous other research endeavors, both large and small. Some of these studies focus on the resolution of particular methodologic issues; others have attempted to break new ground by increasing our knowledge concerning the epidemiology of mental disorders. My own growing skepticism about our hypothetical explanation of our findings as well as the validity of the findings per se determined the design of my second large epidemiologic study which was published as *Community and Schizophrenia* 26 years after the publication of *Mental Disorders in Urban Areas.* This second epidemiologic study focused on one psychosis, schizophrenia, under the assumption that it was a bona fide disease resulting from the interaction of a specific genetic structure and selected sociocultural factors. This is the beginning of another story. I conclude by referring to it, for it represents a spin-off from our original study and an attempt on my part to get at some of the puzzling issues of that study which were not for me satisfactorily resolved.

Summary

Mental Disorders in Urban Areas was conceived and executed during my graduate student days at the University of Chicago. The study has a dual theoretical focus. On one hand, the investigators purport to deal with the reciprocal influence of spatial distribution patterns of mental disorders on urban social organization. On the other hand, they suggest a hypothetical explanation for schizophrenia based on an inference that in high rate areas persons who develop schizophrenia experience extreme social isolation. Human ecological theory is the model at the beginning of the research; socialization theory is the model at the end.

The significance of this study is recognized particularly on two counts. First, it has been a stimulus for numerous spin-off studies by both psychiatrists and sociologists. Second, its publication initiated a dialogue between psychiatrists and social scientists which has continued to this day.

References

Clausen, J. A. & Kohn, M. (1955), Social isolation and schizophrenia. *American Sociological Review*, pp. 265-273.

Dunham, H. W. & Weinberg, K. (1960), *The Culture of the State Mental Hospital.* Detroit: Wayne State University Press.

Dunham, H. W. (1965), *Community and Schizophrenia.* Detroit: Wayne State University Press.

Dunham, H. W. (1966), Epidemiology of psychiatric disorders as a contribution to medical ecology. *Arch Gen Psychiatry.* 14:1-19.

Leighton, A. (1956), A Proposal for Research in the Epidemiology of Psychiatric Disorders. In: *Epidemiology of Mental Disorders.* New York: Milbank Memorial Fund, pp. 128-135.

Levy, L. & Rowitz, L. (1973), *The Ecology of Mental Disorder.* New York: Behavioral Publications.

Myerson, A. (1926), The Inheritance of Mental Diseases. In: *The Psychology of Mental Disorders.* Baltimore: Williams and Wilkins Co.

Myerson, A. (1927), *The Psychology of Mental Disorders.* New York: Macmillan Co.

Myerson, A. (1940), Review of mental disorders in urban areas. *Am J Psychiatry* 16:995-997.

Park, R. E. (1931), Human ecology. *Am J Sociol* 42:1-15.

Park, R. E. (1926), The urban community as a spatial pattern and moral order. In: *The Urban Community,* ed. E. W. Burgess. Chicago: University of Chicago Press, pp. 5-18.

Proceedings: First Colloquium on Personality Investigation 1928, and Second Colloquium on Personality Investigation, 1929. Held under joint auspices of the American Psychiatric Association and the Social Science Research Council. Baltimore: The Johns Hopkins Press, 1930.

Robinson, W. D. (1950), Ecological correlations and the behavior of individuals. *Am Sociol Rev* 15:351-357.

Watson, J. D. (1968), *The Double Helix.* New York: Atheneum.

Chapter 5

The Midtown Manhattan Longitudinal Study: Aging, Generations, and Genders

LEO SROLE
ANITA KASSEN FISCHER

Among the enduring thematic strands that weave through the long fabric of Western thought is the conviction that contemporary man is in a condition fallen from an earlier height of simplicity, virtue, and well-being. This retrospective vision harks back to the innocence of Scriptural Eden, the serenity in the Golden Age of Hellenic mythology, then to chivalric security in the medieval literature, to quintessential harmony in the Rousseauian "state of nature," and to the earthy wholesomeness of our more recent agrarian past. Embodied in these and other variations on the same theme is a nostalgic philosophy of history, which views the complexities, heterogeneity, and associated bedevilments of the present human estate as debris accumulated from the long sweep of social change.

A Psychiatric Philosophy of History

From Benjamin Rush and Phillipe Pinel onward, prominent psychiatrists, out of primary fixation on individual behavioral regressions, have joined others to advance this philosophy in their assumptions about the social etiology of, and preferred forms of care for, mental derangements. Among prime examples are the following: (1) The 19th century alienists who, to treat mental disorders, followed the "back to idyllic nature" path in siting their new "asylums" and "retreats." (2) Their colleagues of the period who arraigned the democratic advances carved into the American Constitution with the charge, typically expressed by one early psychiatric epidemiologist, that our "free institutions promote insanity" (Hayden, 1844). The identical flat claim of factuality was used by their contemporaries who opposed the

Based on the article "The Midtown Manhattan Longitudinal Study vs. 'The Mental Paradise Lost' Doctrine" by Leo Srole and Anita K. Fischer (1980), *Arch Gen Psychiatr* 37:209-221.

abolition of slavery. (3) The very same theme was still being elaborated a century later in Erich Fromm's works, which probably represent the ultimate in the neoutopian, "turn the clock back" tendency in Western historiography.

One key tenet in this ideology is the pervasive conviction, often accepted as prima facie axiom, that mental health in the population at large has long been deteriorating, and at an accelerating tempo during the modern era. Fromm, for example, writes that postmedieval man, . . . having lost the sense of unity with men and the universe, is overwhelmed with a sense of his individual nothingness and helplessness. Paradise is lost for good. . . . The new freedom is *bound* [emphasis added] to create a deep feeling of insecurity, powerlessness, doubt, aloneness and anxiety" (Fromm, 1941). Following Fromm and others, we will refer to this trend in the psychiatric literature as the "Mental Paradise Lost" doctrine.

In a more recent book, Fromm goes much farther in mass diagnosis, and attributes to people in contemporary societies, "schizoid or schizophrenic qualities . . . of a chronic, low-grade type . . . common to a vast part of the population: clerical workers, salesmen, engineers, physicians . . . and especially many intellectuals and artists . . . in fact, one may surmise, to most of the *urban* population [emphasis added]." Thus, to him "it is legitimate to speak of an 'insane society' . . . in which modern man has lost the capacity for subjective experience" (Fromm, 1973). These surmised "facts" doubtless must have come as a belated surprise not only to mental health professionals, but also to the earth's billions of other urbanites.

Sociologists Goldhamer and Marshall (Goldhamer and Marshall, 1943), to our knowledge, are the only 20th century researchers to have assembled time series data challenging the Mental Paradise Lost credo. Calculating age-specific rates of first admissions of psychotic patients to Massachusetts hospitals between 1840 and 1940, they found that in this industrializing century, no increase in such frequencies occurred among those below the age of 50 years. Restated, for the largest nosological category of hospitalized patients, there was a flat trend, rather than an upward thrust, of annual admission rates within the 90% of the population who, through most of the period covered, were younger than 50 years.

One Achillesian flaw in this otherwise sophisticated Goldhamer and Marshall challenge is that, for purposes of generalizing about the universe of mental illness in the population at large, the psychoses represent only a minute fraction of all psychological disturbances; and, to compound difficulties, hospitalized psychotics comprise only a fraction of all psychotics. Required for a credible challenge of the Paradise Lost doctrine would be a series of surveys of the entire spectrum of psychopathology in the general population, replicated over a period of time measured in generations. None has as yet been attempted.

However, the Midtown Manhattan Mental Health Study, launched in 1952 and fielded in 1954, has evolved from a single point-of-time investigation of a general population, with a cross-section design, into a two-stage follow-up exploration, with a longitudinal, panel design. For purposes of labeling convenience, we here refer to the cross-sectional survey of 1954 as Midtown I, the follow-up field research of 1974 as Midtown II, and the analytic delineation of temporal changes observable between those two stages as the longitudinal Midtown III operation.

With Midtown III, we can now approach the issues underlying the Goldhamer and Marshall challenge from an empirical base more appropriate, at least on a number of key dimensions, than was provided by long-term data from Massachusetts mental hospital records. In fact, since exponents of the Paradise Lost doctrine hold urbanization, and the big city in particular, to be the prime villain behind the presumed trends of deteriorating mental health in recent centuries, Manhattan, having long been tagged "crack-up city" (Esquire, July 1953), might offer the ultimate test case for that view. Midtown III is the first socio-epidemiological analysis of a large, community-based population to uncover a previously undetected change in adult well-being between two successive generations born since the turn of the present century.

Concepts and Methods

Given the potential impact of the new findings both on an old-new philosophy of history and on program thinking for the decades ahead, the conceptual and technical underpinnings on which those data rest must be detailed. The relevant findings will then be presented through a series of tables and elaborations. Our concluding section offers one plausible theory to explain the direction of the new data, based in part on evidence from works on 19th and 20th-century history.

As deputy to directing psychiatrist Thomas Rennie, senior social scientist on the multidisciplinary staff of Midtown I from its inception, and director of both Midtown II and III, the present principal author can clarify the main lines and rationales of the unfolding research design that in time came to bind all three operations into an integral whole. (Parts of this account are given fuller elaboration in the Midtown I flagship volume [Srole et al., 1962] and its revised and enlarged edition [Srole et al., 1978]. For a parallel discussion of Midtown II, see Srole [Srole, 1975].)

First, by way of fixing locus, Midtown is our name for a well-delineated, high density "gold coast and slum" residential area, one that in 1954 sheltered some 175,000 inhabitants, 99% of them white. In demographic terms, these Midtowners were a close approximation of the 1.25 million, otherwise extremely heterogeneous, non-Puerto Rican whites then occupying the island of Manhattan. The former, therefore, could be generalized to the latter as parent universe, and probably to similar populations in counterpart hub areas of America's largest cities. Under scrutiny, in short, was a cross-section slice of the most metropolitan segment of the nation's great communal diversity.

Our 1954 field operation was an enterprise in sociopsychiatric epidemiology, with the descriptive and etiological targets fixed on Midtown and its mother borough. From the long perspectives of anthropology and sociology, we viewed that community generically; that is, as presenting visible precipitates of natural experiments of human nature, but concealing the sociocultural and experiential sources of health differences embedded deeply in its cross-cutting subgroups. We accordingly sought to pinpoint descriptively and dissect analytically those sources.

Beyond such basic research goals, Midtown I's social policy sights were set on providing an epidemiological surveyor's map of the community for (A) guidance in planning the expansion and redeployment of professional helping services that were prompted by World War II experiences with military-aged men, and for (B) moving preventive psychiatry forward from a dead-center position then near ground-zero. (The degree to which these goals were subsequently approached is discussed by Srole et al., 1978.)

The Midtown I researchers primarily focused on a randomly culled, area-type probability sample of 1,660 adults, who were spread across the entire prime-of-life span between the ages of 20 and 59 years. (These particular boundary lines of age coverage were chosen to facilitate demographic calibration with the like-age groups in the Midtown and white Manhattan populations, involving unpublished data that were especially tabulated for us by the United States Census Bureau [Srole et al., 1978].) Funded by the recently activated National Institute of Mental Health, the Midtown I designers were faced with adapting a new and relatively untried post World War II sample survey technology. In this connection, Kenneth Boulding, writing on the recent evolution of science, calls attention to:

> . . . two methods which have been developed in the social sciences and have profoundly improved man's power of perception of social systems. In this sense they may be compared with the development of the telescope and microscope. The first of these methods is the sample survey, by which information can be drawn at relatively low cost from large populations or social universes. . . . The other is the technique of indexing information . . . that enables us to see some essential characteristics of a very large and complex system (Boulding, 1964).

Midtown II and III

Nevertheless, with some trepidation about individually confronting a large sample of people from a segment of perhaps the most complex metropolis on earth, and totally preoccupied with the "here and now," the Midtown I designers did not foresee or prepare for a possible restudy of our intended target subjects at some distant date. Several years later, however, while wrestling with refractory analytical problems of a cross-sectional study (Midtown I), one of us (L.S.) began to monitor the highly productive, prevention-relevant follow-up investigation of cardiovascular disease in a sample of Framingham, Massachusetts men (Gordon and Kannel, 1970).

As a result, he was drawn into a commitment ultimately to convert the original Midtown data set, although not specifically framed for the purpose, into the baseline of a two-stage restudy of a large subsample of the same people. More than a decade was to pass before this could begin to come about, in part because we had not systematically built into Midtown I the connecting informational tie-lines that, after a substantial time interval, could help us pick up the trails to the current addresses of an "on-the-move" population element. Given skepticism that our Midtown I sample could, years later, be tracked and corralled in adequate numbers, it was first indispensable to establish follow-up feasibility. With the full support of the National Institute of Mental Health, in 1970 we started a systematic "bureau of missing persons" search to locate the nomads among our Midtown I respondents.

Of course, the fundamental principle of probability sampling for a new investigation is that every person in its population universe must be given an equal chance of being drawn, a principle rigorously applied in Midtown I with, to us, uncanny results. For Midtown II, Richard Remington, our epidemiology consultant (now dean of the University of Michigan School of Public Health), suggested the following adaptation of that principle for follow-up studies: manage your search efforts so as to give all missing members of the stage I sample the same chance of being located for possible restudy in stage II.

Accordingly, we applied the same sequence of search modalities to every one of our Midtown I "address unknown" respondents (or surviving kin) without exception. At completion of this all-inclusive detective sweep (A. K. Fischer and R. Biel, unpublished data, August 1979), we had verified the current whereabouts of 1,124 members (67.7%) of our baseline sample, 858 of them alive and 266 certified as deceased. (Mortality, its causes, and its baseline predictors were target variables of Midtown II and III (Singer et al., 1976.)

Of course, the hazard hanging over all longitudinal sample studies is the certainty of sizable attrition, i.e., loss to follow-up, with the magnitude of losses, other things being more or less the same, tending to be a function of (A) the extent of the tracking information secured in the baseline interviews, (B) the number of years intervening, and (C) the degree of residential turnover in the sample's community base. In all three respects, the attritional risks for the Midtown I sample had been maximal. It might be mentioned that our total unlocated loss of 32.3% figures to an average annual loss of 1.6%, which compares favorably with the rate for most other longitudinal studies focused on career-launched adults. An example is the recent follow-up investigation of 3,224 military personnel exposed to an atmospheric nuclear test in 1957. Despite the uncommon advantages of baseline military records, by 1979 the unlocated loss was 40%, or an average annual loss of 1.8% per year (*Morbidity Mortality Weekly Report,* 1979).

Located Subsample

We ended our search with 858 baseline respondents located alive, plus 266 certified as dead and a residual 536 as terminally unlocatable. By actuarial estimate, approximately 100 of the latter were deceased. Drawing on our baseline data bank, we could also estimate another 100 to have been never-married women, mainly aged 20 to 39 years, who predictably soon married and abandoned their former identifying surname and home precincts, for search purposes becoming anonymous "needles" in our megalopolitan "haystack."

The 858 located survivors, then, comprised the Midtown I subsample finally accessible for approach to be reinterviewed after a lapse of two decades. At minimum, we can in principle generalize from them as their own 20-year controls. Beyond that, we emphatically did not expect to generalize from them to the entire Midtown sample of 1954. However, we can, potentially at least, generalize from them to their living population universe of 1,294 survivors, located and unlocated, in 1974 at age 40 to 79 years, and probably to other similarly constituted populations of like history as well. Practically, however, we could so generalize only if the 858 survivors of known address are an approximately representative subsample, in demographic and other respects recorded in our Midtown I information bank, of all 1,294 Midtown I survivors.

We can determine representativeness, to a large degree, by assessing the fit between the characteristics in 1954 of (A) the 858 visible survivors and (B) those of the 1,394 comprising the 1,294 survivors, unlocated and located, plus the 100 estimated but unidentified deceased (probably elderly, lower-status men in the main), who are numerically too few to significantly diminish the appropriateness of the 1,394 aggregate as a reference population universe. Some may call for a comparison here of the located and the unlocated, i.e., of subsample A and subsample B. This would be relevant if we were interested in the determinants of locatability and nonlocatability. However, for purposes of generalization, the prerequisite is an answer to the question of the part-whole relationship; more specifically, how representative is subsample A of the inclusive A/B population aggregate that is of primary interest here? A secondary, technical issue is: How successful were our efforts to rigorously implement the Remington principle of equal-chance search for all the missing members of the original sample?

Results of comparing the 858 and 1,394 on the hundreds of characteristics reported in the baseline interviews cannot be documented here, but can be briefly summarized as follows: with relatively few exceptions, the accessible subsample entity did not deviate from its stated parent universe by much more than a small known margin of chance variability. Thus, the subsample of accessible survivors passed the initial test necessary to qualify as representative of that parent universe (and probably of counterpart universes of like provenance and age elsewhere), demonstrating that Midtown II was feasible.

With their qualifying test met, those 858 survivors were still a target sample on a list, whom we next had to approach individually for reinterview, without any predefined exclusions, no matter where their homes now happened to be. For this climactic, cliff-hanger purpose, we retained and cosupervised a cadre of experienced health survey interviewers on the staff of the University of Chicago's National Opinion Research Center (NORC). At closure of field work, they had conducted a total of 695 interviews with respondents scattered throughout New York City (62%), its surrounding metropolitan region (22%), 28 states beyond (14%), and while vacationing, with 14 of 18 respondents located outside the continental United States (2%), two as distant as Morocco and Greece.

With the exception of a few who were beyond interview reach, either geographically or by reason of a verified serious physical or mental condition, the nonparticipants had declined several written and phoned (or house call) requests for a home interview appointment communicated by NORC staff members, and as final try in every case, by the Study Director in person. Such extraordinary efforts succeeded in converting 96 (11%) of the located survivors from resisters or refusers into reinterviewees.

The 695 persons interviewed in both 1954 and 1974 comprised 81% of our accessible target sample, compared with our Midtown I 87% participation frequency. The Midtown II 81% rate can be regarded as a satisfactory achievement in light of the fact that, in recent decades, sample surveys have experienced sharp, and bias-threatening, increases in nonparticipation, with the increase largest by far in big cities and among the elderly, where Midtown II on both counts was most vulnerable. (It is revealing that among our 858 located survivors, the nonparticipation rate varied inversely with residential distance from New York City.) On the basis of the 163 nonparticipants' known heterogeneous (although hardly random) baseline characteristics, representing a relatively small proportion of the 858 total, we infer as follows: had all of the nonparticipants been reinterviewed, the findings on the main variables of Study interest would probably not have deviated markedly from those yielded by the 695 panelists.

This abbreviated account of how, and with what results, our Midtown II reinterviewees were painstakingly reassembled for potentially large scientific and history-illuminating purposes has been offered to meet challenges to that panel on the ground that it cannot be representative of the entire Midtown I sample of 1954. Our answer is that the panel is not unrepresentative of its appropriate population universe, that is, the Midtown I sample members surviving to 1974, now advanced to the range of 40 to 79 years of age.

General Mental Health Classification Process

Before proceeding to our panel data, a final level of procedural scaffolding must be sketched to anticipate relevant questions as to the substantive comparability of the key Midtown I and II variable, namely general mental health. The 1954 interview systematically reviewed the presence or absence of an expert-picked sample of some 120 manifestations of mental disturbance. These were principally drawn from such established symptom collocations as the Minnesota Multiphasic Personality Inventory, the Cornell Medical Index (CMI), and the World War II military screening Neuropsychiatric Adjunct (NSA). The symptom questions of the CMI and NSA (Stouffer et al., 1949), in particular, have been established as reliable and, moreover, as valid by the measure of their power to discriminate between diagnostically heterogenous psychiatric patient (criterion) and nonpatient (comparison) groups.

Thomas Rennie, the Midtown I study director and senior psychiatrist (until his untimely death in 1956), chose 83 of those items for their clinical relevance and their time reference to the period of the interview, and the remainder, which referred to the preadult period, only to lend temporal perspective to the currently visible manifestations of mental health status. Detailed presentations of the inclusive Midtown I symptom questions and the procedures for structuring them are given in *Mental Health in the Metropolis* (Srole et al., 1962, 1978).

Several decisions guided Rennie's selection process. (1) The symptom questions were chosen to represent the manifest currents of behavioral disturbance that generally reflect the emotional substrate underlying most of the many narrowly circumscribed patient syndromes to which psychiatrists try to attach a specific diagnostic tag. In Midtown I's single home interview (average duration, 135 minutes), the sample of symptoms covered was intended not for the impossible task of discriminating among those numerous syndromes, (especially in cases falling outside the clinical range of full blown pathology, as most do), but to mark, as does a physician's thermometer, progressive grades of deviation in emotional "fever" and disability, from an asymptomatic state of presumptive wellness. Among the scorable symptom dimensions represented in the interview with multiple items were the following: generalized psychophysiological "body language" that bespeaks varying intensities of tension; a series of organ-specific, often psychogenic, dysfunctions; expressions of diffuse or circumscribed anxieties and phobias; manifest states of depression and their reactive corollaries; tendencies to withdraw from others; paranoid ideations; excessive intakes of liquor and food; signs of maladaptive rigidity and sociopathic orientations; and the interviewer's observations of the respondent along a series of behavioral dimensions. (2) This large and diverse corpus of information from each subject was reviewed and evaluated in its entirety, i.e., as a configuration, by two Study psychiatrists under Rennie's supervision. By judgments of relative severity of symptom formation and degree of explicit or implied impairment in social role functioning, each psychiatrist independently classified each respondent on a six-fold continuum of general mental health, which consisted of two major categories, namely the Unimpaired and the Impaired, each with three classes. The former category included (A) the nonsymptomatic "Well," (B) the "Mild," and (C) the "Moderate" classes of symptom development. The latter category included the following symptomatic grades: (A) the "Marked," (B) the "Severe," and (C) the "Incapacitated" (or "Near-Incapacitated"), who, except for care-giving kin, would be hospitalized. It must be emphasized that this six-grade ordinal schema spanned the entire gamut of general mental health differences in a noninstitutional population, a comprehensive coverage attempted by no other study of community epidemiology known to us at the time. (3) Rennie held the position that no firm consensus had emerged in psychiatry to demarcate reliably the lower, indistinct or ragged, and historically elastic boundary line of "mental illness," or so-called "caseness." In that predicament, after all 1,660 Midtowners had been classified without thought of such nominal demarcation, he chose the category of the "Impaired" as his own operational criterion of functionally significant psychopathology. Parenthetically, the Study's senior social scientist was no less interested in the class of asymptomatic Wells, its prevalence relative to that of the Impaired, and the etiological and community health implications of contrasting numerical balances between these two classes in any population or its component subgroups. The consequences of such a contrast are apparent in comparing the affective "tinderbox" atmosphere found in the slum and the even tenor of the middle class neighborhood as two "worlds" with vastly different mental health "climates."

To place Rennie's unidimensional, step-wise schema of mental health classification in appropriate historical perspective, we would emphasize that (A) it had direct antecedents in the thought and clinical practice of Adolph Meyer and a more recent group of World War II military psychiatrists (Wittson and Hunt, 1955), and coincided in time with the development of a cognate "health-sickness" scale by Karl Menninger and his associates for use with their Topeka Clinic patients (Luborsky, 1962).

Moreover, such a unidimensional framework is a direct parallel of general medicine's own long-standing practice of differentiating progressive grades of "clinical severity" in patients of diverse symptomatologies (Sartwell, 1953). The latter mode of classification has been useful in following patient changes under treatment, and is indispensable as a yardstick for the longitudinal investigator's observation of his subjects' shifts in health status, whatever their original diagnostic rubric. (The diagnosis of a subject could be "neurotic" both at time X and time Y, yet he could fall into the "moderate" category of severity at time X and the "incapacitated" category at Y.)

To the criticism of some psychiatrists (still heard today) that the gradient schema of classifying mental disturbances is "primitive," in the sense that it is nosologically nonspecific, Rennie, a distinguished teacher of clinical psychiatry of the Adolph Meyer school, replied in words (with which many still concur) to approximately the following effects: (1) Diagnostic specificity and symptomatic severity are, of course, indigenous to the clinical information-eliciting context of treating patients. (Not to be overlooked however, are the continuing reservations of psychiatrists that "diagnostic specificity may, in fact, not conform to the clusterings of symptoms as they actually appear in large populations" [Kiev, 1978]. Therefore, they generally concede the definitional "looseness" and arbitrariness of nosological labels.) (2) Moreover, in the epidemiologist's operating milieu of interviewing randomly drawn men and women on their home ground, eliciting the necessary symptom information is feasible for classifying grades of severity of disturbance. This carries the proviso, however, that extreme care must be taken to set the stage for the interview, and arrange its question contents, with major emphasis on somatic and other nonpsychiatric facets of the life history, a requirement essential to minimize the defense-evoking effects of an unexpected, heavy-handed, frontal intrusion into highly defended sectors of the nonpatient respondent's psyche (Srole et al., 1962, 1978). (3) However, procuring the mass of symptom information necessary for differential diagnostic decision-making is not possible under the latter circumstances; that is so primarily because the unrelenting, massive concentration of the structured clinical-type interview on psychopathology, up to the rarest kinds, often generates resistance in the sample subject. The accuracy of information volunteered under such circumstances can be seriously questioned. (4) Implied, therefore, is the research principle that health examinations and classifications must be realistically scaled, to what is humanly and temporally possible within the constraints (A) of each major kind of examinee, i.e., the positively motivated-for-recovery, cooperative institutional patient vs. the more or less neutrally motivated, randomly selected nonpatient, (B) of each major kind of examination setting, i.e., the mental hospital vs. the subject's home base, and (C) the time available to the examiner. (To our dismay, a number of recent epidemiological studies, pressed by increasing demands for diagnostic specificity from clinicians and third-party payers, are appropriating interview instruments clinically developed specifically for mental patients, and are applying them to general population samples.)

Midtown II Mental Health Classifications

From Rennie's classification decisions of 1954, we can now move to their replication in 1974, in which both of us were centrally involved. For purposes of assessing general mental health in 1974, we repeated with identical wording the 83 "current" symptom items used in 1954, excluding as redundant those that referred retrospectively to the respondent's preadult period.

To accurately discern mental health changes since the 1954 baseline, we might have considered having the Midtown panel's 1974 general mental health status classified by the same psychiatrists and judgmental processes as 20 years earlier. Unfortunately, the Study's psychiatrists of 1954 were no longer available. And, even if they had been present to repeat their classification function of 1954, the likely evolution in their professional perspectives would probably have undermined confidence in the objective reproducibility of their subjective judgmental processes of 20 years earlier.

This dilemma presented us with Midtown III's most formidable procedural impasse, which was fortunately resolved by the availability of a surrogate "classifier" not on the scene 20 years before: the computer. As first step, with multiple regression methods applied to the 1954 Midtown corpus of adult symptom information, the computer could be programmed with an equation that parsimoniously reproduced the psychiatrists' six-grade judgmental ratings of 1954 general mental health, with an accuracy suggested by a Pearson correlation of .83. (This compares favorably with a correlation of .75 between the 1,660 independent judgmental classifications of the two Study psychiatrists with each other in 1954. Moreover, that the psychiatrists' ratings could be predicted by multiple regression methods with such a high degree of accuracy suggests that they had been made with very considerable consistency.) The .83 coefficient assures us that the computer-generated ratings of 1954 were an acceptable surrogate for the psychiatrists' judgmental classifications of that year (Singer et al., 1976).

Since we asked the identically worded battery of current symptom questions in 1974, we could next apply the identical regression methods to these later symptoms to produce follow-up mental health ratings that are strictly standardized to the reference model of the computerized 1954 general mental health classifications. In effect, such standardization has ensured that the degree of concordant reliability between the computerized 1954 and 1974 classifications, hereafter referred to as GMH I and GMH II, is 100%.

However, such perfect reliability offers no a priori assurance that GMH II in 1974 is as valid a measure of general mental health as was GMH I in *1954.* The predictive validity of the latter measure can be retrospectively judged against two related outcome measures in 1974: (1) Panelists in 1974 were asked consecutive questions about a "nervous breakdown" experienced, or felt to be "approaching." (The interviewer defined "nervous breakdown" to the respondent as "a halting for some time of your usual work and activities because of nervous and emotional troubles.") If the risk of such a development occurring by *1974* in the *1954* GMH class of Wells is transformed into a value of 1, then the comparable risk escalates to magnitudes of 1.5 in the Mild class, 3.6 in the Moderate class and 4.5 in the Impaired category. (2) The power of GMH I to predict GMH II is expressed by a

Pearson correlation of .45. Our colleague-consultant, Dr. Jean Endicott, out of experiences in constructing, testing, and evaluating a large series of clinical interview instruments, has assessed that coefficient as follows: "If I had been asked beforehand what correlation you could expect between your panel's 1954 and 1974 mental health assignments, I would have replied that .30 was about the most you could expect." We can speculate that the unexpectedly high correlation of .45 implies a greater durability in the emotional substrate measured by GMH I and GMH II than could have been inferred from the volatility of nosologically specific symptom syndromes.

The issue of a possible shift in validity between GMH I and GMH II must still be confronted. After all, the Midtown panel members had aged by 20 years, and the sampled symptoms may be less appropriate for older than for younger people. Moreover, in the intervening two decades, semantic and other forms of sociocultural "drift" could have altered the meanings of symptoms through which mental disturbance is projected and/or verbalized. The latter have been designated as a "time of measurement effect" that can intrude into measures of individual change over time, and the former as an "aging effect." These effects will be more fully discussed below.

To test these possibilities, we have made a series of parallel checks of GMH I and GMH II, including their separate correlations with (among others) a number of classic demographic characteristics, such as age order, sex, and socioeconomic and religious origins. If these time-separated pairs of correlations with the same set of fixed background variables prove to be approximately alike, then the inference would be tenable that GMH I and GMH II have measured mental health status in essentially the same way. To a striking degree, these and other kinds of checks have supported the plausibility of that inference. Such evidence suggests that GMH II is as valid in 1974 as GMH I had been in 1954, in the special sense of validity as measuring the same construct, free of significant time-of-measurement and aging effects, at two distant points of time (Singer et al., 1976).

Thus, satisfying criteria of reliability as well as of predictive and construct validity (Leighton et al., 1966), the computer and multiple regression statistics have given us a standardized, stable yardstick, one that allows us to measure and compare the general mental health status of our Midtown panel members with consistency over a considerable expanse of the adult life cycle. On the technical level, this may be not the least of Midtown III's contributions.

In this connection, parenthetically, to convert a synchronic, cross-sectional survey into a diachronic followup investigation, especially if conversion was not preplanned, is to multiply the technical and substantive complications exponentially. Thus, the Midtown longitudinal effort, working at baseline on relatively unexplored frontiers, with new instruments, was at especially high risk of stumbling into one or more quicksand points of empirical "no return." We are still somewhat disbelieving that none of these possible mishaps has as yet surfaced, and that all of the succession of procedural "pieces" have so far fallen into place in a manner more assuring than we could have expected on the basis of Murphy's Law ("If anything can go wrong, it will.") To successors, we pass on the suggestion that such an outcome does not emerge unless the baseline stage provides the follow-up with a robust foundation.

Up to the present juncture this section must be slightly reminiscent of the lengthy prologue of a George Bernard Shaw "drama of ideas," which usually leaves his characters little space to carry out his great Elizabethan predecessor's dictum that "the play's the thing." Yet the "prologue" in this instance has been written for a critical audience that asks to delineate for them the conceptual and technical scaffolding of Midtown I and II at potentially its most vulnerable points. (In the research literature of psychiatric epidemiology, this canon of public accountability is largely observed in the breach.)

The Findings

This accomplished, we can now open the curtain to Midtown III proper, and the results of re-examining its panel members as a crucial test of the Paradise Lost view of recent general mental health history. First, in Table 1 we set out the panel's full distributions in 1954 and 1974 on the general mental health six-grade continuum. Although by 1974 there are improvements in both a lower Impaired frequency and a higher Well rate, neither of these differences is statistically significant.

TABLE 1
Midtown Manhattan Follow-Up Panel (N=695).
General Mental Health Distributions in 1954 and 1974.

Symptom formation grades	*GMH I (%)*	*GMH II (%)*
1. Well	21.9	25.0
2. Mild	42.6	42.0
3. Moderate	21.3	21.1
4. Marked	9.3	7.5
5. Severe	4.3	3.5
6. Incapacitated	0.6	0.9
4-6 Impaired	14.3	11.9
	100.0	100.0

It must also be emphasized that the seeming near-identity of these two distributions, around the modal class of Mild symptom formation, does not imply predominant individual fixity in mental health status between the two occasions of measurement. On the contrary, only 40% of the entire panel fell into the same GMH grade in 1974 as in 1954, with another 28% of its members slipping one or more classes on that continuum, and 32% improving by moving one or more steps upward.

Thus, the panel's 20-year distribution shifts can be conveyed graphically by the image of a six-step staircase flanked on each side by an escalator. Occupying the same step on the staircase in 1974 as in 1954 are a two-fifths plurality of the panel, while on the escalators one-third of their fellow members have ascended and slightly more than one-fourth have descended. Around the large core of fixity, then, there has been a considerable circulation of mental health changers. (For the same reasons, in the tables to follow, GMH figures for 1974 should be understood to be the net distribution resulting from the panel's post-1954 two-way shifts.)

The findings are hereafter presented in terms of differential frequencies of Impaired GMH, but we emphasize that trends in Well frequencies are usually the direct mirror image of the Impaired trend; that is, bypassing the numerically more or less unvarying intermediate Mild and Moderate classes of symptom formation, the Impaired rates tend to be high where the Well frequencies are low, and vice versa. Thus, although we must largely confine our discussion to group Impaired frequencies, their apparent epidemiological importance is considerably enhanced when they are viewed in tandem with the reversed trend of the Wells.

Age, Generation, and Gender Groups

Because of our overriding interest here in trends over time, adult age differences, divided into four ten-year groups, are necessarily our first-line independent variable, to which general mental health stands as a dependent variable. To summarize the entire Midtown I sample's Impaired frequencies among its separate age groups in 1954, we can report that compared to the rate of the youngest group (20 to 29 years of age), the frequencies in the 30 to 39 and 40 to 49 years of age strata were both half again larger, and in the oldest group (50 to 59 years of age) fully twice as high (6,7). Therefore, except for the similarity of the two intervening age groups with each other, the Impaired rates described a three-step trend line of progressive increments upward on the age hierarchy.

Two different interpretations can be offered to account for this clear-cut trend in the entire Midtown I sample of 1954: (1) The trend reflects the deteriorating consequences of life-cycle aging. On such reasoning, if this (or any other) adult sample's youngest segment were thereafter followed at ten-year intervals, its Impaired (and Well) rates would progressively approximate those of the successively older groups of the Midtown I sample. Indeed, one of us (L.S.) actually so predicted in *Mental Health in the Metropolis* (Srole et al., 1978). (2) Purists of the Mental Paradise Lost school could offer this alternative interpretation: the Midtown I sample's age trends in 1954 reflect only the deteriorating consequences of progressively longer exposure to contemporary civilization, and to the big city environment as its most extreme expression.

Toward mediating this dialectic, we can now turn to Table 2 for a comparison of the Midtown panel's four age groups and their Impaired proportions in 1954 and in 1974. In Table 2, the panel's four age groups are labeled A, B, C, and D, and appear with decade of birth below, next with the number

TABLE 2
Midtown Manhattan Follow-Up Panel (N=695).
GMH Impaired Rates in Decade-of-Birth Groups.

	Decade of birth			
	1900	*1910*	*1920*	*1930*
No.	134	199	195	167
Age in 1954	(50-59)	(40-49)	(30-39)	(20-29)
Rate (GMH I)	22%	16%	14%	7%
Age in 1974	(70-79)	(60-69)	(50-59)	(40-49)
Rate (GMH II)	18%	12%	10%	8%
Difference	−4%	−4%	−4%	+1%
Significance	NS[a]	NS	NS	NS

[a]NS = not statistically significant.

of panel members in each, then with their pairs of Impaired rates, first in 1954 (GMH I) and just below, in 1974 (GMH II). By reading the frequencies horizontally from right to left in each row, we see immediately that in both 1954 and 1974 there is an incremental progression in the rates across the successively older groups to the left of D (the youngest), thereby seeming to confirm the direction of the age trend finding reported in *Mental Health in the Metropolis.* Interestingly, both of the mutually exclusive interpretations of the 1954 age trends in effect predicted that by 1974 the general mental health in all age groups would have slipped further into more unfavorable Impaired frequencies. To test those consensual predictions, we can now examine the *vertical* pair of rates in each Table 2 column, where each age group can be compared with itself after a span of 20 years.

Both interpretations are rejected by the fact that in none of the four groups is the difference between the GMH I and GMH II percentages statistically significant. The contending interpreters justifiably demand an explanation for the apparent contradiction between the vertical, intragroup null differences in Impaired rates after the passage of two decades, and the intergroup horizontal trend, both in 1954 and 1974, toward elevation of those rates at each progressively older stratum.

To resolve the seeming contradiction, we call attention in Table 3 to a rearrangement of Table 2, with focus only on two pairs of cohorts, where age differences have been analytically controlled. The first pair juxtaposes cohort A's Impaired rate in 1954 (GMH I) at age 50 to 59 years, with cohort C's rate in 1974 (GMH II), also at age 50 to 59 years, with contrasting frequencies of 22% and 10%, respectively. Thus, paired cohorts A and C are of identical age-since-birth, but were born 20 years apart, i.e., ±1900 and ±1920, an interval large enough for us to consider them as discrete, successive historical generations; in life-cycle terms, when the latter were ar-

TABLE 3
Midtown Manhattan Follow-Up Panel (N=695).
GMH Impaired Rates by Generation-Separated
Pairs of Like-Age Cohorts.

Cohort	*Rate*
Cohort A (N=134)	
(Age 50-59 in 1954)	
GMH I rate	22%
Cohort C (N=195)	
(Age 50-59 in 1974)	
GMH II rate	10%
Difference	−12%
Significance	$p < 0.01$
Cohort B (N=199)	
(Age 40-49 in 1954)	
GMH I rate	16%
Cohort D (N−167)	
(Age 40-49 in 1974)	
GMH II rate	8%
Difference	−8%
Significance	$p < 0.05$

riving as neonates, the former were passing into adulthood. For present purposes, we can turn to an old English phrase to identify the time gap between one generation and the next as spanning a "score of years." (This does not, of course, denote the conventional parent-offspring, kin sequence of generations.) The second pair in Table 3 includes cohort B in 1954 at age 40 to 49 years and cohort D in 1974, also at age 40 to 49 years, the two presenting generation-specific mental impairment rates of 16% and 8% respectively, a difference statistically significant at the .05 level of confidence.

The vertical pairs of rates in Table 2 show that neither of the alternative interpretations of the 1954 sample's age trends commands any semblance of support in the Midtown II panel, and Table 3 now seems to reveal that the horizontal intergroup rate differences in Table 2 do not reflect the postulated consequences of cumulative individual "wear and tear" from 20 years of open commerce with life-in-environment processes. Rather, Table 2 seems to reflect exclusively the consequences, at least among Midtown mid-life adults in matched age-since-birth pairs, of being born into successive *generation-separated cohorts.*

According to the Paradise Lost school, the later-arrived of two generations should predictably harbor more psychopathology than its predecessor. Up to this point, Table 3 seems to testify that in the Midtown II panel, quite the opposite has been the case, with the later-born cohort in both like-age pairs registering an Impaired rate that is less by one half that of the earlier generation. By the standardized yardstick we have applied to these particular age-matched cohorts, general mental health seems to have improved rather than to have slipped.

Men vs. Women

This new finding demands further elaboration in terms of other constituent groups in the Midtown population, certainly the most salient being the sexes. First, we would recall that, in the Midtown I sample, women and men of like age did not differ in their GMH distributions (Srole et al., 1962, 1978). Second, for the Midtown panel we can summarize the 1974 counterpart of Table 2, dichotomized by gender, as follows: in none of the four age groups has either sex, on balance, changed significantly in its GMH Impaired rate after the 20-year passage between 1954 and 1974. Life-cycle progression across those decades has not been discriminatory in its effects on the genders.

What emerges, however, when we next scan Table 4 as the counterpart of Table 3, with both sexes represented in the contiguous cohort-generations? To judge from the sexist tenor in many of its writings, the Mental Paradise Lost school would probably have predicted this table to show a more pronounced intergeneration decline in GMH among the women. If so, Table 4 could flatly contradict that prognosis.

Examining cohort A's horizontal row, at age 50 to 59 years in 1954, we can see that the Impaired frequency is 15% for its men, and an appreciably higher 26% for its women. In the next row, however, we have cohort C, at like-age (50 to 59 years) in 1974, where the Impaired rates for its two gender groups have both dropped from cohort A's levels, but with a significantly greater decrease among the women, toward virtual parity with men.

Comparison next of the sexes in cohorts B and D, both at age 40 to 49 years, reveals parallel differential intergeneration changes in impairment, from horizontal male-female disparity (9% and 21%) in earlier cohort B to intergender identity (9% and 8%) in the like-age, but later, cohort D. It seems, therefore, that, by a speedometer scaled to the relatively fast-moving age segments of the adult life-cycle, individual mental health status-shifts balance out at net in the same way for the panel's sexes. However, by the scale of the relatively slow-moving procession of generation units, time has dealt rather better with women's mental health than with that of men of the same life-cycle age. For us, these unexpected diversities came as a case of complete serendipity. However, the strength of that new case would be substantially enhanced if Midtown III could marshall evidence of similar diversities on dimensions related to the panel's general mental health.

For this purpose, we can probe a second kind of index of well-being, used with similar wording in both stages of the Midtown investigation, namely a query to the respondent whether his/her "general physical health now is excellent, good, fair or poor?" Two clarifying points about this particular indicator deserve mention. Although the Study's psychiatrists in 1954 did not regard respondent-judged general physical health status (GPH) as a substantively primary component of general mental health, and therefore

TABLE 4
Midtown Manhattan Follow-up Panel (N=695).
GMH Impaired Rates by Generation-Separated Pairs of Like-Age Cohorts and Gender Subgroups.

	Rate	
Cohort	*Men*	*Women*
Cohort A		
(Age 50-59 in 1954)		
GMH I rate	15%	26%
Cohort C		
(Age 50-59 in 1974)		
GMH II rate	9%	11%
Difference	−6%	−15%
Significance	NS	$p < 0.01$
Cohort B		
(Age 40-49 in 1954)		
GMH I rate	9%	21%
Cohort D		
(Age 40-49 in 1974)		
GMH II rate	9%	8%
Difference	0%	−13%
Significance	NS	$p < 0.02$

gave it little weight in their judgmental classifications, Midtown III would probably have surprised them in showing that GPH I (1954) had come up with a zero-order correlation of 0.42 vis-à-vis their 1954 classifications of respondents' general mental health.

On the other hand, Midtown III would hardly have surprised them in also reporting this finding: by methods of multiple regression analysis, applied to verified post-1954 deaths in the entire Midtown I sample, GPH I had significant, discrete power to predict mortality, and to do so independently of (that is, over and above the combined power of), all four of the better known mortality predictors of gender, marital status, socioeconomic status, and the strongest by far: age. Implied is that respondent-rated GPH may predict mortality where age does not, namely premature deaths. In any case, although our GPH question has discrete predictive validity as an indicator of physical durability and mortality risk, we can also consider it as a corollary dimension of subjective well-being.

By way of preliminary, the panel's combined self-judged "fair-poor," i.e., "less than good," responses rose from 16% in 1954 to 23% in 1974, an increase of almost half again over the Midtown I frequency, with the increase almost entirely concentrated in the panel's oldest group that was at age 70 to 79 years in the latter years.

Turning to Table 5, we see that cohort A's women have an unfavorable ("less than good") GPH I frequency that is almost three times that of their like-age men. However, by later cohort C, the male unfavorable rate (GPH II) remains virtually identical with that of cohort A's men, whereas the frequency for cohort C's women has dropped to almost half that of cohort A's women. The gender progressions of GPH I and GPH II in cohorts B and D (both age 40 to 49 years) parallel those observed in cohorts A and C (both age 50 to 59 years).

TABLE 5
Midtown Manhattan Follow-Up Panel (N=695).
General Physical Health:
"Fair-Poor" Frequencies (GPH) by Generation-Separated Pairs of Like-Age Cohorts and Gender Subgroups.

	Frequency	
Cohort	***Men***	***Women***
Cohort A		
(Age 50-59 in 1954)		
GPH I rate	13%	34%
Cohort C		
(Age 50-59 in 1974)		
GPH II rate	14%	18%
Difference	+1%	−16%
Significance	NS	$p < 0.02$
Cohort B		
(Age 40-49 in 1954)		
GPH I rate	16%	24%
Cohort C		
(Age 40-49 in 1974)		
GPH II rate	11%	9%
Difference	−5%	−15%
Significance	NS	$p < 0.01$

Stated differently, in the succession of our like-age but generation-separated cohorts, self-evaluated general physical health has on the average not changed significantly among panel men. However, among counterpart age and generation women, unfavorable GPH rates have fallen from levels higher than those of their male peers in cohorts A and B to nearly identical levels with the men in cohorts C and D.

A third indicator of subjective well-being, developed prior to Midtown I, was an item in the principal author's "Anomia" scale (Srole, 1956) to represent a cognitive, life-devaluing expression of latent suicide potential (LSP), phrased in terms of the following agree-disagree statement: "You sometimes can't help wondering whether anything is worthwhile any more." This was intended to be a somewhat less stark equivalent of "life is no longer worth living."

That item was used in both the Midtown I and II interviews, with about one fourth of the panelists of both sexes agreeing with the statement in both years. We have now analyzed the "agree" responses along lines identical with those followed and just reported on general mental health and self-rated physical health, with parallel results. That is, like-age men in successive generation pairs (A and C, B and D) are similar in their "nothing worthwhile" frequencies.

The women, on the other hand, repeat what we have already reported about their GMH and GPH responses. Table 6 pins down their evidence. Again, both later cohorts of women, C and D, have moved to substantially fewer "nothing worthwhile" outlooks than their earlier age counterparts in cohorts A and B.

TABLE 6
Midtown Manhattan Follow-Up Panel Women (N=401).
"Nothing Worthwhile" (LSP) Frequencies by
Generation-Separated Pairs of Like-Age Cohorts.

Cohort	*Frequency*
Cohort A	
(Age 50-59 in 1954)	
LSP I rate	33%
Cohort C	
(Age 50-59 in 1974)	
LSP II rate	16%
Difference	−17%
Significance	$p < 0.01$
Cohort B	
(Age 40-49 in 1954)	
LSP I rate	31%
Cohort D	
(Age 40-49 in 1974)	
LSP II rate	19%
Difference	−12%
Significance	$p < 0.05$

Thus, there are strikingly consistent, mutually reinforcing trends in the reported intergeneration differences across each of the following sets of variables: (1) across the two genders; (2) across our three different (but intertwined) indicators of subjective well-being; and (3) across our two different, generation-separated midlife age segments, namely 40 to 49 and 50 to 59 years.

To rephrase our data in more specific historical terms, we have discerned significant and consistent differential improvements, among women only, on all three of our indicators of subjective well-being, between the cohorts born in the first two decades of this century and those born in the two decades following. (We shall at times hereafter merge our A and B cohorts as the earlier, or "senior," of the panel's two generations, and C and D as the later, or "junior," generation.)

We recall from the earlier discussion of our pre-1974 trace operation that among our unlocatables in the 1954 sample were a disproportionate number of unmarrried women (then principally 20 to 39 years of age), most of whom probably soon married, changed their surnames, and thus were beyond our search net. In mental health composition, they were then appreciably better off than their single male age-peers (Srole et al., 1962, 1978). Hence, had we been able to locate them as successfully as we had the latter, these women would probably have had a larger representation in our panel cohorts C and D (ages 40 to 59 years in 1974), where their presence would likely have produced an even greater intergender contrast on our three well-being measures.

Further Questions

Before moving on to consider the historical implications of the data, three final questions warrant consideration. First, to start with general mental health, are not the reported age and generation differences confounded with what are called "time of measurement effects?" Referred to are the consequences that can follow from the fact that a measure of construct A employed at time Y, as repeated from previous use at time X, may be invalid in the sense that it no longer measures the earlier underlying construct in the same way. Such an artifactual intrusion has often been extremely difficult to isolate from other kinds of effects operating concurrently across time. Nevertheless, this issue was partially addressed earlier in this article. We there reported on our checks to determine whether or not GMH I and GMH II behaved in the same ways relative to a series of fixed background variables represented both in 1954 and 1974. We there shared the assurances generated by this methodological exercise that GMH II is as valid a measure of the same construct as was GMH I before it. Also, it seems most unlikely that our replicated one-item indicators of general physical health and latent suicidal potential, on their face content, could be significantly more vulnerable to time-of-measurement distortions than apparently was our multi-item GMH yardstick. Moreover, it is unlikely that all three measures in concert are vulnerable to such distortions in one gender and not in the contemporaneous other. Such inferences seem to be reinforced by the parallels found in the trend patterns of all three measures of well-being. Of course, the possibility of such artifacts intruding in our longitudinal change measures remains open and will continue to be explored further.

However, given that those future probes are unlikely to nullify the direct and circumstantial kinds of evidence just discussed, we can next turn to a second question. Across the life span, individual microaging inputs and historical macrosocial inputs are inextricably interwoven, and their separate effects are therefore difficult to identify. Have these in fact been adequately segregated?

We can reply that in part our data tables have already done so. On the one hand, we have observed that 20 years of aging registered no net distributional changes in the three measures of well-being among any of the panel's four age groups (except self-judged physical health in the oldest stratum only). On the other hand, holding the age variable constant by comparing only like-age cohorts, we isolated significant intergeneration differences on all three well-being indicators between cohorts born in different segments of the 20th century.

The final question is this: Are there intergenerational differences in demographic composition that could account for the sex-linked pattern of distributions on the three subjective well-being measures? Foreign or US birth is one of those demographic factors, and for purposes of illustration might be briefly discussed here. The foreign-born, who are predominately of lower socioeconomic origin, comprise 27% of the Midtown panel and are principally concentrated in the two earlier generation cohorts (A and B). Therefore, if we shift the analysis to the US-born only, we find that the difference in Impaired rates between successive like-age cohorts A and C narrows somewhat from -12% to -8.6%, but the difference between cohorts B and D remains -8%, both differences being statistically significant ($P < .05$). Again, these differences among the US-born are almost wholly confined to the women of the respective cohorts. Clearly, this illustrative demographic variable fails to account for the intergeneration pattern of female-only advances in general mental health that will continue to be our overriding interest here.

Summary, Explanatory Theory, and the Future

The Midtown Study has confronted the Mental Paradise Lost protagonists with their arch-villain, New York City, and on that most strategic testing ground favorable to their own position, has put two of the school's three major articles of faith under systematic empirical scrutiny.

(1) They have held that mental health in the general population has been on the downgrade over time. To this keystone of their thinking, Midtown III has responded in two parts: (A) After exposure to 20 years of living mainly in or around the City (Srole, 1978), the Midtown panelists show no significant net change in mental health composition among any of their four decade-of-birth groups. (This holds irrespective of their post-1954 residential distance

from New York.) (B) On the other hand, by the temporal measure of two generation units, mental health in the later generation, with age controlled, is not worse than it had been in the earlier generation, but significantly better.

(2) Those ideologues in many cases have entertained a view of women as the constitutionally and psychologically fragile gender, implying that, compared to men, their mental health over time has been more vulnerable to erosion. Again Midtown III has countered with two generalizations: (A) After 20 years of living, the Midtown panel women of all age groups have changed no more in mental health makeup than did their male peers. (B) On the time scale of generation units, the Midtown panel's intergeneration improvement in mental health is found to be exclusively concentrated in its female ranks.

Earlier, we cautiously defined the specific population universe to which the Midtown panel's findings can be generalized, and reiterate that caution here. However, we would add that there are grounds for the hypothesis that Midtown's differential intergender progression in well-being between successive generations (A) may be underrepresented in rural and other small communities, and conversely, (B) may be principally concentrated in the big cities (Fass, 1977). If the Midtown-specific generalizations are in due course confirmed in other populations, it is predictable that the Mental Paradise Lost doctrine, spun from strands out of a long tradition of nostalgic legend and folklore, will take its place with the Ptolemaic cosmology and other intuitive prescientific formulations that evolved quasiscientific supports to sustain their popular acceptance for centuries.

Change Over Generations

The longitudinal reach of the Midtown Study enabled us to sort out the discrete changes between successive generations in the subjective well-being of their members. It is our final charge to offer a theory that might plausibly articulate the interconnections between (A) the Midtown collectivity units called generations, (B) the overarching macrosocial shifts that occurred in the separate periods of history they passed through, and (C) the sex-specific patterns of changes in well-being.

In a ground-breaking essay published prior to World War II (1936), social scientist Karl Mannheim elaborated the concept of generations as of fundamental, crosscutting importance to sociology, psychology, and history. In a later work, he asked: "Why did the Middle Ages and the Renaissance produce entirely different types of men?" He there urged behavioral scientists to "study the changes of the human mind in an historical setting, in close connection with the changes in the social structure (Mannheim, 1940).

Of course, the concept of generations is one of the most multidimensional constructs in the entire repertoire of the human sciences. That it refers to a terrain of potentially bewildering proportions is documented by the huge literatures of fiction, autobiography, and biography, where it has been the scene of endless contention. An excellent 18th century illustration of the cumulative divergences of two successive generations is to be found in Washington Irving's hard-drinking character, Rip Van Winkle. To recall that classic tale, Rip was a temporally displaced person, jolted by the overwhelming changes he encountered in his home village on return after an unbroken sleep of 20 years in the mountains. Implying a comparison of New York City past and present, novelist Saul Bellow has written in a related vein, "Not even Walt Whitman could today embrace it emotionally: the attempt might capsize him" (Srole et al., 1978; p. 5).

The notion of human generations embraces a reality with enormously complex entanglements in the structures of, and the unceasing interactive processes between individual biological givens and the protean, far more volatile sociocultural realm, extending out into geographic space, into life-cycle trajectories, and into historical time. More concretely, in a century of accelerating social and economic changes, interspersed with major macrosocial convulsions speeding up that tempo, successive generation groups have maturated in, and navigated through, different temporally definable segments in that 100-year stream of history, each segment a cycloramic milieu, each with its own characteristic mix of benign and noxious ingredients. The different sections of that "engulfing stream" at different stages of the life cycle, contribute to the proverbial "communication gap" that marks off one generation, with its own uniquely timed sequence of common experiences, from the next.

Mannheim underscores the difficulties field researchers face in trying (within the span of a single professional career) to encompass that order of behavioral universe. "It is not easy," he writes, "to bring [research] to bear in analyzing historical experiences and in diagnosing the symptoms of the present time [thereby foreshadowing Midtown II by about 40 years]. The generation factor...which at the biological level operates with the uniformity of a natural law...becomes the most elusive one at the social and cultural level, where its effects can be ascertained only with great difficulty and by indirect methods (Mannheim, 1936).

Yet our reported Midtown data insist that we address this question: How are we to explain the differential intergender shifts in well-being between the Midtown A/B generation, born in the two decades before 1915, and the C/D generation appearing during the two decades following? Because this question did not surface for us until the Midtown III stage of the study, we had not sought answers in the preceding stages. Nevertheless, in a retrospective, gender-oblivious way, Midtown II did systematically explore macrosocial and purely individual episodes, major and minor, that had marked the life course of our panelists, most episodes dating since the Midtown I interviews of 1954, some predating that occasion by ten years (e.g., World War II) or as far back as two decades (e.g., the Great Depression).

Stratification of Experience

These relatively recent life-history intrusions on a panel-wide basis remain to be analyzed for their gender-differential connections, and will be reported in a sequel article. In the meantime, toward considering the question just posed, two influences have forced us to look for empirical leads to new hypotheses at a farther reach back into time than we have probed heretofore. The first influence, as already implied, has been the crystallizing impact of Mannheim's thought. He refers to the "phenomena of the 'stratification of experience'" in a generation group, arising from exposure to the chronological ordering of imprinting macrosocial configurations. He then emphasizes the critical distinction between the experiences of preadulthood that "happen to make those all important 'first impressions'...and [those] which follow to form the second, third and other 'strata'Early impressions tend to coalesce into a *natural view* of the world. All later experiences then tend to receive their meaning from this original setThe continuous shift in objective conditions has its counterpart in a continuous shift in the oncoming new generations which are first to incorporate the changes in their behavioral systems" (Mannheim, 1936).

We can elaborate these important insights in terms of five propositions: (1) Given the macrosocial and microsocial changes between one historical period and the next, we can designate the behavioral milieus of the separate periods as subcultures in flux. (2) The several age-ordered generations present in a given period of time, A, can be envisaged metaphorically as dominoes superimposed in a stratified ziggurat pattern, the youngest cohort at the bottom and the oldest at the top. (3) Dominant carriers of the subculture prevailing in period A are usually the cohorts in midlife who are its models. (4) The changes imminent and emergent during period A that foreshadow the subculture of period B will leave varying imprints on the hierarchy of cohorts present during period A. In specific terms of values, goals, life-styles and lifecourse pathways, the impacts of period-A changes will be greatest on the youth cohorts (adolescents and young adults, as in the Vietnam War years), with progressively diminishing effects on the successively higher (i.e., older) cohorts. (5) The midlife models of subculture A and the youth-stage, forthcoming models of subculture B are in a relationship of contention that can be characterized as "the muted battle of the generations," across what the French call *fosse,* meaning "ditch" or "moat."

The point of key relevance here is the paramount importance of the subculture milieu during the formative stage of a generation's development. Although that stage was by no means untapped in the Midtown I and II interviews, we lacked the prescience to try to conceptualize and systematically recapture it retrospectively, if indeed that would have been possible at those times in terms relevant for present purposes.

The second influence to push the inquiry back into time, anecdotal in nature, was the coincidence that one of us (L.S.) happens to be a contemporary of the Midtown panel's cohort B, timing him to be a schoolboy hearsay witness of World War I, and a participant in its aftermath. In the midst of those social upheavals, he was himself caught up in the tradition-shattering changes that were sweeping through the arena of intergender relationships, of course without any insight as to their historical significance or foresight as to their future long-range consequences. Those experiences remained vivid in memory, but lacked an adequate historical perspective until the surprising Midtown cohort data were in hand, sending us to documentary works on that period and the decades immediately before and after. This literature fortunately has been highly relevant for a credible theoretical response to our question about the possible main sources of the Midtown panel's intergeneration-cum-intergender differences in well-being, compelling us here to share its illuminations and implications for an historically grounded social psychiatry.

Women in the Victorian Era and After

To face our question adequately, we must turn back to the last decades of the 19th century, which was the temporal habitat of the parents of Midtown's cohorts A and B. The distinguished historian J. H. Plumb needs only two sentences to summarize the predicament of women in that culminating period of the Victorian Era: "Except in the highest ranks of the aristocracy, women...were as securely locked in the prison of their households as any convict...condemned to a daily treadmill of toil.... Husbands could be and were tyrants" (Plumb, 1973).

Kinder, Kucher, Kirche fixed the specific confines of a woman's life, with children one-after-the-other pressing the limits of her gestation cycles and emotional reserves. To that image of crowded confinement, illuminating details are added by Gunnar Myrdall, the Swedish sociologist, in an interesting appendix to his magisterial work on American society, subtitled, "The Negroe Problem and Modern Democracy" (Myrdall, 1940). He there emphasizes the striking similarities in the antebellum blacks' position vis-à-vis their masters, and that of white wives vis-à-vis their own "keepers." Both were harnessed to a yoke under "the paternalistic idea which held the slave to be a sort of family member and...placed him beside [the white] women and children under the power of the paterfamilias." Myrdall quotes one 19th century author's norm that "there is no deformity of human character from which we turn with deeper loathing than from a woman forgetful of her [inferior] nature and clamorous for the vocaton and rights of men."

Myrdall adds: "The myth of the 'contented women' who did not want to have suffrage or other civil rights and equal opportunities, had the same social function as the 'contented Negroes'.... In drawing a parallel between the position of, and feeling toward, women and Negroes we are uncovering a fundamental basis of our culture." That "basis" was (and partially still is), of course, the paradox of (A) constitutional guarantees of unqualified equality of rights, and (B) de facto abridgement of those rights. In elementary legalistic terms, this contradiction represents a systematic miscarriage of justice and personal insult and injury to the uncounted victims of that double bind. Stated historically, the advances of democratic principles generated during the 18th century were stopped at the doorstep of "the man's castle," preserving thereby his feudal role as "lord of the manor."

However, that contravention of the guarantee of civil rights to women was compounded by the second and far more penetrating contradiction: women then were placed as cult symbols of sexless purity on a public pedestal but privately were locked into a chastity belt, so to speak, of tight moral proscription of sexual expression and impulse; all of this while they were also forced to give silent lip service to the unwritten double standard tacitly enabling men to give their sexuality free rein in or out of the marital bed.

A more pathogenic, culturally patterned design for intergender relationships can hardly be imagined, a point confirmed by Professor Plumb's reference to the period's "agonizing preoccupation with sin, combined with a Jehovah-like inflation of the figure of the father ... Fearful repression of sex was followed, as might be expected, by life-destroying neuroses.... The whole Victorian scene is littered with broken minds, broken lives and broken careers" (Plumb, 1973). Students of hysteria (Hinsie and Campbell, 1970,

Freedman et al., 1975) during the late 19th century emphasized that it was "a disease of the female sex almost exclusively...[that] its prevalence reached almost epidemic proportions during the reign of Queen Victoria," and that far from being wholly a middle or upper class phenomenon, "it occurred frequently [among the poor], and chiefly among the more respectable poor who, 'resisting the normal effects of passion, fall victim to the abnormal' " (Veith, 1965). Sigmund Freud himself was a product of this period of history, turning in the 1890's to a preoccupation with hysterias and their underlying, repressed sexual conflicts that were one of the prime forces impelling his subsequent breakthrough into the depths of the human psyche and psychoanalytic theory.

It was this Victorian generation, concludes Plumb, that carried "enormous burdens of anxiety that within this last [20th] century...have been lifted off the shoulders of men and women, particularly in the highly industrialized West, to a degree that they can scarcely appreciate" (Plumb, 1973). It is therefore plausible to infer, with Plumb, that during this Victorian period, mental disturbance in the general population had been at higher levels of frequency and more severe levels of intensity, above all among its submerged women, than were to ever prevail thereafter.

Parenthetically, balancing all the pluses and the many remaining minuses of the present period, we hold the considered opinion that both the average man and average woman beyond the age of 40 years are objectively and subjectively healthier than ever before in the history of this Republic. We were able to put this view to a partial test in 1974, by asking our Midtown panelists the following question: "Your parents grew up to adulthood in a very different period from the young people of today. In your opinion, which generation grew up in a better period to enjoy life: Your parents' generation, your generation, or today's younger generation?" In choosing among these alternatives, only 22% of our panel members replied "my parents' generation," fully twice as many (43%) declared "my own generation," and another 35% chose "today's younger generation" as growing up in the best period. In other words, almost 80% of the panel members perceive progress in the quality of the social worlds that have emerged at least since the generation of their grandparents. It is of particular interest that whereas significantly more panel men than women prefer parents' generation (28% to 19%), valuing "my own generation" most were only 33% of the men, and 50.3% of the women. In any case, members of the last Victorian generation were contemporaries and counterparts of the parents who brought up the Midtown panel's own cohorts A and B, offspring appearing, as we have seen, with disparities on all three indicators of subjective well-being that were manifestly unfavorable to their women.

Plumb goes on to report how the social and psychological currents began to shift on behalf of women in the Edwardian decade (1901 to 1910) to be accelerated by "that great liberator, World War I." Milestones of female progress were marked by their first entrance into male-monopolized sectors of the labor force (Hesse, 1979) and, by 1920 and the 19th Amendment, into voting booths, representing a long delayed, partial whittling down of previous barriers to female economic and political equality.

In her recent widely acclaimed monograph, social historian Paula S. Fass (1977) documents that during the "free-wheeling" decade of the "roaring 20s," "American culture was remade...by social transformation of major proportions. It was the change in female behavior that underlined the overall changes that had taken place."

Young women now, writes Fass, "defined equality not as political rights or economic opportunities, but as something more subtle: freedom...the right to self-expression, self-determination and personal satisfaction." In short, they intended to steer the life course primarily by their own lights and not, as in the past, exclusively by those of their men. With this shift, notes Fass, there followed "a democratization of family relations between husband and wife, parents and children, and more latitude for emotional expression for each member of the family."

A related consequence was "an expanded view of children's welfare," including "a trend toward more equal involvement with, and affection for each child, regardless of sex." In light of the fact that the Victorian family had previously regarded the preadult son as "a man still growing," and the daughter in effect as "ever a little girl," this new parental "promotion" of the latter toward equality with her brothers probably represented a definite eugenic gain, especially in her own eyes, of socially valued status and personal self-esteem.

This, then, was the context of the generation that emerged during and after World War I, which was first socialized in the "derigidified" family and age-peer milieus of the 1920's, and appeared decades later in the Midtown Study panel as adult cohorts C and D. We find an exemplar of the women of this generation in Rosalyn Yalow, in 1921 born of immigrant parents in a working class New York City environment that could prompt her, at age 8 years, to announce her awareness that she could become not only a wife and mother, but also a career scientist. She, of course, achieved all three goals, and more, becoming a researcher in the almost *Frauen-frei* field of physics, and at age 56, a Nobel Laureate in Medicine *(New York Times Magazine,* April 9, 1978).

This is the generation that in the last two decades had emerged as a "new breed of women," who in growing numbers have been cutting through the barriers to university graduate schools, into male-dominated professional, semiprofessional, and other occupational strongholds, to launch the revived feminist movement and to enlarge their presence and voice in political forums at all levels (Kirkpatrick, 1976).

All of the above post-World War I milieu developments can be considered sociologically isomorphic with our observed cohort C and D women's quantum jumps in subjective well-being, representing advances over that of their A and B "preliberated" predecessors at like age, and probably even more over that of their late Victorian grandmothers who had suffered the fate of a culturally contrived "iron maiden" confinement.

Midtown Results and the Future

It is a credible hypothesis that isomorphisms on such a three-generation time scale are not mere chance coincidences of the play of history, but reflect a cause-and-effect connection between the partial emancipation of women from their 19th century status of sexist servitude, and their 20th century advances in subjective well-being. Our "control subjects" in this "experiment of human nature" on the psychological consequences of social change are the Midtown panel men who had no comparable sexist "chains to lose," and showed no comparable progress on our three measures of subjective well-being. Thus, we are led to suggest the following law of sociopsychology: Improvements in a group's social position and role in a society's objective system of status allocations are conducive to improvements in that group's subjective well-being and other dimensions of health. Implicit here is the notion of relative self-fulfillment as a eugenic, socially generated counterpart of the sociopathogenesis-denoting concept of relative deprivation.

Unless unexpected technical artifacts of both sex-specific and generation-specific kinds should turn up to suggest otherwise, the magnitude of our cohort C and D women's gains in subjective well-being must be seriously assessed for their potential social policy implications. Our figures, as they now stand, support estimates, that may be conservative, of a cut of 50% to 60% in the cohort C and D female mental impairment rates below the levels of their A and B counterparts, and a roughly corresponding increase in their Wellness frequencies. Consistent with these tentative estimates, one of us (L.S.) has elsewhere mounted strong circumstantial evidence that parallel long-term trends of liberation from the demeaning deprivations of poverty have had similar eugenic mental health effects.

To suggest the further implications of such separate kinds of evidence, we hold that a substantial part of the psychopathology at large in the population is precipitated by long refractory, discriminatory dysfunctions that are foisted on specific, power-weak community subgroups, damaging their members and subverting the most basic Judeo-Christian canons of a democratic society. Since these social pathologies are legally and politically correctable, it can hardly be denied that in the calculus of both humanist and cost/benefit values the surest primary preventive medicine lies in a general policy of making accessible larger dosages of social equality to groups where it is in less than health-sustaining supply. (Most immediately, this emphatically includes those unyielding points of female second-class citizenship that remain to be corrected through the instrument of the unconscionably stalled Equal Rights Amendment to the American Constitution.)

However, if our findings have challenged the Mental Paradise Lost doctrine, we are not implying an expectation that the broad policy goal just recommended can alone bring about a Mental Paradise Regained in our enormously complex society, although it can help the latter advance much farther from its "dystopia" antecedents in the 19th century. Even so, there will still remain a large reservoir of (A) discordances between individual psychic capacities and the marketplace of demanding adult roles, and (B) circumscribed intrafamily pathologies that are destructive for children. Both of these will, of course, require the interventions of secondary preventive psychiatry, of established and newer modalities, toward fostering improved intrapsychic and interpersonal functioning. Also relevant here is the recent warning of Erik Erikson (*New York Times*, Aug. 4, 1979) that "just as sexual repression characterized the Victorian era, there is a real danger that a new kind of repression may become a mark of adult life, namely repression of the urge to have children."

Nowhere, we believe, are the massive behavioral impacts and imprints of objectively changing social conditions more clearly manifest than in the procession of successive generations, each marching, like Mannheims's medieval and Renaissance people to its "own music." Prompted by our compelling longitudinal findings, we have reached into the historians' archives going back more than a century to the decade that began about 1870. Looking toward the future, we project two further sets of follow-up interviews: Midtown IV, focusing on our cohorts C and D, to intensively test and elaborate the theory offered above, and alternative hypotheses toward explaining the gender's differential intergeneration advances in subjective well-being.

Midtown V will follow up the 1,160 adult children of our four cohorts, their births spanning the years 1920 to 1960. As preparation, in the 1974 interviews with their parents, we systematically secured eight items of recent life-situation information (including psychiatric episodes) about each of those children. With such new baseline information already stored in our growing data bank, we will be able to cover four generations since the Midtown panel's earliest births in 1895.

Envisaged thereby is furtherance of an epidemiological nucleus for the crystallization of the specialty multidisciplinary field of sociopsychiatric history. On its agenda would be research questions such as the following: Will the newer adult generations of the 1980s change in levels of well-being, relative to the baselines of their parents, in a linear or cyclical, pendulum, fashion? When is a predominantly affluent society based on eugenic freedom at risk of slipping into a pathogenic, self-destructive system of narcissistic license, an outcome not without historical precedents? At least speculatively, what might be the mechanisms inherent in a specific historical macrosocial universe, for differentially potentiating the gene pool of the preadult generation engulfed in it?

Acknowledgments

This article is the fifth in a continuing series of published research reports from the Midtown Manhattan Longitudinal Study, and carries the identity number RS/5. The Midtown follow-up investigation has been conducted under National Institute of Mental Health (NIMH) grant 13369, and is sponsored jointly by the Columbia University Department of Psychiatry and the New York State Psychiatric Institute, Leo Srole, Principal Investigator. Supplementary funding has been provided by a special grant of the Foundations Fund for Research in Psychiatry, Fritz Redlich, MD, President. The Study draws its baseline data from the investigation launched on July 1, 1952, under NIMH grant M515 to the late Thomas A. C. Rennie, MD, Professor of Psychiatry, Cornell University Medical College. Supplementary support is acknowledged from the Grant Foundation, the Littauer Foundation, the Milbank Foundation, the Rockefeller Brothers Fund, and the

Samuel Rubin Foundation. Access to the Midtown I data bank has been made possible through the cooperation of Stanley Michael, MD, and Robert Michels, MD, Chairman, Cornell Department of Psychiatry. Special acknowledgments are owed to our consultants, Louis Linn, MD, Jean Endicott, PhD, Steven M. Cohen, PhD, Donald Treiman, PhD, Richard Remington, MD, and W. Edwards Deming, PhD. Robert Markush, MD, Ben Locke, MS, and Shirley Reff-Margolis, PhD, of the NIMH Center for Epidemiological Studies and the CES Review Committees have been pillars of support throughout. E. Joel Millman, PhD, study statistician, engineered the pool of computer runs from which this article's six tables have been drawn.

The Midtown Longitudinal Study through May 31, 1981 was carried out under grant 32794 from the NIMH Center for Epidemiological Studies and Center for Aging Studies.

References

Boulding, K.E., (1964), *The Meaning of the Twentieth Century.* New York: Harper & Row, pp. 70-71.

Erikdon, E., (1979), In an Address to the International Psychoanalytical Association, reported in the *New York Times,* August 4.

Fass, P.S., (1977), *The Damned and the Beautiful: American Youth in the 1920's,* Oxford, England: Oxford University Press.

Fischer, A.K. & Biel, R., Tracing urban adults for follow-up: The Midtown Manhattan Longitudinal Study, 1954-1974. In press.

Freedman, A.M., Kaplan, H.I., Sadock, B.J. (1975), *Comprehensive Textbook of Pyschiatry II,* Baltimore: Williams & Wilkins Co., pp. 264-265.

Fromm, E., (1941), *Escape from Freedom.* New York: Rinehart & Co., pp. 62-63.

Fromm, E. (1973), *The Anatomy of Destructiveness.* New York: Holt, Rinehart & Winston, pp. 350-356.

Goldhamer, H. & Marshall, A., (1943), *Psychosis and Civilization.* Glencoe, Illinois: Free Press.

Gordon, T. & Kannel, W.B., (1970), The Framingham, Massachusetts Study, Twenty Years Later, *The Community as an Epidemiological Laboratory,* eds. I.J. Kessler & M.I. Levin, Baltimore: Johns Hopkins University Press, pp. 122-148.

Hayden, D.C., (1844), On the distribution of insanity in the United States. *Third Literary Messenger,* 10:178.

Hesse, S.J., (1979), Women Working: Historical Trends. In: *Working Women & Families,* ed. Feinstein, K.W,, Beverly Hills, CA: Sage Publications.

Hinsie, E., and Campbell, R.J., (1970), *Psychiatric Dictionary,* New York: Oxford University Press, pp. 366-369.

Kiev, A.,(1978), The Role of Expectancy in Behavioral Change, *Controversy in Psychiatry,* eds. Brady J.P. & Brodie, H.K. Brodie, Philadelphia: W.B. Saunders Co., pp. 579-590.

Kirkpatrick, J., (1976), *The New Presidential Elite: Men and Women in National Politics*, New York: Russell Sage Foundation.

Lawrence, H., (1953), "New York: Crack-up City," *Esquire Magazine*, July.

Leighton, A.H., Leighton, D.C., (1966), Validity in Mental Health Surveys. *Can Psychiat Assn J*, 167-168.

Luborsky, L., (1962), "Clinicians' judgements of mental health: A proposed scale," *Arch Gen Psych* 7:407-417.

Mannheim, K., (1936), *Ideology and Utopia: An Introduction to the Sociology of Knowledge*, translated by L. Wirth & E.A. Shils. New York: Harcourt, Brace, and Co.

Mannheim, K., (1940), *Man & Society in an Age of Reconstruction*. New York: Harcourt, Brace, and World, Inc.

Morbidity and Mortality Weekly Report, U.S. Center Disease Control, Vol. 28, p. 36, August 10, 1979.

Myrdall, G., (1940), *An American Dilemma*. New York: Harper & Brothers.

Plumb, J.H., (1973), *In the Light of History*. Boston: Houghton Mifflin & Co.

Sartwell, P.E., (1953), Problems of identification of cases of chronic disease. *Milbank Mem Fund Quart*, Vol. 31.

Singer, E, , Garfinkel, R., Cohen, S.M. & Srole, L., (1976), Mortality and mental health: Evidence from the Midtown Manhattan Restudy. *Soc Sci Med*, 10:517-525.

Singer, E., Cohen S., Garfinkel, R. & Srole, L.,(1976), Replicating psychiatric ratings through multiple regression analysis: The Midtown Manhattan Restudy, *J Health Soc Behav*, 17: 376-387.

Srole, L., (1956), Social integration and certain corollaries. *Am Soc Rev* 21:709-716.

Srole, L., Langner, T.S., Michael, S.T., Kirkpatrick, P.& Rennie, T.A.C. (1962), *Mental Health in the Metropolis: The Midtown Manhattan Study*, New York: McGraw Hill, pp. 3-66; 388-407; 408-410; 39-66; 44-45; 174-189; 178.

Srole, L., (1975), "Measurement and classification in socio-psychiatric epidiemiology: The Midtown Manhattan Study (1954) and Midtown Manhattan Restudy (1974)," *J Health Soc Behav* 16:347-364.

Srole, L., Langner, T.S., Michael, S.T., Kirkpatrick, P. & Rennie, T.A.C. (1978) In: *Mental Health in the Metropolis*, Revised and Enlarged Edition, eds., Srole, L. & Fischer, A.K., New York: New York University Press, pp. 113-180; 161-180; 508-514; 156-157; 220-228; 240-258; 5-19; 145-146.

Srole, L. (1978), The city versus town and country: New evidence on an ancient bias. eds. Srole, L. & Fischer, A. In: *Mental Health in the Metropolis*, New York: New York University Press, pp. 433-459.

Stone, E., (1978), A Mme. Curie from the Bronx. *New York Times Magazine*, April 9.

Stouffer, S. et al. (1949), *The American Soldier*, Princeton, NJ: Princeton University Press, Vol. II, pp. 411-455, and Vol. IV, pp. 486-567.

Veith, I., (1965), *Hysteria: The History of a Disease*, Chicago: University of Chicago Press, pp. 199-242.

Wittson, C.L. & Hunt W.A., (1955), A rationale for psychiatric selection, *Am Psychol* 10:199-204.

Chapter 6

Social Class and Mental Illness

AUGUST B. HOLLINGSHEAD

Thirty years have elapsed since the research reported here was undertaken. Although the main purpose of this chapter is to present the findings of that research, I shall also endeavor to share with the reader the rationale for such research at that time. The comprehensive report of this study is published in Hollingshead and Redlich (1958) and Myers and Roberts (1959). This research grew out of the work of a number of investigators, who have demonstrated that the social environment in which individuals live is connected in some way, as yet not fully explained, to the development of mental illness (Rosanoff, 1916; Stern, 1913; Sutherland, 1901; White, 1903). Physicians have approached this problem largely from the viewpoint of epidemiology (Braatoy, 1937; Gerard and Siegel, 1950; Hyde and Kingsley, 1944a, 1944b; Hyde and Chisholm, 1944; Malamud and Malamud, 1943; Malzberg, 1940; Roth and Luton, 1943; Ruesch, Jacobson and Loeb, 1948; Tietze et al., 1941, 1943). Sociologists, on the other hand, have analyzed the question in terms of ecology (Dunham, 1947; Faris and Dunham, 1939; Felix and Bowers, 1948; Green, 1939), and of social disorganization (Faris, 1934, 1944). Neither psychiatrists nor sociologists have carried on extensive research into the specific question we are concerned with, namely, interrelations between the class structure and the development of mental illness. However, a few sociologists and psychiatrists have written speculative and research papers in this area (Clark, 1948, 1949; Davis, 1938; Dollard and Miller, 1950; Parsons, 1950; Ruesch, 1949; Warner, 1937).

The present research, therefore, was designed to discover whether a relationship does or does not exist between the class system of our society and mental illnesses. Five general hypotheses were formulated to test some dimension of an assumed relationship between the two. These hypotheses were stated positively; they could just as easily have been expressed either negatively or conditionally. They were phrased as follows:

1. The *expectancy* of a psychiatric disorder is related significantly to an individual's position in the class structure of his society.
2. The *types* of psychiatric disorders are connected significantly to the class structure.

3. The type of *psychiatric treatment* administered is associated with a patient's position in the class structure.
4. The *psycho-dynamics* of psychiatric disorders are correlated to an individual's position in the class structure.
5. *Mobility* in the class structure is neurotogenic.

Each hypothesis is linked to the others, and all are subsumed under the theoretical assumption of a functional relationship between stratification in society and the prevalence of particular types of mental disorders among given social classes or strata in a specified population. The present paper is limited to a discussion of hypotheses 1, 2, and 3.

Methodologic Procedure

The research was done by a team of four psychiatrists (F. C. Redlich, B. H. Roberts, L. Z. Freedman, and L. Schaffer), two sociologists (A. B. Hollingshead and J. K. Myers), and a clinical psychologist (H. A. Robinson). The data were assembled in the New Haven urban community, which consists of the city of New Haven and surrounding towns of East Haven, North Haven, West Haven, Hamden, and Woodbridge. This area had a population of some 250,000 persons in 1950. The population of each component was as follows: New Haven, 164,443; East Haven, 12,212; North Haven, 9,444; West Haven, 32,010; Hamden, 29,715; and Woodbridge, 2,822. The New Haven community was selected because the community's structure has been studied intensively by sociologists. In addition, it was served by a private psychiatric hospital, three psychiatric clinics, and 27 practicing psychiatrists, as well as state and Veterans Administration facilities.

Four basic technical operations had to be completed before the hypotheses could be tested. These were the delineation of the class structure of the community, selection of a cross-sectional control of the community's population, the determination of who was receiving psychiatric care, and the stratification of both the control sample and the psychiatric patients.

August B. Hollingshead and Jerome K. Myers took over the task of delineating the class system. Fortunately, Maurice R. Davie and his students had studied the social structure of the New Haven community over a long period (Davie, 1937; Kennedy, 1944; McConnell, 1937; Myers, 1950; Minnis, 1951). Thus we had a large body of data we could draw upon to aid us in blocking out the community's social structure.

The community's social structure is differentiated vertically along racial, ethnic, and religious lines; each of these vertical cleavages, in turn, is differentiated horizontally by a series of classes. Around the sociobiological axis of race two social worlds have evolved: a black world and a white world. The white world is divided by ethnic origin and religion into Catholic, Protestant, and Jewish contingents. Within these divisions there are numerous ethnic groups. The Irish hold aloof from the Italians, and the Italians move in different circles from the Poles. The Jews maintain a religious and social life separate from the gentiles. The horizontal strata that transect each of these vertical divisions are based on the social values that are attached to occupation, education, place of residence in the community, and associations.

The vertically differentiating factors of race, religion, and ethnic origin, when combined with the horizontally differentiating ones such as occupation, education, and place of residence, produce a social structure that is highly compartmentalized. The integrating factors in this complex are twofold. First, each stratum of each vertical division is similar in its cultural characteristics to the corresponding stratum in the other divisions. Second, the cultural pattern for each stratum or class was set by the "Old Yankee" core group. This core group provided the cultural mold that has shaped the status system of each subgroup in the community. In short, the social structure of the New Haven community is a parallel class structure within the limits of race, ethnic origin, and religion.

This fact enabled us to stratify the community, for our purposes, with an Index of Social Position. This index used three scaled factors to determine an individual's class position within the community's stratificational system: ecological area of residence, occupation, and education. Ecological area of residence is measured by a six-point scale; occupation and education are each measured by a seven-point scale. To obtain a social class score on an individual we must therefore know his address, his occupation, and the number of years of school he has completed. Each of these factors is given a scale score, and the scale score is multiplied by a factor weight determined by a standard regression equation. The factor weights are as follows: ecological area of residence, 5; occupation, 8; and education, 6. The three factor scores are summed, and the resultant score is taken as an index of this individual's position in the community's social class system.

The index enabled us to delineate five social strata. The principal strata or classes may be characterized as follows:

Class I. This stratum is composed of wealthy families whose wealth is often inherited and whose heads are leaders in the community's business and professional pursuits. Its members live in areas of the community generally regarded as "the best." The adults are college graduates, usually from famous private institutions, and almost all gentile families are listed in the New Haven *Social Directory*, but few Jewish families are listed. In brief, these people occupy positions of high social prestige.

Class II. Adults in this stratum are almost all college graduates. The males occupy high managerial positions, many are engaged in the lesser ranking professions. These families are well-to-do, but there is no substantial inherited or acquired wealth. Its members live in the "better" residential areas. About half of these families belong to lesser ranking private clubs, but only 5% of Class II families are listed in the New Haven *Social Directory*.

Class III. This stratum includes the vast majority of small proprietors, white-collar office and sales workers, and a considerable number of skilled manual workers. Adults are predominantly high school graduates, but a considerable percentage have attended business schools and small colleges for a year or two. They live in "good" residential areas. Less than 5% belong to private clubs, but they are not included in the *Social Directory*. Their social life tends to be concentrated in the family, the church, and the lodge.

Class IV. This stratum consists predominantly of semiskilled factory workers. Its adult members have finished the elementary grades, but the older people have not completed high school. However, adults under 35 have generally graduated from high school. Its members comprise almost half of the community, and their residences are scattered over wide areas. Social life is centered in the family, the neighborhood, the labor union, and public places.

Class V. Occupationally, Class V adults are overwhelmingly semiskilled factory hands and unskilled laborers. Most adults have not completed the elementary grades. The families are concentrated in the "tenement" and "cold-water flat" areas of New Haven. Only a small minority belong to organized community institutions. Their social life takes place in the family flat, on the street, or in neighborhood social agencies.

The second major technical operation in this research was the enumeration of psychiatric patients. A psychiatric census was taken to discover the number and kinds of psychiatric patients in the community. Enumeration was limited to residents of the community who were patients of a psychiatrist or a psychiatric clinic, or were in a psychiatric institution on December 1, 1950. To make reasonably certain that all patients were included in the enumeration, the research team gathered data from all public and private psychiatric institutions and clinics in Connecticut and nearby states, and all private practitioners except a small number in New York City.

Forty-four pertinent items of information were gathered on each patient and placed on a schedule. The psychiatrists gathered material regarding symptomatology and diagnosis, onset of illness and duration, referral to the practitioner and the institution, and the nature and intensity of treatment. The sociologists obtained information on age, sex, occupation, education, religion, race and ethnicity, family history, and marital experience.

The third technical research operation was the selection of a control sample from the population of the community. The sociologists drew a 5% systematic sample of households from the 1951 New Haven City Directory. This directory covers the entire communal area. The names and addresses in it were compiled in October and November, 1950, a period very close to the date of the Psychiatric Census. Therefore, there was comparability of residence and date of registry between the two population groups. Each household drawn in the sample was interviewed, and data on the age, sex, occupation, education, religion, and income of family members, as well as other items necessary for our purposes were placed on a schedule.

Our fourth basic operation was the stratification of the psychiatric patients and of the control population with the *Index of Social Position*.

Selected Findings

Before we discuss our findings relative to Hypothesis 1, we emphasize that this study is concerned with diagnosed or treated prevalence rather than total prevalence. Our psychiatric census included only *psychiatric cases* under treatment, diagnostic study, or care. There are undoubtedly many individuals in the community with psychiatric problems who escaped our net. If we had true prevalence figures, many findings from our present study would be more meaningful, perhaps some of our interpretation would be changed.

Hypothesis 1, as revised by the nature of the problem, stated: *The diagnosed prevalence of psychiatric disorders is related significantly to an individual's position* in the class structure. A test of this hypothesis involves a comparison of the sample population with the psychiatric population. If no significant difference between the distribution of the sample population and the psychiatric patient population by social class is found, Hypothesis 1 may be abandoned. However, if a significant difference is found between the two populations by class, Hypothesis 1 should be entertained until more conclusive data are assembled. Pertinent data for a limited test of Hypothesis 1 are presented in table 1. The data included show the number of individuals in the normal population and the psychiatric patients. What we are concerned with in this test is how these two populations are distributed by class.

TABLE 1
Distribution of Normal and Psychiatric Population by Social Class.

	Sample Population[a]		*Psychiatric Population*	
Social class	*No.*	*Percent*	*No.*	*Percent*
I	358	3.1	19	1.0
II	926	8.1	131	6.7
III	2,500	22.0	260	13.2
IV	5,256	46.0	758	38.6
V	2,037	17.8	723	36.8
Unknown[b]	345	3.0	72	3.7
TOTAL	11,422	100.0	1,963	100.0

Chi-square = 408.16, $p < 0.001$.

[a]These figures do not include Yale students, transients, institutionalized persons, and refusals.

[b]The unknown cases were not used in the calculation of chi-square. They are individuals drawn in the sample, and psychiatric cases whose class level could not be determined because of paucity of data.

When we examined these population distributions by the use of the chi-square technique, we found a significant relation between social class and the prevalence of treated psychiatric patients. A comparison of the percentage distribution of each population by class readily indicates the direction of the class concentration of psychiatric cases. For example, Class I contains 3.1% of the community's population but only 1.0% of the psychiatric cases.

Class V, on the other hand, includes 17.8% of the community's population, but contributed 36.8% of the psychiatric patients. On the basis of our data Hypothesis 1 should be accepted as tenable.

Hypothesis 2 postulated a significant connection between the type of psychiatric disorder and social class. This hypothesis involves a test of the idea that there may be a functional relationship between an individual's position in the class system and the type of psychiatric disorder that he may present. This hypothesis depends in part on the question of diagnosis. Our psychiatrists based their diagnoses on the classificatory system developed by the Veterans Administration *(Psychiatric Disorders and Reactions,* 1947). For present purposes, all cases are grouped into two categories: the neuroses and the psychoses. The results of this grouping by social class are given in table 2.

TABLE 2
Distribution of Neuroses and Psychoses by Social Class.

	Neuroses		*Psychoses*	
Social class	*No.*	*Percent*	*No.*	*Percent*
I	10	52.6	9	47.4
II	88	67.2	43	32.8
III	115	44.2	145	55.8
IV	175	23.1	583	76.9
V	61	8.4	662	91.6
TOTAL	449		1,442	

Chi-square = 296.45, $p < 0.001$.

Table 2 shows that the neuroses are concentrated at the higher levels and the psychoses at the lower end of the class structure. Our team advanced a number of hypotheses to explain the sharp differences between the neuroses and psychoses by social class. One suggestion was that the low percentage of neurotics in the lower classes was a direct reaction to the cost of psychiatric treatment. But as we accumulated a series of case studies, we became skeptical of this simple interpretation. Our detailed case records indicate that the social distance between psychiatrist and patient may be more potent than economic considerations in determining the character of psychiatric intervention.

Hypothesis 3 stipulated that the type of psychiatric treatment a patient receives is associated with his position in the class structure. A test of this hypothesis involves a comparison of the different types of therapy being used by psychiatrists on patients in different social classes. We encountered several forms of treatment but they may be grouped under three main types: psychotherapy, organic therapy, and custodial care. The patient population, from the viewpoint of the principal type of therapy received, was divided roughly into three categories: 32.0% received some type of psychotherapy; 31.7% received organic treatments of one kind or another; and 36.3% received custodial care. The percentage of persons who received custodial care was greatest in the lower classes. The same finding applied to organic treatment. Psychotherapy, on the other hand, was concentrated in the higher classes. Within the psychotherapy category there were sharp differences between the types of psychotherapy administered to the several classes. For example, psychoanalysis was limited to Classes I and II. Patients in Class V who received any psychotherapy were treated by group methods in the state hospitals. The number and percentage of patients who received each type of therapy is given in table 3. The data clearly support Hypothesis 3.

TABLE 3
Distribution of the Principal Types of Therapy by Social Class.

	Psychotherapy		*Organic therapy*		*No treatment*	
Social class	*No.*	*Percent*	*No.*	*Percent*	*No.*	*Percent*
I	14	73.7	2	10.5	3	15.8
II	107	81.7	15	11.4	9	6.9
III	136	52.7	74	28.7	48	18.6
IV	237	31.1	288	37.1	242	31.8
V	115	16.1	234	32.7	367	51.2

Chi-square = 336.58, $p < 0.001$.

Neurotic Patients

We turn now to presentation of the data on treatment among the 449 persons diagnosed as neurotic in the psychiatric census.

In this analysis we are concerned with a single question: Is a neurotic patient's position in the community's class structure related significantly to the treatment he receives for his disorder? The data will be viewed from six perspectives: *(a)* how the patients came into treatment; *(b)* how their problems were diagnosed; *(c)* where they were treated; *(d)* the type of treatment they received; *(e)* the intensity of treatment; and *(f)* the length of treatment.

Sources of Referral

The circumstances involved in the initial contact of each patient with a psychiatric agency were ascertained. These data were grouped into four categories called "sources of referral." The principal ones are: medical doctors; self, family, and friends; police and courts; and other professional persons. The data on sources of referrals are summarized in table 4.

TABLE 4
Percentage of Neurotic Patients by Source of Referral and Class.

	Class			
Source of referral	*I and II (n=98)*	*III (n=115)*	*IV (n=175)*	*V (n=61)*
Medical doctors	61.2	56.5	57.7	36.0
Self, family, friends	33.7	29.6	23.5	11.5
Other professional persons	4.1	7.8	9.1	29.5
Police and courts	1.0	6.1	9.7	23.0

Chi-square = 61.2184, $p < 0.001$.

The chi-square of 61 + shows significant differences between the patients' class positions and the ways they are referred to psychiatrists. Medical doctors are responsible for over half of the referrals in the four higher classes, but only slightly more than a third of the Class V patients. In Class V, over 90% of the medical referrals come from physicians in the outpatient clinics of the New Haven Hospital. In the four higher classes they are made largely by private physicians. Professional persons other than physicians play minor roles in bringing patients into the treatment process. Lawyers and clergymen make a few referrals, mainly in Classes I, II, and III. In Classes III and IV, teachers play major roles in the category of "Other professional persons." In Class V, almost three patients out of five are involved in some type of difficulty that calls them to the attention of police officers, social workers, or teachers.

Diagnostic Groups

The patients were diagnosed by the team psychiatrists in terms of their symptomatology. The specific diagnoses were then combined into six groups: character and behavior disorders; phobic and anxiety reactions; mixed psychoneuroses; depressive reactions; somatization reactions; conversion and obsessive-compulsive reactions. The distribution of the patients by diagnostic group and class is presented in table 5.

The significant association between class position and the diagnostic groups shown in table 5 is an interesting finding of theoretical import, but our concern here is primarily with treatment. Thus the pertinent question is: How is diagnosis related to treatment?

TABLE 5
Percentage of Neurotic Patients by Diagnostic Group and Class.

	Class			
Diagnostic group	*I and II (n=98)*	*III (n=115)*	*IV (n=175)*	*V (n=61)*
Character and behavior disorders	20.4	29.6	20.6	36.1
Phobic and anxiety reactions	16.3	19.1	30.9	16.4
Mixed psychoneuroses	36.7	24.3	13.1	16.4
Depressive reactions	13.3	12.2	10.3	8.2
Somatization reactions	6.1	8.7	13.1	11.5
Conversion and obsessive-compulsive reactions	7.1	6.1	12.0	11.5

Chi-square = 37.6120, $p < 0.01$.

We began with the assumption that race, sex, age, psychiatric history, diagnosis, place of treatment, and class position might be related to the kind of treatment a patient received. However, no relationship was found between the type of therapy administered to the patients and race, sex, age, psychiatric history, or diagnostic group. These findings enabled us to focus the analysis of the treatment process on the two significant variables of class position and place of treatment for the patient population as a whole.

Treatment Agencies

Where persons suffering from mental difficulties receive help depends upon a number of different factors: their understanding of their problem; what they know about psychiatric theories; the reputation of psychiatrists and psychiatric agencies; the availability of treatment facilities; their social position; the size and condition of their pocketbook; as well as their relationship to nonpsychiatric institutions in the community, such as the police, social welfare agencies, churches, and schools. How these facilities are utilized by the several classes is depicted in table 6.

Ninety percent of Class I and II patients are cared for in private facilities. When the use of private psychiatric facilities is examined from the viewpoint of who pays the bill, the class gradient becomes even sharper. One hundred percent of the Class I and II patients treated in private facilities pay for their own treatment; but such payments are made by only 63% of the Class IIIs, 39% of the Class IVs, and none of the Class Vs. Patients in Classes III and IV who are treated by private practitioners and do not pay their own bills are financed entirely by the Veterans Administration.

TABLE 6
Percentage of Neurotic Patients by Class and Agency of Treatment.

	Class			
Agency	*I and II (n=98)*	*III (n=115)*	*IV (n=175)*	*V (n=61)*
Private practitioners and private hospitals	89.8	73.0	62.9	18.0
State and Veterans Administration hospitals	3.1	6.1	13.7	27.9
Clinics	7.1	20.9	23.4	54.1

Chi-square = 87.5613, $p < 0.001$.

In Class V, the private patients' bills are paid either by the VA or by compensation insurance carried by employers. Were it not for patients sent to private practitioners by the VA and by employers, the association between treatment agency and class position would be even greater. In short, if the typical Class V neurotic patient receives treatment it is at public expense in either a public or a private agency. This generalization is applicable also to some 60% of the Class IV patients.

Type of Treatment

The four principal types of treatment administered are: individual psychotherapy; group psychotherapy; shock and operation; and drugs and sedation. The percentage of patients by class who receive each of the specified types of treatment is given in table 7.

TABLE 7
Percentage of Neurotic Patients Who Receive a Specified Type of Treatment, by Class.

	Class			
Type of treatment	*I and II (n=98)*	*III (n=115)*	*IV (n=175)*	*V (n=61)*
Individual psychotherapy	96.9	83.5	74.8	59.0
Group psychotherapy	1.0	2.6	2.9	8.2
Shock and operation	1.0	5.2	8.6	8.2
Drugs and sedation	1.0	8.7	13.7	24.6

Chi-square = 41.3613, $p < 0.001$

Although individual psychotherapy is the predominant type of treatment in all classes, a definite gradient is associated with it. All Class I patients and 97% of the Class IIs receive individual psychotherapy. Only a relatively small number receive group psychotherapy, but the largest concentration is in Class V; these are all state hospital cases. Organic treatments are minor forms in all classes. However, the lower the class of the patient the higher the probability that he receives one of the organic therapies: shock, operation, or drugs. When the organic therapies are combined the following differences appear: Class II, 2%; Class III, 14%; Class IV, 23%; and Class V, 33%.

When the interrelations between class position and the principal forms of treatment were found, specific types of individual psychotherapy were examined to see if a particular type was associated with different class positions in given treatment agencies. By controlling for places of treatment it was possible to determine whether class position was an independent variable in the treatment process within a particular type of agency. This point is demonstrated in table 8.

Twenty-three percent of the patients treated by a form of individual psychotherapy are clinic patients. Within the clinic group there is a definite association between class position and the type of psychotherapy administered. Analytic psychotherapy is related most directly to class position; the higher the class the greater the percentage of patients treated by this form. Eclectic psychotherapy is equally distributed in each class except Class II. Relationship therapy is concentrated most highly in Class V.

The significant association of individual psychotherapies with class position within the clinics is of interest. Here the treatment of patients is independent of payment. The patients are treated free of charge or for nominal fees determined by social workers who have no direct connection with the therapy process. We may infer, therefore, that the type of therapy given to clinic patients is related more to social factors than to economic costs. Private practitioners administer 75% of the individual psychotherapy given to neurotic patients. Psychoanalysis is limited entirely to Classes I and II. Analytic psychotherapy is also confined, in large part, to the same strata, but is received in addition by 21% of Class III. Relationship therapy is inversely related to class position, increasing from 24% in Class II to 100% in Class V. The inference is clear from the data in table 8 that the type of individual psychotherapy given to patients both in clinics and in private practice is related very definitely to class position.

Intensity of Treatment

The intensity of the treatment process among patients who receive individual psychotherapy was measured by two variables: *(a)* the number of times patients saw their therapists per month; and *(b)* the length of each visit. The data on the number of treatments per month are summarized in table 9. The number of visits patients made to their psychiatrists each month differs significantly from one class to another. However, there are no clear-cut class gradients except among patients receiving intensive psychotherapy. These patients see their therapists more than twice a week.

TABLE 8
Percentage of Patients Receiving Different Types of Psychotherapy[a] by Treatment Agency and Class.

Private Practitioners[b]	*Class*			
Type of psychotherapy	***(n=7)***	***(n=19)***	***(n=34)***	***(n=21)***
Analytic	71.4	42.1	20.6	9.5
Eclectic	14.3	52.6	50.0	47.6
Relationship	14.3	5.3	29.4	42.9

Chi-square = 13.9437, $p < 0.01$

Clinics	*Class*		
Type of psychotherapy	***I and II (n=87)***	***III (n=76)***	***IV and V[c] (n=105)***
Psychoanalysis and analytic psychotherapy	46.0	21.1	1.9
Eclectic	30.0	23.7	14.3
Relationship	24.1	55.3	83.8

Chi-square = 78.2014, $p < 0.001$

[a]The four types of individual psychotherapy may be categorized as follows: (1) Psychoanalysis is the orthodox Freudian method practiced by a member, an advanced student, or an approved institute of psychoanalysis; (2) analytic psychotherapy follows psychoanalytic principles, including insight into unconscious forces, transference, resistance, defenses, and so on, and is practiced by analytically trained psychiatrists but does not include full analysis; (3) eclectic therapy is any combination of the analytic and relationship approaches; (4) relationship therapy includes three subtypes: *(a)* supportive, in which the treatment aim is primarily to maintain the current level of personality integration, *(b)* directive, which involves deliberate manipulation of the social and personal environment, and *(c)* suggestive, in which the patient is manipulated by the physician in less open and direct ways than in directive therapy.

[b]Includes eight patients in private hospitals.

[c]Eleven Class V patients were combined with Class IV. All the Class V patients received relationship therapy.

About one third of Class I and II receive intensive individual psychotherapy, whereas only 4% of Class III, 2% of Class IV, and none of Class V are treated by intensive individual psychotherapy.

The data on the length of each visit are presented in table 10. Approximately 94% of the Class I and II patients pay for a 50-minute hour and receive this amount of their therapist's time. At the other end of the class scale, only 45% of Class V receive treatment for 50 minutes. Some 36%

TABLE 9
Percentage of Neurotic Patients by Class and Number of Individual Psychotherapy Sessions Per Month.

	Class			
Number of sessions	*I and II (n=94)*	*III (n=95)*	*IV (n=128)*	*V (n=32)*
1-3	31.2	42.4	60.0	50.0
4	24.7	35.9	32.8	37.5
5-8	12.9	17.4	4.8	12.5
9 and over	31.2	4.3	2.4	

Chi-square = 72.6290, $p < 0.001$

TABLE 10
Percentage of Neurotic Patients by Class and Length of Psychotherapy Sessions.[a]

	Class			
Length of sessions	*I and II (n=87)*	*III (n=76)*	*IV (n=91)*	*V (n=11)*
50-60 minutes	94.3	81.3	75.8	45.5
30-49 minutes	3.4	17.3	20.9	18.1
15-29 minutes	2.3	1.4	3.3	36.4

Chi-square = 47.0909, $p < 0.001$
[a]Private practitioners' patients only are included here.

are treated for less than 30 minutes. In contrast, only 3% or less of the patients in the higher ranking classes are treated by "short time." Thus we may conclude that the intensity of treatment, as measured by the number of visits per month to the private psychiatrist, and the length of the visits are variables that differ significantly from one class to another. The same tendency is present in the clinics, but the differences from one class to another are not significant.

Duration of Present Treatment

The final aspect of the treatment process is the length of time the patients have been in therapy. The data on this point are summarized in table 11.

TABLE 11
Percentage of Neurotic Patients by Class and Duration of Present Treatment.

	Class			
Duration of treatment	*I and II (n=98)*	*III (n=115)*	*IV (n=175)*	*V (n=61)*
Less than one year	44.2	61.4	61.5	73.8
One year to two years	22.1	11.4	10.3	11.5
Two and three years	27.4	17.5	16.7	11.5
Four years and over	6.3	9.6	11.5	3.3

Chi-square = 23.5222, $p < 0.01$

Like other phases of the treatment process, the length of time the patients have been in psychiatric care differs significantly from one class to another. Some 74% of Class V have been in treatment less than a year. The corresponding figure in Classes I and II is 44%. However, there is no difference between Classes III and IV; in both classes some 61% have been in treatment less than a year. The patients in treatment from one year through three years do not reveal significant class differences except in Classes I and II. Patients in treatment 4 years and longer tend to be concentrated in Classes III and IV. These are chronic cases in need of more or less continuous support. They tend to be "hangers on" in the clinics, or severe cases who are hospitalized in state and VA hospitals.

This analysis has been concerned with the presentation of empirical data on interrelations between social class position and the treatment process among neurotic patients in the New Haven community. Very definite interrelations have been found. We have not discussed what may be a more important question: How can interrelations between class position and the treatment process be explained?

A number of different social and cultural factors operate on the psychiatrist, the patient, his family, and in the community to produce the relationships reported here. The principal ones appear to revolve around the evaluation of psychiatry by different class groups, the attitudes psychiatrists hold toward patients in the several classes, the attitudes of patients toward psychiatrists, and the abilities of persons in the several classes to pay for psychiatric care. Another major factor is the different ways members of the several classes conceive of the nature and treatment of mental disorders. Finally, differing perceptions create communication problems for both the doctor and his patient.

Schizophrenia and Social Class

The association between social class and the distribution of diagnosed schizophrenia in the community's population was measured by an Index of Prevalence so constructed that if the number of patients in a class was proportionate to the total population of the class in the community the index would be 100. Instead of an equal distribution of patients by class the following pattern was found. In Class I the index figure was 23; in Class II, 33; in Class III, 48; in Class IV, 84; and in Class V, 246. This distribution posed the question we shall discuss here, namely, how can these differences be explained?

Discussion of this problem gave rise to the formulation of two tentative explanatory hypotheses: *(a)* Schizophrenic patients are downwardly mobile; hence the concentration of patients in Class V; *(b)* The class differences in the Index of Prevalence reflect differences in treatment and rehabilitation.

Presentation of Data

Downward Mobility

We first approached the problem of the wide difference in prevalence, between the several classes from the viewpoint of mobility, because this has been a controversial point in both psychiatric and sociological literature. Our data enabled us to examine mobility from the standpoint of both geographic movement and movement within the class structure. Our examination of mobility was divided into four steps. First, the native and foreign-born patients were compared with the corresponding population of the community to see if there were a significant relationship between foreign birth and schizophrenia. The results are given in table 12.

TABLE 12
Native-Born and Foreign-Born Schizophrenics
Over 21 Years of Age Compared with Total Population
in the Community Over 21 Years of Age.

	Schizophrenics		*Population*	
Nativity	*No.*	*%*	*No.*	*%*
Native-Born	643	76.9	135,568	79.5
Foreign-born	193	23.1	34,900	20.5
TOTAL	836	100.0	170,468	100.0

Chi-square = 3.4871, $p < 0.05$

The data in table 12 were tested by the chi-square technique and no significant differences appeared between the native and foreign-born categories. The second step was a comparison of where the native-born patients had been born and reared. The data are summarized in table 13. The low chi-square for table 13 shows that there is no significant relationship between schizophrenia by class, birthplace, and place reared for the native-born patients.

TABLE 13
Place Reared for Native-Born Schizophrenics, by Class.

	Class							
	I & II		*III*		*IV*		*V*	
Place born and reared	*No.*	*%*	*No.*	*%*	*No.*	*%*	*No.*	*%*
Community	12	44.5	51	63.8	212	70.4	153	61.2
New England	7	25.9	14	17.5	49	16.3	46	18.4
United States	8	29.6	15	18.7	40	13.3	51	20.4
TOTAL	27	100.0	80	100.0	301	100.0	250	100.0

Chi-square = 11.8971, $p < 0.05$.

The third step was an examination of the residential histories of the patients who had been born and reared in the community. This operation showed that the Class I and II patients had lived in the "best" residential areas all their lives; and the Class V patients had always lived in New Haven's "slums." The other classes were more widely scattered, but there was no perceptible movement of patients and their families from the better to the poorer residential areas.

By social mobility we mean actual movement from one class to another, not "mobility aspirations" or slight intraclass changes through the years. Movement within the class structure was tested by an examination of the family histories of all patients to determine if their class position was the same as or different from the family of orientation. The patient's class position at the time of first contact with a psychiatrist, as well as at the time of present hospitalization, was noted. The results of our comparison of the class positions of patients and of their families in two generations are summarized in table 14.

The data in table 14 furnish little evidence of downward mobility. The significant facts here are: *(a)* that most patients were in the same class as their parental families; and *(b)* there is greater mobility upward than downward within the small minority who do change their class positions. Clearly the data do not support the hypothesis that downward mobility can account for the concentration of patients in Class V.

TABLE 14
Evidence of Social Mobility Among Schizophrenics Through Two or More Generations, by Class.

	Class							
	I & II		*III*		*IV*		*V*	
Evidence of mobility	*No.*	*%*	*No.*	*%*	*No.*	*%*	*No.*	*%*
Patient upward from family	7	24.0	19	22.9	6	1.7		0.0
Patient downward from family	1	3.0	2	2.4	3	0.8	4	1.0
Patient and family stable	20	70.0	54	65.1	332	91.5	340	88.8
Insufficient family history	1	3.0	8	9.6	21	6.0	39	10.2
TOTAL	29	100.0	83	100.0	352	100.0	383	100.0

The hypothesis that differential responses to treatment might be an explanation of the disproportionately large number of cases in Class V was stimulated by our analysis of the ages of the patients at the time they first came into psychiatric treatment in comparison with their present ages. We were impressed by the finding that the upper classes reach a psychiatrist earlier in life than the lower classes. But what started us on the trail of an analysis of the treatment process was the finding that the present mean ages of the patients in the different classes were different from their ages at first psychiatric contact. For example, the differences between mean age at first contact and present mean age in Classes I and II (table 15), is only 11 years, whereas in Class V the mean age difference is 17 years. Briefly, this increased differential suggested an accumulation of chronic patients in the lower classes.

After we found the wide differences between age at contact and present age, we constructed an index of prevalence by duration of psychiatric contact. This index is constructed in such a way that if each class were proportionately represented in the patient group by duration of contact the index figure would be 100. The crucial data bearing on duration of professional contact with psychiatrists are presented in table 16. If the duration of contact, i.e., treatment and care, in all classes were equal through the years, the index should be the same as current prevalence given at the bottom of table 16.

Instead of a stable index by duration of treatment we found a variable set of figures. The index numbers for patients in treatment for less than a year are inversely proportional to class. In Class V the proportion of patients in treatment for one year or less is twice as high as in Classes I and II. But at the other extreme of the table, that is, patients under care for 21 years

TABLE 15
Mean Ages of Schizophrenics by Class at First Psychiatric Contact and at Present.

	Mean ages	
Class	*First contact*	*Present*
I & II	29	40
III	31	44
IV	32	45
V	33	50

TABLE 16
Index of Prevalence by Duration of Treatment in Each Class.

	Class			
Years in treatment	*I & II*	*III*	*IV*	*V*
1	84	43	102	176
2	102	52	105	144
3-5	26	71	101	175
6-10	25	60	101	194
11-20	26	20	86	280
21 and above	10	40	70	308
Current prevalence	29	48	84	246

and more, the index is 31 times higher in Class V than in Classes I and II. Furthermore, there is a steady decrease in the index numbers as treatment lengthens for all classes except Class V. In Class V the index increases steadily from the second year. The data of table 16 show that Class V is a reservoir of chronicity.

We examined the treatment process for clues to help us understand the accumulation of chronic patients in Class V. Table 17 compares referrals of patients to psychiatrists and psychiatric agencies by class. It is impressive that schizophrenics of the upper classes are referred for treatments predominantly through medical channels, while schizophrenics of the lower classes are referred by legal authorities such as police, criminal, and probate courts. And it is surprising that referrals through social and educational institutions and through the initiative of private individuals are comparatively rare.

Since a very large proportion of chronic patients in Classes IV and V receive only custodial care, we tabulated types of treatment for 5 years' dura-

TABLE 17
Source of Referral for Schizophrenics, by Class.

	Class							
	I & II		*III*		*IV*		*V*	
Source of referral	*No.*	*%*	*No.*	*%*	*No.*	*%*	*No.*	*%*
Medical								
Psychiatrist	4		2		4		6	
Psychiatric clinic			3		12		1	
Psychiatric hospital	7	55.2	7	24.1	25	13.9	37	12.3
Physician	5		7		7		3	
Medical clinic	—		1		1		—	
Legal								
Police or court	1		3		52		105	
Probate commitment	7	27.6	55	69.9	233	81.0	224	85.9
Social agency and school	1		—		5		3	
Self, relatives, friends	4	17.2	5	6.0	13	5.1	4	1.8
TOTAL	29	100.0	83	100.0	352	100.0	383	100.0

tion and less by class (table 18): We found that the "no treatment" category is absent in Classes I and II. Organic treatment and custodial care are more frequent at the lower class levels. Individual psychotherapy is concentrated disproportionately in Classes I and II; whereas group psychotherapy is limited to the three lower classes.

Table 19 demonstrates that schizophrenics in the higher classes are hospitalized, on the average, a significantly greater number of times than the lower-class patients. This is additional proof that the chances of an upper-class schizophrenic leaving a mental hospital are better than those of a lower-class schizophrenic.

From table 20 one may conclude that schizophrenics of the upper classes are more likely to be treated as ambulatory patients before they are hospitalized than those of the lower. Also lower-class ambulatory patients are more likely to break contact with psychiatrists and psychiatric agencies than are higher class ones.

Discussion

Our data show significant class differences in the prevalence of treated schizophrenics in the New Haven community. But are these differences valid? They are valid for our population, but whether they reflect true prevalence

TABLE 18
Type of Therapy for Schizophrenics in Treatment for 5 Years and Less, by Class.

	Class							
	I & II		*III*		*IV*		*V*	
Type of therapy	*No.*	*%*	*No.*	*%*	*No.*	*%*	*No.*	*%*
None			3	12.5	7	7.8	7	12.3
Organic	2	16.7	13	54.2	59	65.6	40	70.2
Psychotherapy								
Individual	10	83.3	4	16.7	16	17.8	5	8.8
Group	—	0.0	4	16.7	8	8.9	5	8.8
TOTAL	12	100.0	24	100.0	90	100.1	57	100.0

Chi-square = 38.9143, $p < 0.001$.

TABLE 19
Mean Number of Psychiatric Hospitalizations, by Class.

Class	*Mean No. of hospitalizations*
I & II	2.7
III	2.2
IV	2.0
V	1.7

in the total population, rather than in a treated one, is problematic. Only an epidemiologic study of prevalence in the total population, or a large stratified sample, could answer this question decisively.

Although our data deal with prevalence in a population under psychiatric care, we feel justified in assuming that class differences in the schizophrenic group might hold in a true prevalence study. First, class differences in the incidence of acute schizophrenia are so marked that the chance is that these differences are not fortuitous. We do not believe we overlooked the large number of cases in Classes I and II which would be necessary to explain the differences we have found; neither can we assume that the number of schizophrenics in the higher social classes who do not enter treatment would equal the proportion we found in Class V. Second, schizophrenics in the upper classes who have entered treatment are less prone to break contact

TABLE 20
Schizophrenics' Experience with Treatment, by Class.

	Class							
	I & II		III		IV		V	
Treatment experience	*No.*	*%*	*No.*	*%*	*No.*	*%*	*No.*	*%*
First admission to hospital	3	10.3	22	26.5	126	35.8	214	55.9
Re-admission to hospital	14	48.3	45	54.2	182	51.7	153	40.0
Ambulatory treatment before hospitalization	6	20.7	3	3.6	18	5.1	9	2.3
Ambulatory treatment after hospitalization	5	17.2	8	9.6	18	5.1	1	.3
Ambulatory treatment; no hospitalization	1	3.4	5	6.0	8	2.3	6	1.6
TOTAL	29	99.9	83	99.9	352	100.0	383	100.1

Chi-square = 102.0021, $p < 0.001$.

with a psychiatrist than lower-class patients. It is with the lower-class patient that treatment contact breaks unless the patient is hospitalized.

The index of prevalence in Class III is of interest, but we can only speculate as to its meaning. It has been suggested that in Classes I and II families seek treatment for mentally ill relatives and that in Class V, on the other hand, schizophrenics get entangled with the law. Neither condition prevails in Class III. Possibly, the stable conditions of living in Class III may provide an answer.

If we view the data from the perspective of incidence we are still faced with the task of explaining why Class V has an index figure approximately twice that of Classes I and II. Although we have no answer to this question, one might speculate that certain factors in lower-class living are responsible.

A second question arises: What possible explanations can be given for the class differences we have found in the prevalence of treated schizophrenia? We have no definite answer, but from our material it is clear that the patient population of New Haven is not geographically mobile, and immigrants are not more frequent among our patients than in the total population of the community. Furthermore, there is little evidence of a drift into socially and economically underprivileged areas; rather we have significantly more upward than downward mobility among our patients.

Clearly there is a concentration of chronic patients in the lower social classes, particularly in Class V. But why? Certain tentative conclusions may be drawn. First, schizophrenics in Class I enter treatment earlier. This early treatment may be extremely important, especially if the upper-class schizophrenic receives better treatment than the lower-class one. Second, the upper-class schizophrenic enters treatment through medical channels; the lower-class schizophrenic through legal ones. Stated more dramatically: the upper-class mental patient rests on a therapist's couch, the lower-class one on a prison or hospital cot.

Treatment is markedly different in the upper and lower classes. However, the differences during the acute phases of the illness are less marked than in the more chronic stages. The most striking difference is the administration of psychotherapy to upper-class schizophrenics and the lack of any systematic treatment of chronic lower-class schizophrenics.

Once in a mental hospital, the lower-class schizophrenic is less likely to leave; he rarely has more than one chance in the community. If he does not make the grade he becomes a permanent resident of the institution. This fact, coupled with more or less impressionistic observations, particularly in studying rehabilitation of lobotomized patients, makes us assume that the role of the community and its most important unit, the family, is of enormous importance in determining who stays in a hospital and who becomes reintegrated with the family. We believe that forces operating within the family are as powerful a determinant for recovery as early casefinding and the right type and quality of treatment. The combination of late casefinding, inadequate treatment, and serious obstacles in rehabilitating the lower-class schizophrenic into an already poorly integrated family may account for the increase of chronic patients at the lowest class level. More research into prognosis and, particularly, into the factors determining rehabilitation into the patient's family are indicated.

In short, our second hypothesis, that the distribution of schizophrenic patients reflects class differences in the processes of treatment and rehabilitation as well as responses to treatment, seems valid. Implications of this conclusion for better casefinding, better treatment in our mental hospitals, and the intelligent use of rehabilitation techniques are obvious for psychiatry, social work, and public health administration.

Summary

We found treated prevalence of schizophrenia in the lowest social class two times more frequent than in the upper class. From our data it may be concluded that the difference is not due to downward social mobility. Tabulating approximate treated incidence of schizophrenics (patients in treatment for less than one year) we found that approximately twice as many schizophrenics occur in Class V than in Class I and II combined. At the more chronic levels the ratio between upper- and lower-class schizophrenics is much higher. We found 31 times as many schizophrenics in Class V as in Classes I and II. This increase of chronic patients in Class V appears to be related to significant differences in treatment. Our data demonstrate that schizophrenics in the upper and middle classes enter treatment earlier than those in the lower class. Upper- and middle-class schizophrenics are referred for treatment through medical channels; lower-class schizophrenics through legal ones.

Schizophrenics of the upper and middle classes are more likely to be treated by psychotherapy, while lower-class patients are more likely to receive organic treatment and in many cases are not treated at all. Patients in the upper and middle classes have a greater chance of being discharged to family and community than lower-class schizophrenics.

References

Braatoy, T. (1937), Is it probable that the sociological situation is a factor in schizophrenia? *Psychiat Neurol* 12:109-138.

Clark, R. E. (1948), The relationship of schizophrenia to occupational income and occupational prestige. *Am Sociol Rev* 13:325-330.

Clark, R. E. (1949), Psychoses, income, and occupational prestige. *Am J Sociol* 44:433-440.

Davie, R. (1937), The pattern of urban growth. In: G. P. Murdock (ed.), *Studies in the Science of Society*, ed., G. P. Murdock. New Haven: Yale University Press, pp. 133-162.

Davis, K. (1938), Mental hygiene and the class structure. *Psychiatry* 1:55-56.

Dollard, J. & Miller, N. *Personality and Psychotherapy*. New York: McGraw-Hill, 1950.

Dunham, H. (1947), Current status of ecological research in mental disorder. *Social Forces* 25:321-326.

Faris, R. E. L. (1934), Cultural isolation and the schizophrenic personality. *Am J Sociol* 39:155-169.

Faris, R. E. L. (1944), Reflections of social disorganization in the behavior of a schizophrenic patient. *Am J Sociol* 50:134-141.

Faris, R. E. L. & Dunham, H. W. (1939), *Mental Disorders in Urban Areas*. Chicago: University of Chicago Press, 1939.

Felix, R. H. & Bowers, R. V. (1948), Mental hygiene and socio-environmental factors. *The Milbank Memorial Fund Quarterly* 26:125-147.

Gerard, D. L. & Siegel, J. (1950), The family background of schizophrenia. *Psychiat Quart* 24:47-73.

Green, H. W. (1939), *Persons Admitted to the Cleveland State Hospital, 1928-1937*. Cleveland Health Council.

Hollingshead, A. B. & Redlich, F. C. (1958), *Social Class and Mental Illness*. New York: John Wiley & Sons.

Hyde, R. W. & Kingsley, L. V. (1944A), Studies in medical sociology. I: The relation of mental disorders to the community socio-economic level. *New Engl J Med* 231:543-548.

Hyde, R. W. & Kingsley, L. V. (1944B), Studies in medical sociology. II: The relation of mental disorders to population density. *New Engl J Med* 231:571-577.

Hyde, R. W. & Chisholm, R. M. (1944), Studies in medical sociology. III: The relation of mental disorders to race and nationality. *New Engl J Med* 231:612-618.

Kennedy, R. J. R. (1944), Single or triple melting-pot: Intermarriage trends in New Haven, 1870-1940. *Am J Sociol* 39:331-339.

McConnell, J. W. (1937), *The Influence of Occupation Upon Social Stratification.* Unpublished Ph.D. thesis, Yale University.

Malamud, W. & Malamud, I. (1943), A socio-psychiatric investigation of schizophrenia occurring in the Armed Forces. *Psychosomat Med* 5:364-375.

Malzberg, B. (1940), *Social and Biological Aspects of Mental Disease.* Utica, N.Y.: State Hospital Press.

Minnis, M. (1951), *The Relationship of Women's Organizations to the Social Structure of a City.* Unpublished Ph.D. thesis, Yale University.

Myers, J. K. (1950), Assimilation to the ecological and social system of a community. *Am Sociol Rev* 15:367-372.

Myers, J. K. & Roberts, B. H. (1959), *Family and Class Dynamics in Mental Illness.* New York: John Wiley & Sons.

Parsons, T. (1950), Psychoanalysis and the social structure. *Psychoanal Quart* 19:371-384.

Psychiatric Disorders and Reactions, Technical Bulletin 10A-78, October 1947. Washington, D.C.: Veterans Administration.

Rosanoff, A. J. (1916), *Report of a Survey of Mental Disorders in Nassau County, New York.* New York: National Committee for Mental Hygiene.

Roth, W. F. & Luton, F. H. (1943), The mental health program in Tennessee: Statistical report of a psychiatric survey in a rural county. *Am J Psychiat* 99:662-675.

Ruesch, J. (1949), Social technique, social status, and social change in illness. In: *Personality in Nature, Society, and Culture.* eds., C. Kluckhohn and H. A. Murray. New York: Alfred A. Knopf, pp. 117-130.

Ruesch, J., Jacobson, A. & Loeb, M. B. (1948), Acculturation and illness. Psychological Monographs: General and Applied, Vol. 62, No. 5, Whole No. 292. Washington, D.C.: American Psychological Association.

Stern, L. (1913), *Kulturkreis und Form der Geistigen Erkrankung.* (Sammlung Zwanglosen Abshandlungen aus dem Gebiete der Nerven-und-Geites-krankheiten), X, No. 2, Halle a. S:C Marhold, pp. 1-62.

Sutherland, J. F. (1901), *Geographical Distribution of Lunacy in Scotland.* Glasgow: British Association for Advancement of Science.

Tietze, C., Lemkau, P. & Cooper, M. (1941), Schizophrenia, manic depressive psychosis and social-economic status. *Am J Sociol* 47:167-175.

Tietze, C., Lemkau, P. & Cooper, M. (1943), A survey of statistical studies on the prevalence and incidence of mental disorders in sample populations. *Publ Health Rep 1909-27,* 58.

Warner, W. L. (1937), The society, the individual and his mental disorders. *Am J Psychiat* 94:275-284.

White, W. A. (1903), Geographical distribution of insanity in the United States. *J Nerv Ment Dis* 30:257-279.

Chapter 7

The Stirling County Study

JANE M. MURPHY

The objective of this chapter is to summarize the psychiatric methods and findings of the Stirling County Study in its baseline phase (1952). Attention is directed to the kind of rate chosen for measurement, the data from which it was derived, the methods of analysis leading to it, and the percentage of the population to whom it referred. The Stirling Study made use of the first *Diagnostic and Statistical Manual* (DSM-I) (American Psychiatric Association, 1952). In view of this, comparisons will be drawn between the early manual and its contemporary successor, DSM-III (American Psychiatric Association, 1980). Because the Stirling and Midtown Studies took place in the same era of community epidemiologic studies and have frequently been grouped together in the light of several similarities, contrasts between the two studies will be pointed out where this offers clarification (Srole et al., 1962; Langner and Michael, 1963).

Area and Sample

In keeping with most community-based epidemiologic studies, a geopolitical entity was the unit of study—in this case, a county located in eastern Canada which was given the pseudonym of Stirling. This area of towns and countryside has maintained a population of approximately 20,000 from 1952 to the present.

Early decisions of research design were to focus on adults and to lay the foundation for generalization through sampling. The main sample consisted of 463 men and 547 women, ranging in ages from 17 to 88. These 1,010 subjects were chosen as alternating male and female heads of households. Sampling rates were variable for different districts composed of communities that were roughly homogeneous in cultural and economic terms. On the average, one of every four to five households was selected. The sample was found to compare favorably with the age and sex breakdowns for household heads reported in the 1951 Canadian census. The effect of variable sampling rates was assessed by using weighted and unweighted frequencies. The differences in the derived percentages were found to be negligible, and the weighting system was considered expendable (D. Leighton et al., 1963a, p. 142). In this chapter, findings will be presented using unweighted frequencies.

Type of Epidemiologic Rate Selected For Study

The epidemiologic rate used to characterize the distribution of psychiatric disorder in this sample was *prevalence*. While recognizing that *incidence* would have been superior, it appeared likely that information regarding the onset date of untreated disorders, though necessary for the latter, would be subject to considerable error in a baseline field study (D. Leighton et al., 1963a, pp. 34-35).

The goal was to count all instances of psychiatric disorder that had occurred in the lives of the sample members up to May 1, 1952. This latter date was chosen to coordinate with data-collecting procedures. The rate was described as "total reportable prevalence." Since current status was better represented in the data than lifetime evidence due to matters of recall, the rate was further defined as "more than current prevalence," and "less than lifetime prevalence" (D. Leighton et al., 1963a, p. 118). Actually, the Stirling researchers thought that the rate was dominated by current and chronic cases (D. Leighton et al., 1963a, p. 355).

Six Points of Methodological Orientation

The psychiatric methods leading to the prevalence rate took shape in the light of six main points.

1. *Psychiatric disorder consists of many categories of psychiatric cases (A. Leighton, 1959, pp. 93-129).*—The goal of the study was to identify the full range of different diagnostic types of psychiatric disorders. Recognizing that "it is possible to be exceedingly obscure—if one talks about psychiatric disorders in general" (A. Leighton, 1959, pp. 94, 352-388), it was decided to use DSM-I as the nosological guide. It had just been published and was then the most up-to-date version of a standard nomenclature for statistical reporting in North America. The definition of psychiatric disorder adopted was in essence "what the *Manual* catalogues." "The phenomena of reference in this definition are, to say the least, heterogeneous; psychiatric disorder is not an 'it' but a 'they' " (D. Leighton et al., 1963a, p. 172). Although a structure for classifying disorders was seen as essential, DSM-I itself was viewed as unsatisfactory in many ways, especially in its failure to indicate criteria for case counting other than through the nature of symptoms. Because it lacked specifications for many decisions that had to be made, a handbook was developed to spell out how to use the Manual for evaluating the kind of data available.

   While the Stirling group thus took the approach of adapting DSM-I, the Midtown researchers decided to follow the model of the United States National Health Survey concerned with somatic illness and to attempt to place each subject on a "linear scale of functional impairment" (Srole et al., 1962, p. 63). This single dimension was concerned with classifying individuals "according to the severity of their symptoms and the disability they entail" (Srole et al., 1962, p. 135). The choice of such a classificatory scheme was motivated by some of the same reservations regarding traditional diagnostic procedures as was expressed by the Stirling researchers in their modifications of DSM-I. The Midtown group, however, affiliated their classification decisions with the trend at that time to "see mental health and mental illness as differing in degree rather than kind" as expressed by Felix and Bowers (1948, p. 130) and as being similar to the "unitary concept of mental illness" described by Menninger (1959).

2. *Because the Stirling research was concerned with exploring social factors as possible causes of psychiatric disorders, etiologic attributes should not be assumed in the diagnostic classification (A. Leighton, 1959. p. 357).*—DSM-I was variable in terms of the degree to which etiology was specified in its categories, but the description for "psychoneurotic depressive reaction" illustrates the problem posed for social research:

The anxiety in this reaction is allayed, and hence partially relieved, by depression and self-depreciation. *This reaction is precipitated by a current situation* (italics added), frequently by some loss sustained by the patient, and is often associated with a feeling of guilt for past failures or deeds... The term is synonymous with "reactive depression" and is to be differentiated from the corresponding psychotic reaction (APA, 1952, pp. 33-34).

If one followed this description, psychoneurotic depressive reaction could only be used when it was known to be a reaction to social circumstances. The only other way to register the presence of depressive symptomatology was to employ one of the categories of affective reaction listed under psychotic disorders. Subscription to this scheme would have ruled out the possibility of testing associations with social factors and would have enforced a dubious definition of the difference between psychotic and neurotic depression. Thus it was decided to use DSM-I categories in a nonetiologic sense so that in later analyses it would be possible to determine whether these psychiatric phenomena appeared to be a reaction to life experiences or not. The DSM-I category of "adult situational reaction" was discarded on these grounds and the rest of the classification system was used as an aid for the accurate recognition of the manifestations of psychiatric disorders rather than as a commitment to a presumed etiology. The organic brain syndromes were the only categories where etiology retained its defining role.

Had the DSM-I been organized in the way DSM-III has emerged, it probably would have been possible to use it with relatively little adaptation for this point. The principle of organization for DSM-III involves three classes of disorders: those for which there is a known necessary organic etiology; those which share descriptive features; and those with known or presumed necessary psychosocial etiology (Spitzer et al., 1977, pp. 6-7). Most of the DSM-III classification involves categories built on shared features, and it is possible to use a category like Depressive Disorder under circumstances when it is a reaction to psychosocial stresses or physical illness *and* when it is not. Thus, while DSM-III is intended to reflect the current state of knowledge about the causes of psychiatric disorders, it is not bound to etiological suppositions. "When the etiology of a disorder is not known, as is the case with most of the mental disorders, the classification should facilitate systematic inquiry" (Spitzer et at., 1977, p. 3).

Lacking such recognition of the limits of etiological knowledge and believing that the word "diagnosis" implied that etiology *was* known, the Stirling researchers decided to emphasize the nonetiologic use of DSM-I categories by employing a different term. The phrase "symptom pattern" was adopted to replace the term "diagnosis." "Symptom pattern" was illustrated by the concept of an "anxiety attack" as it might appear under "diagnostic impression" on a referral form filled out by a general practitioner (D. Leighton et al., 1963a, p. 117). It comprehends the pattern or configuration of symptoms which a physician might list under "complaints": "An acute and circumscribed attack. . . of palpitations, tachycardia, dyspnoea, sensations of choking. . . . Marked fear of dying and concern about the heart" (A. Leighton, 1959, p. 35). Thus "symptom pattern" was used to mean a diagnosis in the sense of identifying a constellation or syndrome of symptoms perceived by a clinician as being what he would customarily call anxiety reaction, schizophrenia, mental retardation, etc., but not to mean a diagnosis in the sense of including etiology.

3. *Multiple category designations from DSM-I may be needed to describe a person over his life span or even at one point in time (D. Leighton et al., 1963a, pp. 68, 160).*—The prevailing use of the Manual discouraged the employment of multiple categories, and certain combinations of categories were disallowed in an effort to achieve a primary diagnosis. It seemed wiser to the Stirling researchers to avoid the procrusteanism often involved in forcing each subject to be classified in one and only one category. Thus, if evidence existed that a subject was mentally retarded but also had periods of psychoneurotic depression, the objective was to record both types of disorder without rank ordering.

   Unlike its predecessor, DSM-III encourages the use of multiple categories "when necessary to describe the current condition" (APA, 1980, p. 24). If the new manual were to be modified for community research oriented to life time prevalence, the need for multiple categories would undoubtedly be put in even stronger terms. Also DSM-III is more than a classification in which multiple categories can pertain; it is also a multiaxial classification which requires that "every case be assessed on each of several axes" (APA, 1980, p. 23). The five axes involved are: 1) Clinical Psychiatric Syndromes; 2) Personality

Disorders; 3) Non-Mental Medical Disorders; 4) Psychosocial Stressors; and 5) Functioning in Recent Year. The fact that DSM-III divides the former classification into its first two axes with the second to be used for longstanding and possibly less florid patterns of maladaptation means that multiple categories are not only allowed but that at least two categories must receive some kind of evaluation. A manual like DSM-III would have obviated some of the DSM-I modifications employed by the Stirling group regarding this point.

4. *A conservative position should be taken with regard to psychophysiologic and sociopathic disorders (D. Leighton et al., 1963a, p. 46).* —Where the margins of psychiatric disorder may be blurred and where confusion may arise about what is psychiatric, what is organic, and what is deviance, the Stirling group tried to avoid being overinclusive.

DSM-I specifications called for the acceptance of a fairly large number of physiological disorders as countable in a psychiatric framework "when emotional factors play a causative role." For example, the specifications for psychophysiologic skin reactions include "neurodermatoses, pruritus, atopic dermatitis, hyperhydrosis, and so forth" (APA, 1952, p. 30). Further, the DSM-I section on psychophysiologic disorders is patterned on the ICD, *The International Classification of Diseases* (WHO, 1948). With the exception of infectious and parasitic diseases, neoplasms, complications of pregnancy, and congenital abnormalities, each of the major morbidity categories in the ICD is represented in DSM-I. If one interpreted the phrase "when emotional factors play a causative role" in a multifactorial way allowing emotion to be one among several causes, almost any disorder except cancer, infectious diseases, and congenital abnormalities could be classified in DSM-I. The intent was clearly not so broad as this, however, and the purpose was to identify the classical psychosomatic disorders when, presumably, the emotional contribution was strong and had been demonstrated. It is noteworthy that in reports emanating from the use of DSM-I in psychiatric hospitals and clinics these categories were so rarely employed that they are subsumed under "all other diagnoses" (Kramer et al., 1972). This probably relates to the fact that psychosomatic disorders are mainly dealt with in primary care settings, which in turn probably stems from the difficulty in demonstrating the degree to which emotional factors are indeed implicated in any given case.

In view of the nonetiologic use of DSM-I in the Stirling Study, it should be pointed out that employing the psychophysiologic categories without assuming an emotional etiology was a somewhat different kind of adaptation than to use depression without commitment as to whether it was endogenous or reactive. While one could be relatively certain that the syndrome of symptoms characterizing depression was present as a clinical entity while reserving judgment about its cause, one would question the relevance of counting hypertension in a psychiatric classification at all unless emotional factors were known to contribute substantially. In view of this it seemed wise to develop special analytic conventions for these categories so that they would not contribute to the case count in the absence of evidence of emotional factors which were classifiable in the psychoneurotic or other clearly psychiatric categories (D. Leighton et al., 1963a, p. 120).

Another adaptation of DSM-I was to separate the sociopathic disorders from the section on personality disorders and to view them as distinctive in the feature of being socially disruptive and out of keeping with social norms (A. Leighton, 1959, p. 127). The sociopathic categories included alcoholism, antisocial and dyssocial behavior, as well as sexual deviations.

A similarly conservative attitude was taken toward these categories as toward the psychophysiologic disorders, and the analytic rules prevented these disorders being counted as clear-cut psychiatric disorders in the absence of other evidence. This conservatism represented the kind of consideration that led to removing homosexuality from the official psychiatric nomenclature in 1973. The effect of this decision was not, however, of much relevance to the total reportable rate in the Stirling Study— simply because there was little evidence of sexual deviation in the data. Its main effect concerned alcoholism which was the most commonly used category in the sociopathic section. In this regard, the Stirling Study was out of step with the course of history. The analytic scheme involved a conscious underrepresentation of a category which has come into increasing prominence as a disorder for which psychiatry has responsibility and which in DSM-III has been broadened to include alcohol abuse over and above alcohol addiction.

5. *The professional best equipped by training and experience to recognize the phenomena to be catalogued in DSM-I is a psychiatrist (D. Leighton et al., 1963a, pp. 45-49).*—This principle led to a situation in which the health-related information about the sample members was processed in the minds of research psychiatrists. The findings reported represent their clinical judgments.

   In developing the analytic plans for the Stirling Study, an attempt was made to maintain a balance between the dual objectives of using standardized techniques and of applying a clinical approach; that is, of having the obvious research advantage of systematic principles being applied to uniform data but without robbing the procedure of the factor of clinical judgment. One way to achieve this would have been for the research psychiatrists to interview each subject using a standard but flexible interview format. Although this approach was employed with subsamples in later phases of the Stirling Study, such a method of data gathering was not used regarding the sample of 1,010 adults who form the core of the baseline study. In contrast, the procedure used for this sample may be called an *approximated clinical assessment,* and it involved the psychiatrists as readers and evaluators of a written protocol about each sample member.

The concept of "confidence" played a vital role in the clinical judgment procedures (A. Leighton, 1959, pp. 362-381). Confidence was considered to be a unilinear continuum applicable to the decision-making process. It represented the psychiatrists' assessments of the quality and quantity of data pointing to phenomena of psychiatric import. "Complaints about and appearance of low spirits, for instance, are not necessarily a symptom pattern with psychiatric significance" (A. Leighton, 1959, p. 370). Thus the confidence ratings served the purpose of reflecting the decision that evidence should be classified within a psychiatric framework and that it matched the descriptions in DSM-I.

6. *The presence of a psychiatric disorder is distinct from the impairment which may flow from it; and those cases which give evidence of impairment in work, family, or community roles are among the ones to be counted in a prevalence rate if such a rate is to be clinically meaningful (D. Leighton et al., 1963a, pp. 134-170).*—This principle takes cognizance of the fact that two individuals might have very similar patterns of anxious or depressed mood but one might be unable to work, have periods of sleep difficulty, need medication, and be confined to the house, while the other might function in a way almost indistinguishable from other similar age and sex persons in his social environment. Thus the position was taken that "illness stands for more than the presence of symptoms; it means a certain intensity of them and usually also a certain amount of interference with ordinary functioning" (D. Leighton et al., 1963a, p. 73).

The diagnostic categories of DSM-I spelled out what kinds of symptoms were to be recognized but they lacked criteria for intensity, duration, and impairment by which the symptoms could be translated into clinical entities. The presence of such criteria in DSM-III is one of the major contrasts between it and its predecessors.

The DSM-I diagnostic category of anxiety reaction is a case in point:

> In this kind of reaction the anxiety is diffuse and not restricted to definite situations or objects, as in the case of phobic reactions. It is not controlled by any specific psychologic defense mechanism as in other psychoneurotic reactions. This reaction is characterized by anxious expectation and frequently associated with somatic symptomology. The condition is to be differentiated from normal apprehensiveness or fear (APA, 1952, p. 32).

Compare this to the operational criteria of a Panic Disorder paraphrased from DSM-III: *(a)* At least three panic attacks in three weeks unrelated to physical exertion or life-threatening situations; *(b)* At least four of the following symptoms present during each attack: dyspnea, palpitations, chest pain, choking, dizziness, feelings of unreality, paresthesias, hot/cold flashes, sweating, faintness, trembling, or fear of dying; *(c)* Not due to a physical disorder or another mental disorder; and *(d)* Not meeting the criteria for agoraphobia (APA, 1980, pp. 231—232). When used in conjunction with the Research Diagnostic Criteria, the operational criteria also include a component on impairment in which social functioning, use of medication, seeking or being referred for help, or drug abuse are taken into consideration (Spitzer et al., 1975, 1978).

It would be misleading if these comments suggested that DSM-I neglected impairment altogether. DSM-I called for a rating of degree of psychiatric impairment among other elements to be evaluated. It did not, however, factor impairment into the diagnostic categories and it provided almost no specification about how to make the impairment ratings. This is illustrated by the fact that the definitions of diagnostic terms were contained in 31 pages while the section on impairment consisted of three.

The impairment rating scheme of DSM-I was conveyed mainly by an abstract scale of percent of disability divided by arbitrary cutting points into five units: *(a)* no impairment; *(b)* minimal impairment (up to 10%); *(c)* mild impairment (20%-30%); *(d)* moderate impairment (30% to 50%); and *(e)* severe impairment (more than 50%). This percentage scale referred to "the degree to which the individual's total functional capacity is affected by the psychiatric condition" (APA, 1952, p. 49). Quite aside from the fact that "functional capacity" was not defined in terms of its component parts, it was unclear whether the percentage scale referred to a person's total functional capacity during a week, a year, or the person's whole life in the cumulative sense.

Despite the special inadequacies of this part of the *Manual*, the Stirling group believed that an assessment of impairment was imperative. They decided that disorder and impairment should be measured separately and then joined. The final product of the Stirling method of analysis was a paradigm of *need for psychiatric attention* that took into account both the type of disorder and impairment. The development of this paradigm, through which prevalence was reported, was intended to affiliate the results of the study with the clinical practice of psychiatry and it represented the effort of the Stirling group to compensate for one of the greatest weaknesses they perceived in DSM-I.

The major problem of DSM-I for community epidemiology was that it did not give a definition of what should be counted as a case in a prevalence or incidence rate. It had been developed to describe individuals in treatment; that is, individuals about whom the need for psychiatric attention had already been established, but it did not give the community epidemiologist a standard for determining to whom among the untreated the classification should be applied. The purpose of the Stirling typology of need for psychiatric attention was to make explicit for community epidemiology what was implicit in DSM-I when it was used solely in hospitals and clinics.

Of these six points which give orientation to the psychiatric methods of the Stirling Study, the fifth (using psychiatrists as evaluators of the data) is the one that the Midtown and Stirling Studies shared in a fundamental sense, and the sixth by virtue of the fact that both took impaired functioning into account. While the result of such analysis in the Midtown Study was a linear rating of psychiatric impairment, the product in the Stirling Study was an assessment of need for psychiatric attention.

Nature of the Data

Three types of information were brought together for the approximated clinical assessments: *(a)* Hospital records, *(b)* General practitioner records, and *(c)* Self report by the subject in response to an interview that involved a health questionnaire and a standardized screening instrument.

Hospital Records

Searches were carried out in six hospitals. Records available from the main provincial mental hospital date back to 1868, but taking all hospitals together, there was quite a consistent coverage from 1940 onwards to the prevalence date (D. Leighton et al., 1963a, p. 62). For the sample of 1,010, a total of 466 records was located. Only 10 of these contained a psychiatric diagnosis in traditional DSM-I terms. Due to the fact that up to five hospital records had been found for a few people and two records for a sizeable number, the proportion of subjects who had one or more hospital records was 21%.

General Practitioner Records

In 1952, 10 primary care physicians were in practice in Stirling County. These physicians were interviewed by psychiatrists concerning each of the sample subjects who lived in their catchment areas. The interview was semistructured and had three basic aspects of coverage: medical history, psychiatric history, and social adjustment (D. Leighton et al., 1963a, p. 41). The physicians were asked to convey the duration and level of their knowledge about each subject and to describe each medical and psychiatric episode as fully as possible in terms of when it occurred, how long it lasted, symptomatic manifestations, treatment, referral, and impairment. The number of general practitioner records available for each sample member ranged from 0 to 6, with an average of nearly 2 per subject. Only 49 subjects were unknown to all the physicians, thus the proportion of subjects who had one or more general practitioner record was 95%.

Self Report in Response to a Medical Checklist and a Standardized Screening Instrument

The sample was surveyed using a questionnaire interview that contained a large number of questions relevant to social experience; questions about general health organized mainly as a checklist; and a screening instrument. This questionnaire was administered verbally in a face-to-face session by trained interviewers.

The questions and responses from the health section of the questionnaire and the screening instrument along with the interviewer's marginal record of the subject's verbal elaborations were later copied into the written protocol. This unit of self-report data consisted of answers to 56 questions: 28 medical checklist items, 24 items from the screening instrument, 2 items on impairment, and 2 general health questions. The latter were employed in an open-ended fashion as, "Do you have any particular physical or health trouble at present?" and "What sorts of serious illnesses have you had?" The checklist items covered the systems of the body but with special attention on disorders often thought to involve a psychogenic component, such as asthma and hypertension. Each checklist query was dated for occurrence and the subject was asked for his estimate of severity. The questions on impairment dealt with work; one was, "have you ever had to go easy on your work because of poor health?" and the other, "have you ever had to change your work?" Both of these were dated for onset, and duration was requested.

The screening instrument, called the Health Opinion Survey (HOS) was derived from work carried out as a preparatory phase of the Stirling Study (Macmillan, 1954; Macmillan, 1957). Its purpose was to detect persons who, if subsequently examined by a psychiatrist, would with high probability be found to be psychoneurotic cases. Twenty of the 24 questions used in the Stirling Study discriminated between 93 patients diagnosed as psychoneurotic and an identified normal group at or beyond the 0.01 level of significance. The qualities of this screening instrument have been assessed in several ways within the framework of continuing studies in Stirling County and by independent workers (Murphy, 1981). For the purpose of describing the data utilized in the approximated clinical assessments, it is sufficient to say that this standardized screening instrument comprised about half of the self report data. In more than nine of ten cases the self report data were supplemented by at least one general practitioner record, and in one of five cases by one or more hospital records.

This data base is substantially different from that available in the Midtown Study. The Midtown protocols contained no information of the type provided by general practitioners although they did include the results of searches of psychiatric treatment and social service records. The psychiatric portion of the Midtown questionnaire consisted of 120 items (Srole et al., 1962, pp. 40-43). The Midtown psychiatrists processed about twice as much self-report data from a structured questionnaire as was true in the Stirling Study, and the Stirling questionnaire contained more specification of medical history than did the Midtown instrument.

Approximated Clinical Assessments

These assessments resulted in four cumulative and interlocking units: *(a)* symptom patterns, *(b)* psychiatric caseness, *(c)* overall impairment, and *(d)* need for psychiatric attention. In essence, the symptom pattern recognition led to the caseness recognition; the overall impairment ratings were made next and joined to psychiatric caseness to make the final product of need for psychiatric attention. The approximated clinical assessments were carried out separately by two psychiatrists, and their independent analyses were reviewed in a joint session. The jointly determined products for each of the four units were reported as sets of findings representing steps in a series of successive approximations leading to the final assessment.

Symptom Patterns

These were the building blocks upon which the rest of the assessment stood. The adapted version of DSM-I had 32 detailed categories grouped within the framework of the major categories of organic brain syndromes, psychoses, mental retardation, psychoneuroses, personality disorders, sociopathic disorders, and psychophysiologic disorders. The recognition of symptom patterns represented a "yes" versus "no" decision about whether there was evidence for any of the detailed categories. If something pertinent to a category was assessed as ever having been present, further ratings were made for confidence, time of occurrence, duration, and the impairment associated with that pattern.

The confidence rating was recorded as high, medium, or low. High confidence meant that the psychiatrists believed that the DSM-I descriptions were matched by the data. Medium confidence meant reservation of various kinds, including the adequacy of the data, and low confidence meant doubt.

In view of the nature of the data, an important element of the confidence rating was a matter of discarding organic material from the registering process so that what remained would be clearly psychiatric. DSM-I did not require overt recognition of the medical history or current organic condition of the subjects whose psychiatric status was being catalogued. Thus the interpretative process concerned ruling out organicity. This meant removing symptom reports that could reasonably be associated with an organic process if clear evidence of the latter existed and the disorder was not among those classified in the psychophysiologic section. Thus, if the psychiatrists were evaluating a subject currently under treatment for cancer, some of the checklist items might have been considered its concomitants and some of the HOS responses might have been discarded as lacking psychiatric significance. Thus a wealth of information about nonmental disorders, which would today be taken into account as the third axis in the multiaxial approach of DSM-III, played no role in these assessments except as it referred to the psychophysiologic disorders.

Time of occurrence was recorded as "ongoing in 1952" or "past only," and duration was shown as "up to 6 months," "6 months to 2 years," and "more than 2 years."

The impairment ratings for the symptom patterns were intended to reflect the amount of interference with functioning associated with this particular pattern as well as the duration of this particular episode of impairment. The evidence of impairment given in the general practitioner data was multifaceted and touched on such factors as work history, marriage and family roles, role in the community, and use of medical and legal institutions. When derived only from the self-report data it was limited to the work spheres. To illustrate what would have been assessed as a mildly impairing symptom pattern identified solely from the questionnaire data, it would have required that the person say he was or had been "going easy" on work, that the duration of this was at least several months, and, of course, that it could not be attributed to any symptom pattern other than the one being recognized.

The published analysis of symptom patterns focused on *current* symptom patterns. The confidence, duration, and impairment ratings attached to them were not used at that time. Under these conditions, the most commonly used major category of DSM-I was the psychophysiologic section, with 59% of the sample members having at least one low confidence detailed pattern therein. The next most common was psychoneurosis with 52% (D. Leighton et al., 1963a, p. 74).

The net cast to report these percentages was very loosely woven and included everything the psychiatrists judged to be even conceivably relevant to the epidemiological profile.

Psychiatric Caseness

This rating refers to the confidence held by the psychiatrists that the subject could be considered a psychiatric case *in DSM-I terms.* It involved four categories: "A" meant strong confidence; "B" meant less certainty; "C" stood for doubt; and "D" meant confidence that there was no evidence in any way suggestive of a psychiatric disorder.

Although not analyzed and presented at that time, there was a consistent relationship between the confidence ratings given the detailed symptom patterns and the ABCD ratings. In essence almost every person rated as ever having had the syndrome of symptoms to which high confidence was applied in a detailed category within the major categories of psychosis, mental retardation, brain syndrome, psychoneurosis, and personality disorder was given an "A" rating for Caseness. The psychoneurotic patterns illustrate this. Although 52% of the sample was seen as having a psychoneurotic pattern at some level of confidence, only 26% was so perceived with high confidence. Virtually all of the latter group (250 of 259) were rated as "A" cases. The difference between a high confidence psychoneurotic pattern in an "A" case and one not rated "A" was a matter of discounting a depressive reaction, for example, when it appeared to be normal grief and not therefore a psychiatric case in DSM-I terms. On the other hand, subjects who had high confidence patterns only in the psychophysiologic and/or sociopathic categories were always classified as "B" cases. This was the mechanism whereby a conservative position was taken in regard to the latter patterns. The "A" rating served one other function over and above that of being the repository for cases that matched DSM-I descriptions in the clearly psychiatric categories. This function was to allow the psychiatrists to register their judgment that a subject was a definite psychiatric case even though none of the manifest DSM-I descriptions pertained with certainty.

Among the 1,010 sample members, 30.5% received the rating of "A" (D. Leighton et al., 1963a, p. 121). After the approximated clinical assessments were completed, the psychiatrists provided the research analysts with "guesses" as to what percentage in each of the confidence categories would turn out on more intensive investigation to be psychiatric cases according to the *Manual.* These guesses were 90% for A, 70% for B, 40% for C, and 10% for D, and they led to the suggestion that "57 percent of the adult population in this county would be considered 'psychiatric cases' if diagnosed according to the criteria of the *Manual*" (D. Leighton et al., 1963a, p. 121). This 57% figure is independent in derivation from the actual findings but it happened empirically to be identical to the actual finding that 57% of the sample had been classified as either "A" or "B."

In reporting the findings, this 57% figure and extrapolations from it such as "about half the adults in this county" were routinely qualified by phrases like "according to the criteria of the *Manual.*" This meant, for example, that the psychiatrists were satisfied that they had recognized anxiety in contrast to normal fear and depression in contrast to normal grief but not that such evidence constituted illness in the clinical sense or that it provided an adequate basis for estimating prevalence. Although these DSM-I estimates were considered to be a step forward in the process, they were rejected as the final conclusion. "It seemed more fruitful instead to think in terms of a quantitative variable of 'need for psychiatric attention'" (D. Leighton et al., 1963a, p. 356). This drew heavily on the impairment ratings described in the next point.

Overall Impairment Rating

The overall impairment rating stemmed from the description given above of the impairment for the individual symptom patterns—with one important difference. The time frame was the person's entire life up to the time of interview, while that for the individual symptom patterns was the duration of the episode of impairment related to that particular symptom pattern. "This total was a subjectively weighted average of the detailed symptom pattern ratings, and the weight was based on their duration and severity rather than the extent to which any given pattern represented a psychiatric disorder" (D. Leighton et al., 1963a, p. 126).

This impairment rating can best be understood as having a vertical and a horizontal axis. Severity referred to the amount of impairment at one point in time based on what could be generally thought of as the total functional capacity of persons of similar age and sex in this social environment. Thus inability to work was differentiated from reduced functioning in work. Duration referred to how long such impairment had been in evidence. Considerable attention was given to the demarcation between minimal and mild because the mild category and those for moderate and severe were later grouped as "significant impairment," or simply as "impairment."

It is probably clear from the above that these impairment ratings were difficult to make because they required the research psychiatrists to remember five arbitrary cutting points on a scale with 100 points that supposedly represented the functional capacity of typical people in both the cross-section and the span of their lives. The word "subjectively" in the quotation above was an honest display of how the DSM-I scheme had to be dealt with in the absence of specifications.

In the sample of 1,010, 31.1% received total impairment ratings of mild or more (D. Leighton et al., 1963a, p. 127). This figure includes impairment associated with all kinds of disorders catalogued in the system. Thus a subject impaired by anything classifiable in the psychophysiologic and sociopathic categories was included here even if there was no evidence of an associated psychological component.

Need for Psychiatric Attention

As said earlier, this paradigm attempted to compensate for DSM-I inadequacies and took into account the type of disorder and impairment. Psychoses and Organic Brain Syndromes were the diagnostic types thought most likely to require some kind of psychiatric attention. Psychophysiologic and sociopathic types were excluded from the paradigm unless they were combined with a more clearly psychiatric type of disorder. Impairment at the level of mild or more was considered sufficient to warrant psychiatric attention.

The typology of need for attention had five categories constituted in the following way: Type I contained A cases with psychosis or organic brain syndrome (3% of the sample); Type II included A cases with mild or more impairment and not in Type I (17%); Type III consisted of all other A cases and B cases (37%); Type IV involved C cases (26%); and Type V contained D cases (17%). This typology identified 20% of the sample as needing psychiatric attention. This was considered to be the most satisfactory means of reporting prevalence given the principles and methods which guided the study (D. Leighton et al., 1963a, p. 356).

In summarizing the findings of the study, the Stirling group considered that the 20% estimate was comparable to the 23.4% estimate from the Midtown Study. "In sum, it appears that at least 20% of the general population has definite need for psychiatric help. . . . This corresponds in size with the Midtown group who have serious symptoms and various degrees of impairment" (D. Leighton et al., 1963b, p. 1023). Thus, despite the differences in methods and place of study, the two studies were surprisingly similar in their estimates of prevalence.

Types of Disorders and Current Prevalence

Because the Stirling work was undertaken with an emphasis on the heterogeneity of psychiatric disorders and involved exploratory use of DSM-I, it seems unfortunate now that the 20% total reportable prevalence rate was not described in more detail. Aside from the category that combined psychoses and organic brain syndromes, the remaining 17% was described mainly as containing an unexpected preponderance in the psychoneurotic category (D. Leighton et al., 1963a, p. 357).

The data sets prepared from the approximated clinical assessments provided considerably more categorical description of the types of psychiatric disorder counted in this rate than appeared in the published analysis. In preparation for a longitudinal analysis and as a test of the procedures of replication, the total reportable rate has been converted to an estimate of current prevalence in 1952. This conversion represents two adjustments: *(a)* recovered cases and those with no currently impairing symptom patterns have been removed, and *(b)* definite cases with at least one impairing current symptom pattern have been added. The latter had been excluded earlier because in the cumulative sense their current impairment was not seen as lasting long enough to warrant being put in the mild category in lifetime terms. These additions and deletions involve small and almost equal numbers so that the current prevalence rate thus calculated identifies 20.7% of the sample.

This current prevalence rate is described in table 1 by means of what can be called clear-cut symptom patterns or diagnostic impressions. A clear-cut symptom pattern is one which the psychiatrists recognized with high confidence *and* which was impairing at the time of the survey in 1952. Such patterns had been in evidence for longer than a month, usually much longer and sometimes over a period of many years.

This presentation of findings follows the six points outlined earlier as underlying the Stirling methods.

1. The table shows that psychiatric disorders were recognized not as a general "it" but rather as a heterogeneous "they." In the interests of simplicity, it is organized mainly according to the major categories of DSM-I as adapted for the Stirling Study. Rates for the detailed categories for psychoneurosis are, however, shown in parentheses.
2. With the exception of the organic brain syndromes, this classification can be interpreted as based on descriptive entities rather than etiology.
3. Multiple category designations for one subject are shown where needed. This accounts for the fact that the sum of the category percentages is greater than the percentage of subjects counted in the prevalence rate. The major category most frequently found in combination with another was Personality Disorder, a finding that fits well with the DSM-III principle of making the Personality Disorders a separate axis.
4. A conservative attitude lies behind the psychophysiologic and sociopathic categories. All of the subjects shown in these categories had a symptom pattern in another category, usually the psychoneurotic category, but the latter was not always considered to be as impairing as the psychophysiologic or sociopathic. This rate, however, excludes such conditions as hypertension, asthma, and ulcers, when there was no evidence of anxiety or other emotional factor. The rate also excludes cases of alcohol abuse and should be interpreted as involving underestimation in this regard.
5. The symptom patterns and cases shown here were recognized with firm confidence by the research psychiatrists as belonging in a psychiatric classification.
6. This presentation takes account of the fact that illness was conceived to be more than the presence of symptoms and includes only those patterns currently associated with reduced functioning through the impairment rating.

TABLE 1
Current Prevalence (1952) of Major Categories of Psychiatric Disorder with Detailed Categories for Psychoneurotic Disorders in Rates per 100.[a]

	Males		*Females*		
Psychiatric Disorder	*Under 45 (n=192)*	*45 and over (n=269)*	*Under 45 (n=281)*	*45 and over (n=268)*	*Total (n=1,010)*
Depression	(2.1)	(4.5)	(6.4)	(3.0)	(4.1)
Hypochondriasis	(1.6)	(1.8)	(1.4)	(2.2)	(1.8)
Conversion	(0.0)	(0.0)	(0.0)	(0.4)	(0.1)
Anxiety	(2.1)	(0.7)	(2.5)	(6.0)	(2.9)
Other	(2.1)	(0.7)	(2.5)	(7.5)	(3.3)
Psychoneurotic disorders	7.8	7.8	12.8	19.0	12.2
Psychophysiologic disorders	3.6	7.4	2.8	10.4	6.2
Sociopathic disorders	1.6	3.3	0.7	0.0	1.4
Personality disorders	1.0	0.0	0.7	1.5	0.8
Mental retardation	0.5	1.5	0.7	0.7	0.9
Psychotic disorders	0.0	0.4	0.7	1.1	0.6
Organic brain syndromes	1.0	0.7	0.0	0.0	0.4
No clear cut pattern	1.6	1.8	2.8	4.1	2.7
TOTAL	13.0	17.8	18.1	31.3	20.7

[a]The labels for the major and detailed categories are adapted from DSM-I. The detailed categories of Psychoneurotic Disorders are organized as mutually exclusive categories by counting a subject only in the highest pertaining category of the list as shown. The multiple use of the major categories for one subject means that the sum of the category rates is larger than the total rate.

As forecast in the original publication, the most common patterns were in the psychoneurotic category (12%). Among those with psychoneurotic disorders, 4% were found to be experiencing an impairing episode of depression at the time of the survey. On the other hand, the controls for currency and confidence reduced the use of the categories for psychosis and organic brain syndromes from 3% to 1%. In keeping with the findings published earlier, this current prevalence rate contains more women than men, and more older people than younger.

Validity and Reliability

Within the framework of the baseline study in Stirling County, work was done to assess both the reliability and the validity of procedures. Three small substudies on validity were reported in the original publication. These were based on existing opportunities rather than on a designed plan, but each suggested that the Stirling methods underestimated prevalence (D. Leighton et al., 1963a, pp. 171-199). Later, a larger study of validity was designed and undertaken in which a group of independent psychiatrists visited 122 sample members in their homes after a similar Stirling survey in 1962 (A. Leighton et al., 1966). The agreement between the results of the approximated clinical assessments based on the protocols and the face-to-face assessments based on the home visits was considerably closer than the earlier validity tests and suggested that the Stirling method somewhat overestimated prevalence.

The reliability of the approximated clinical assessments was tested in terms of the agreement between the research psychiatrists (D. Leighton et al., 1963a, pp. 423-435). A correlation of 0.79 for the ABCD ratings was considered to be fairly satisfactory, but the use of the jointly agreed upon results was considered an improvement. Subsequently the issue of reliability was taken up in collaboration with an independent group of researchers, and in a new trial, correlations ranged between 0.70 and 0.80 (Goldfarb et al., 1967). In this latter study, a small experiment in removing the records of the general practitioners pointed to a marked alteration in the results.

The validation and reliability testing efforts carried out by the Stirling group have until recently taken the psychiatric judgment conveyed in the ABCD ratings and the impairment ratings as the assessments to be tested and measured. This stemmed from the fact that these were the units of analysis through which findings were presented. It was also based on the reasonable assumption that the clinical judgment of a psychiatrist is not necessarily valid and reliable and should be tested. However, a procedure that brings diverse types of information together through the means of clinical judgment is only as valid as the data utilized are valid.

Questions about the reliability and validity of self-report data and general practitioner records are as important as those about psychiatric judgment. The documentation from the 1952 approximated clinical assessments did not contain information on which source of information had been used to make a given decision, but it was known that the general practitioners contributed information on all types of disorder while the questionnaire survey contributed, except in very rare instances, only to the psychoneurotic, psychophysiologic, and unclear cases. The findings on prevalence would have been quite different had they been calculated separately on the basis of the different sources of information. From work carried out in preparation for a longitudinal study, it can be indicated that approximately 15.2% was identified as needing psychiatric attention from the questionnaire interviews, 11.1% from the general practitioners, and 1% from the hospital records. Comparison of the results from these independent sources might also have served as a means of estimating validity.

FIGURE 1

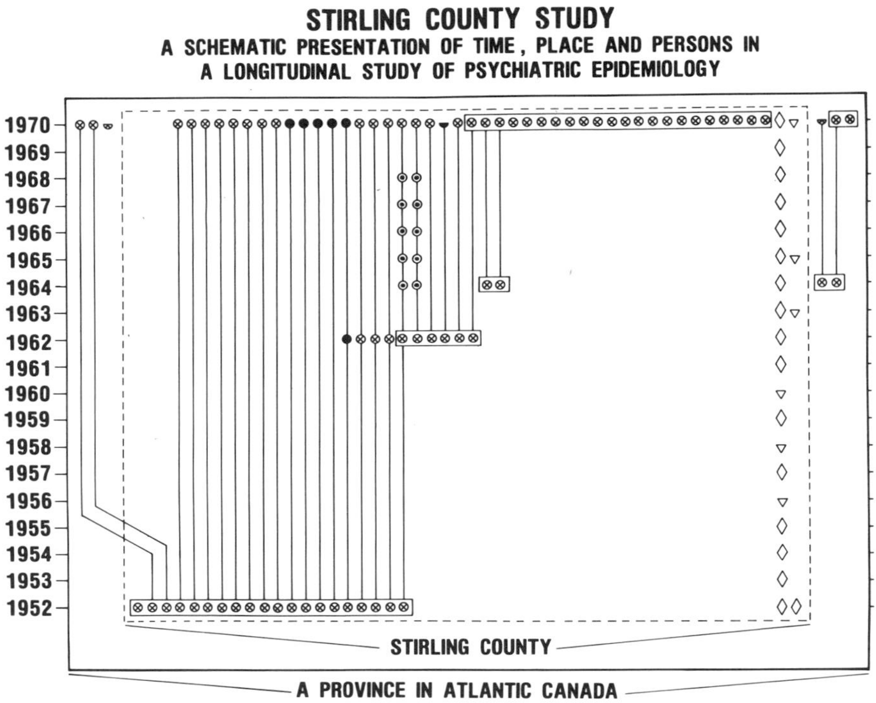

○ Each circle stands for approximately 60 adults.

⊗ Means that the information gathered consists of responses given in structured questionnaire interviews and reports from general physicians who knew these persons.

● Means that the information consists of death certificates and physician reports.

⊙ Means that the information consists in evaluations made by clinical psychiatrists who carried out a semi-structured interview with these persons in their homes.

▭ Each oblong box refers to a probability sample of a defined geographic area. The samples for 1952 and 1970 concern Stirling County as a whole; those for 1962 and 1964 refer to selected communities in the county. In the upper right hand area of the graph, samples are shown for 1964 and 1970. These pertain to communities in other counties that were studied for purposes of comparison.

Each vertical line stands for gathering follow-up information on approximately 60 adults. The length of the lines reflects the duration of each cohort interval. Most of the surviving cohort members were located in the county or in the province as shown; a few were located elsewhere.

◊ Each diamond stands for approximately 75 children and adults of Stirling County who were seen for treatment or referral in the Community Mental Health Centre that serves this area. Demographic and diagnostic information was assembled to assess the provision of psychiatric specialty services in the same place over the same time as the community-based study.

The Stirling Study as a longitudinal investigation now consists of information from general practitioner surveys and structured questionnaire interviews concerning 2848 community residents. These subjects constitute representative samples drawn in 1952, 1962, 1964, and 1969-1970. Each earlier sample was also conceived to be a cohort and was followed up with questionnaire surveys among those still living and death certificate searches among those who died. Figure 1 contains a diagram of the longitudinal study.

Various opportunities exist for evaluating the reliability and validity of the different sources of information taken independently. Over and above the fact that predictive validity can be addressed in a special way in a longitudinal study, a key resource is the fact that subsamples were home-visited and examined annually by clinical psychiatrists from 1964 through 1968 (Beiser, 1971).

Summary

The Stirling County Study in its baseline phase (1952) was an exploration in using DSM-I for community epidemiology. The early *Manual* was found to be inadequate in many ways, especially in its lack of criteria for case identification other than by the nature of symptoms and its lack of specifications for rating impairment. Following DSM-I guidelines, a very high prevalence would have been reported as the conclusion of the study. DSM-I was, however, modified to take account of several principles that now reside in DSM-III. An important adaptation of the *Manual* was the development of a typology of need for psychiatric attention. The customary use of DSM-I concerned its application to patients whose need for psychiatric attention had already been established. This typology was an attempt to make explicit in using DSM-I in a community study what was implicit in its use in hospitals and clinics.

The typology of need for psychiatric attention took into account both the diagnostic category in which the disorder was classified and the amount of impairment associated with the disorder. It was built from evidence drawn from general practitioner records, survey questionnaire responses, and hospital records. Information from these sources was brought together in a written protocol that was read and evaluated by psychiatrists in a procedure intended to approximate a clinical assessment. It was found that 20% of this general population appeared to need psychiatric attention. It was evident at the baseline period of the Stirling Study, and has continued to be true throughout a longitudinal investigation that followed from it, that most of the psychiatric attention directed toward these needs has occurred in the offices of general practitioners rather than in formal psychiatric services.

It is suggested that DSM-III is a far superior manual to its predecessors for community studies as well as the clinical investigations for which it is primarily designed. This interpretation does not lack recognition of the controversies and criticism which have and still surround the new manual. These criticisms do not, however, appear to concern the elements suggested as particularly valuable to community research: *(a)* increased precision in category specifications; *(b)* operational criteria which include essential features, duration, number and kinds of symptoms, and amount and types of impairment; and *(c)* registration of concomitant organic disorders. Futhermore, there is recognition that there has been a fruitful growth of psychiatric interview instruments, especially schedules designed specifically for gathering data appropriate for classification within DSM-III (Spitzer et al., 1977; Endicott and Spitzer, 1978). Such instruments have been effectively used in community research (Weissman and Myers, 1978). The Epidemiologic Catchment Area studies and the Diagnostic Interview Schedule described in this volume give further evidence that the principles and criteria of DSM-III aid research in community surveys of psychiatric epidemiology.

Acknowledgments

The analysis on which this report is based has been supported by National Health Research and Development Projects No. 603-1040-29 and No. 6603-1145-44, Department of National Health and Welfare of Canada, and by the Sandoz Foundation. The original study in Stirling County was funded mainly by the Milbank Memorial Fund, the Carnegie Corporation of New York, the Department of National Health and Welfare of Canada, and the Department of Public Health of the Province of Nova Scotia. The early phase of the longitudinal work was funded mainly by grants MH08180 and MH12892 from the National Institute of Mental Health, U.S. Public Health Service.

References

American Psychiatric Association (1952), *Diagnostic and Statistical Manual, Mental Disorders.* Washington, D.C.: American Psychiatric Association.

American Psychiatric Association (1980), *Diagnostic and Statistical Manual of Mental Disorders.* Washington, D.C.: American Psychiatric Association.

Beiser, M. (1971), A study of personality assets in a rural community. *Arch Gen Psychiatry* 24:244-254.

Endicott, J. & Spitzer, R. L. (1978), A diagnostic interview: The schedule for affective disorders and schizophrenia. *Arch Gen Psychiatry* 35:837-844.

Felix, R. H. & Bowers, R. V. (1948), Mental hygiene and socio-environmental factors. *Milbank Mem. Fund Quart* 26:125-147.

Goldfarb, A., Moses L. E., Downing J. J., & Leighton, D. C. (1967), Reliability of newly trained raters in community case finding. *Am J Publ Health* 57:2149-2157.

Kramer, M., Pollack, E. S., Redick, R. & Locke B. Z. (1972), *Mental Disorders: Suicide.* Cambridge, Mass.: Harvard University Press.

Langner, T. S. & Michael, S. T. (1963), *Life Stress and Mental Health.* New York: Free Press of Glencoe.

Leighton, A. H. (1959), *My Name Is Legion.* New York: Basic Books.
Leighton, A. H., Leighton, D. C. & Danley, R. A. (1966), Validity in mental health surveys. *Can Psychiatr Assoc J* 11:167-178.
Leighton, D. C., Harding, J. S., Macklin, D. B., Macmillan, A. M. & Leighton, A. H. (1963a), *The Character of Danger.* New York: Basic Books.
Leighton, D.C., Harding, J. S., Macklin, D. B., Hughes, C. C. & Leighton, A. H. (1963b), Psychiatric findings of the Stirling County Study. *Am J Psychiatry* 119:1021-1026.
Macmillan, A. M. (1954), Explorations in rural community health with particular reference to psycho-physiological symptoms. Ph.D. dissertation, Cornell University.
Macmillan, A. M. (1957), The health opinion survey: Technique for estimating prevalence of psychoneurotic and related types of disorder in communities. *Psychol Rep* 3:325-339.
Menninger, K. (1959), Toward a unitary concept of mental illness. In: *A Psychiatrist's World.* New York: Viking Press.
Murphy, J. M. (1981), Psychiatric instrument development for primary care research: Patient self report questionnaire. NIMH Contract No. 80M014280101D. Rockville, MD.: Division of Biometry and Epidemiology.
Spitzer, R. L., Endicott, J. & Robins, E. (1975), Research diagnostic criteria (RDC) for a selected group of functional disorders. Instrument 58, NIMH Clinical Research Branch Collaborative Program on the Psychobiology of Depression, mimeographed report.
Spitzer, R. L., Endicott, J. & Robins, E. (1978), Research diagnostic criteria: Rationale and reliability. *Arch Gen Psychiatry* 35:773-782.
Spitzer, R. L., Sheehy, M. & Endicott, J. (1977), DSM-III: Guiding principles. In: *Psychiatric Diagnosis,* eds., V. Rakoff, H. B. Kedward, H. C. Stancer, New York: Brunner/Mazel.
Srole, L., Langner, T. S., Michael, S. T., Opler, M. K. & Rennie, T. A. C. (1962), *Mental Health in the Metropolis.* New York: McGraw-Hill.
Weissman, M. M. & Myers, J. K. (1978), Affective disorders in a US urban community. *Arch Gen Psychiatry* 35:1304-1311.
World Health Organization (1948), *International Classification of Diseases, Sixth Revision.* Geneva: World Health Organization.

Chapter 8

Psychiatric Disorders in a U.S. Urban Community: The New Haven Study

JEROME K. MYERS
MYRNA M. WEISSMAN

Recent estimates of the community-wide prevalence of specific psychiatric disorders that include both treated and untreated persons are unavailable in the United States (Weissman and Klerman, 1978). Prior to World War II, psychiatric cases were usually counted by indirect methods such as interviews with community leaders, and little attention was paid to the reliability of the diagnostic criteria. Following World War II, psychiatric epidemiology took a different direction and there was a surge of community studies. These post-World War II studies derived from the experience of psychiatry in the military and incorporated some of the precise sampling techniques and screening instruments developed during the war (Gurin et al., 1960; Leighton et al., 1963; MacMillan, 1957; Srole et al., 1962). However, in order to avoid nosologic disputes and diagnostic unreliability, these studies used undifferentiated severity measures of psychiatric impairment and derived a mental status measure that was independent of specific diagnosis. The results obtained from these scales obscured the underlying heterogeneity of psychiatric disorders, and could not be easily translated into clinically useful diagnoses. When rates of specific disorders have been collected recently, they are not complete. The National Institute of Mental Health (NIMH) Division of Biometry and Epidemiology has over the years directed an important national effort to survey facilities providing mental health services. This effort has primarily provided rates of persons under treatment (treated prevalence), and it is well substantiated that many, if not the majority, of persons suffering from psychiatric disorders do not seek treatment. Therefore, untreated persons are not included in their rates.

Portions of this chapter were taken from M. M. Weissman and J. K. Meyer (1978), Affective disorders in a U.S. urban community: The use of research diagnostic of criteria in an epidemiological survey, *Archives of General Psychology* 25:1304-1311.

Over the last decade, there has been a resurgence of interest in types of psychopathology and their diagnosis. New techniques for improving diagnostic reliability and validity have been developed (Spitzer et al., 1975), and advances have been made for assessing psychiatric symptoms using dimensional symptoms, multivariate, and categorical approaches. One new technique, a categorical approach, developed by Spitzer, Endicott, and Robins—the Schedule for Affective Disorders and Schizophrenia-Diagnostic Research Criteria (SADS-RDC)—has received attention (Spitzer et al., 1977; Endicott and Spitzer, 1977). This approach handles the criterion, subject, occasion, and information variance of discrete psychiatric disorders through the use of structured questionnaire and operational definitions. It is the most developed diagnostic technique available in the United States and the DSM-III is based on this approach. The availability of improved diagnostic techniques, as well as increasing pressure to have community-wide data on psychiatric disorders for planning health care and manpower needs, have converged to make community surveys more necessary and feasible.

This chapter presents data on the epidemiology of psychiatric disorders in a U.S. community, including both treated and untreated persons, and demonstrates the first application of the SADS-RDC in a community sample.

Method

In 1967, a longitudinal survey of the population of a community mental health center catchment area in New Haven, Connecticut was undertaken. The catchment area has a population of approximately 72,000, which includes a changing inner-city section of 22,000 and a more stable industrial town of 50,000. It represents a cross section of the community's population and includes all ethnic, racial, and socioeconomic groups.

Sampling

A systematic sample of 1,095 households was selected; one adult (18 years of age or over) was chosen at random from each for inclusion in the sample. A personal interview was conducted with each respondent in 1967. Of the 1,095 individuals contacted, 12% refused to be interviewed, 2% could not be reached at home to be interviewed, and 86% (938) were interviewed (Myers et al., 1971).

Two years later, in 1969, the same population was reinterviewed. Of the original 938 interviewees, 8% refused to be reinterviewed, 11% had moved out of the area, 4% had died, and 77% (720) were reinterviewed. With one exception, the reinterviewed sample did not differ significantly ($P < 0.05$) from the original cohort within any of the major categories of the 6 following variables: social class, race, sex, religion, marital status, mental status, and age. The exception cited above was the under-30 age group, which dropped from 25% in 1967 to 19% in 1969 (Myers et al., 1972; Myers et al., 1975).

In 1975 and 1976, the 720 respondents interviewed in 1969 were again followed up. Of this number, 72% (515) were followed up, 9% had died,

8% could not be located, and 11% refused to cooperate. The rates in this chapter are based on 511 respondents as diagnostic data are missing on four persons.

The reinterviewed sample did not differ significantly ($P < 0.05$) from the original cohort within the major sociodemographic categories with the exception of race and class—there were fewer nonwhites and fewer lower social class individuals. Further analysis shows an interaction between these two variables. Among the nonwhites there was no class difference between those who were interviewed and those who were not, but there was a difference among the whites: 84% of whites still living, in social class I through IV, were interviewed, whereas only 73% of class V whites were interviewed. Among the nonwhites, the respective figures were 63% and 62%. Most important, however, when we examined the symptom status in 1967 and in 1969 between persons interviewed and not interviewed in 1975, we found no significant ($P < 0.05$) differences.

Diagnostic Assessment

Information for making diagnostic judgments was collected on the SADS in the 1975-1976 sample only, as this is when the instrument became available. The SADS is a structured interview guide with an accompanying inventory of rating scales and specific items. It records information on the respondent's functioning and symptomatology. Although the name of the instrument suggests that it only includes information on affective disorders and schizophrenia, in fact it is an overall mental status inventory and contains the information necessary for making diagnostic judgments for most major psychotic, neurotic, and personality disorders. This method has been shown to reduce the portion of variance in diagnosis due to differing interviewing styles and coverage. There are several versions of the SADS, depending on the time period assessed—current, past 5 years, or lifetime. We used the lifetime version (SADS-L), which includes an assessment of the respondent's current as well as lifetime mental status.

Based on the information collected on the SADS, the respondents were classified on the RDC, which is a set of operational diagnostic definitions with specific inclusion and exclusion criteria for a variety of nosologic groups. These operational definitions were developed for reducing the variance due to differing criteria, which has been shown to account for the largest source of errors between clinicians. The RDC has evolved from a decade of research on diagnosis. The conditions included have the most evidence of validity in terms of clinical description, consistency over time, familial association, and response to treatment.

Diagnoses on the RDC are made both for the current time period (current point prevalence) and for lifetime (lifetime prevalence) with the exception of several diagnoses that are considered lifetime diagnoses only, regardless of whether or not the respondent is currently manifesting symptoms of the disorder. These lifetime-only disorders are the personality disorders (depressive, cyclothymic, Briquet's syndrome, antisocial) and the bipolar disorders. Psychiatric disorders that cannot be categorized due to limitation of information or absence of diagnostic criteria are listed as "other." All diagnoses can be classified as either "probable" or "definite."

Interviewers' Training and Reliability

There were two raters with college or graduate-level educations and previous clinical experience in psychiatry and interviewing. Both raters underwent a 3-month period of training on the SADS and RDC under the supervision of doctoral-level persons with consultation of psychiatrists. After the training period, interrater reliability was tested between interviewers and supervising staff and found to be excellent. For example, 15 separate interviews per rater were conducted, during which one rater interviewed and the second rater observed the interview and co-rated. The raters alternated in conducting the interviews. For the 15 interviews, there was complete agreement on lifetime diagnosis on 13 of the cases (87%) and partial agreement on the other two cases (13%). In the two cases where there was partial agreement, both raters agreed for two diagnoses each per respondent and disagreed on the third diagnosis. For example, both raters agreed that the respondent had a lifetime diagnosis of Briquet's syndrome and drug abuse. One rater thought the subject also had general anxiety; the second rater did not. In the second case, both raters agreed on the diagnosis of major and minor depression, but one rater thought the respondent was a drug abuser and the second rater did not. Agreement for the current diagnosis was also excellent. There was complete agreement in 14 of the 15 cases (93%) and partial agreement in the 15th case (7%). A separate publication will report on test-retest stability and further interrater reliability.

The RDC diagnoses were also checked against psychiatric treatment records when available and when the person's permission had been received. In 33 of the 35 cases checked, there was agreement between the psychiatrist's description of symptom and diagnosis and the RDC. For the two cases where there was disagreement, one respondent was diagnosed as bipolar on the RDC and as having marital maladjustment by the treating psychiatrist. The second case was diagnosed as schizo-affective on the RDC and as depressed by the treating psychiatrist.

A search of mental health center records for all respondents in the catchment area disclosed that cases reported as not ill had not had psychiatric treatment. However, cases that were treated outside the catchment area or treated before the services were available (1966) could have been missed. In addition, all cases presenting diagnostic problems were reviewed weekly by the supervising doctoral-level staff. If consensus could not be reached, the respondent was reinterviewed by a different interviewer who was blind to the initial findings.

Results

Current Rates of Any Psychiatric Disorder

The interview results (table 1) show that 15.1% of the population had a definite and 2.7% a probable current psychiatric disorder, totaling 17.8% of the population with a probable or definite current diagnosis. These figures include not only the major disorders such as schizophrenia and major depres-

TABLE 1
Current Point Prevalence Rates[a] of Psychiatric Disorders.

Item	*Definite diagnosis (%)*	*Probable diagnosis (%)*	*Total (n=511)(%)*
Current RDC diagnosis			
Major depression	3.7	0.6	4.3
Generalized anxiety	2.3	0.2	2.5
Minor depression	2.0	0.5	2.5
Alcoholism	1.3	1.2	2.5
Phobic disorder	1.2	0.2	1.4
Other psychiatric disorder	1.0	0.2	1.2
Drug abuse	0.0	1.0	1.0
Panic disorder	0.4	0.0	0.4
Schizophrenia	0.4	0.0	0.4
Borderline features	0.2	0.0	0.2
Unspecified psychosis	0.0	0.2	0.2
Schizo-affective (manic or depressed disorder)	0.0	0.0	0.0
Manic disorder	0.0	0.0	0.0
Hypomania	0.0	0.0	0.0
Obsessive-compulsive disorder	0.0	0.0	0.0
Lifetime RDC diagnosis			
Depressive personality	4.5	0.2	4.7
Bipolar disorder	1.2	0.0	1.2
Briquet's syndrome	0.4	0.0	0.4
Cyclothymic personality	0.2	0.2	0.4
Antisocial personality	0.2	0.0	0.2
Any diagnosis	15.1	2.7	17.8

[a]The rates given in this table are not additive because an individual could have one or more probable or definite diagnoses.

sion, but the more minor ones such as anxiety and the personality disorder. Four and one-half percent of the population had multiple diagnoses.

Current Rates of Specific Psychiatric Disorders

Table 1 shows the overall current rates of specific disorders arranged in order of frequency. Major depression is the most frequent, followed by anxiety, minor depression, and alcoholism. The current rate of definite schizophrenia is 0.4%. No current cases of schizo-affective (manic or depressive), manic, hypomanic, or obsessive-compulsive disorders were found. Only probable cases of unspecified psychosis and drug abuse were found. Of the personality disorders, depressive personality was the most frequent (4.7%).

As indicated above, major depression was the most common disorder found in the community. Combined with minor depression, it included 6.8% of the New Haven population. Furthermore, 4.7% of the population had a diagnosis of depressive personality. Because of the high frequency of such disorders and their importance for mental health policy, we shall now focus attention upon the affective disorders.

Affective Disorders

Definitions and Types of Affective Disorders

Affective disorders are a group of psychiatric conditions in which disturbances of mood predominate. This group of disorders is frequently differentiated from disorders of thinking, which conventionally include schizophrenia, paranoia, and similar states. While there is not unanimous agreement as to which affects are included, it is generally agreed that depression and elation are the major affective disorders. Some authorities such as Mapother and Lewis in the past have also included anxiety conditions, but current thinking excludes them (Klerman and Barrett, 1973). The grouping of affective disorders does not imply common etiology or treatment; rather, the similarities in clinical symptomatology probably represent common manifestations of multiple etiologic mechanisms. The RDC includes affective disorders that are episodic and those that are intermittent and chronic. Figure 1 shows the relationship among the affective disorders. The term "episodic" means a period of illness in which there is sustained disturbance clearly distinguished from previous functioning. Included in this group are major depression, minor depression, and manic and hypomanic disorders. The major depressions are further subdivided as to whether they are primary or secondary. Disorders are assessed as being present currently at interview (yielding a current point prevalence rate), as well as ever being present during the individual's lifetime (yielding a lifetime prevalence rate). Persons who have at some time in their lives evidenced both manic episodes and major depression are further classified as bipolar I, and those having evidence of hypomania and major depression are classified as bipolar II. Bipolar disorders are considered as lifetime-only diagnoses. A more recent version of the RDC, dated June 15, 1977, has other subtypes of depression, including a recurrent unipolar category. We did not make these finer subtypings of depression in this study. A third type of episodic disorder, which may or may not be classified under affective disorder because of the mixture of both mood and thought disturbances, is schizo-affective disorder, either depressed or manic type. Since family studies indicate that schizo-affective disorder is a variant of affective disorder, this diagnosis was included as an affective disorder in this survey (Spitzer et al., 1977).

The intermittent disorders refer to chronic disturbances that do not have a clear onset and in which, over a period of years, there are intermittent and recurring disorders of mood lasting for a few hours or days separated by periods of normal mood. Persons with intermittent disorders can be either depressive or cyclothymic, and they are considered lifetime-only diagnoses.

Because of the overlap in presenting symptoms, there is an effort in the

FIGURE 1

Relationship among Affective Disorders.

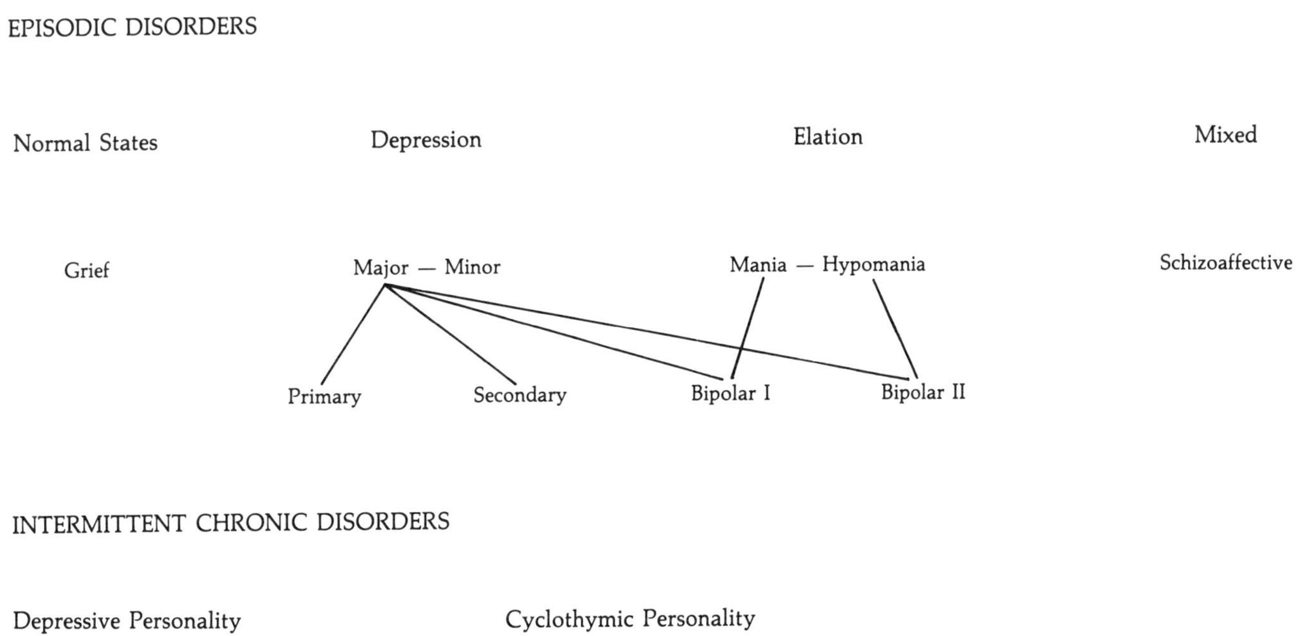

RDC to separate clinical depression from normal grief reactions secondary to the death of a "significant other." Symptoms are considered symptomatic of grief if they met the criteria for major depression but appeared within 3 months of the death of a close relative. Symptoms that lasted more than a year were considered symptomatic of major depression.

Major-Minor Depression

Current Point Prevalence Rates

Table 2 shows the current rates of major (4.3%) and minor (2.5%) depression, yielding a rate of 6.8% for both disorders combined, including both probable and definite categories. When only definite cases are included, the combined rates are reduced to 5.7%. Major depression was highest in whites, social classes III, IV, and V, persons not currently married, women (female-male sex ratio, 1.6:1), and persons over age 45. However, only the relationship with age was significant ($P < 0.10$). Minor depression was higher in non-whites, social class V, persons not currently married, and persons over age 45. Only the social class relationship was significant ($P < 0.05$). The female-male sex ratio for current minor depression was nearly equal (1.2:1). When both current disorders were examined together, only the relationships with marital status and age were significant ($P < 0.10$). The lower rates of minor as contrasted with major depression may be due to the inability of persons in the community to recall minor disorders. This problem requires further exploration.

Lifetime Prevalence Rates

Table 3 shows the lifetime rate (probable and definite diagnoses) of major (20%) and minor (9.2%) depression. The lifetime rate for major and/or minor depression was 26.7%. When only definite cases are included, the lifetime rates are reduced to 24.7%. It should be noted that persons could have more than one diagnosis. Relationships with sociodemographic variables were stronger in the lifetime than in the current rates due to the larger number of cases in the lifetime category. At times, the lifetime trends were opposite of those seen with the current rates, e.g., there was an association ($P < 0.10$) between lifetime major depression and social class (the higher rates were now in the upper social classes) and with age (the highest rates were now in the youngest age group—25 to 45 years). These trends were similar for minor depression. The higher rates in women were consistent with major or minor depression, whether current or lifetime. When the lifetime rates of major and minor depression were examined together, the rates were similar among the various social classes but the relationship with the female sex and younger age group still held. The increased rates of lifetime depression in the younger group may be a cohort effect, an artifact of selective recall, or an artifact of differential mortality.

TABLE 2
Current Rates of Major and Minor Depression[a] by Sociodemographic Characteristics.

	Rates/100		
Characteristic	*Major depression*	*Minor depression*	*Major and minor depression*
Race			
White (n=458)	4.8	2.4	7.2
Nonwhite (n=53)	0.0	3.8	3.8
Significance	NS[b]	NS	NS
Social class			
I and II (n=65)	1.5	0.0	1.5
III (n=98)	3.1	2.0	5.1
IV (n=225)	5.8	1.3	7.1
V (n=123)	4.1	6.6	10.7
Significance	NS	$p < .05$	NS
Currently married			
No (n=136)	6.7	3.7	10.4
Yes (n=375)	3.5	2.1	5.6
Significance	NS	NS	$p < 0.1$
Sex			
Male (n=220)	3.2	2.3	5.5
Female (n=291)	5.2	2.7	7.9
Significance	NS	NS	NS
Age, yr.			
26-45 (n=210)	1.9	1.9	3.8
46-65 (n=190)	6.3	3.2	9.5
≥ 66 (n=111)	5.4	2.7	8.1
Significance	$p < 0.1$	NS	$p < 0.1$
Total (n=511)			
Probable and definite	4.3	2.5	6.8
Definite only	3.7	2.0	5.7

[a]Grief reactions are excluded.
[b]Not significant.

Primary and Secondary Depression

Table 4 shows that the majority (86%) of major depressions were primary. Of those 14 depressions that were secondary, the preceding disorder was

TABLE 3
Lifetime Rates of Major or Minor Depression[a] by Sociodemographic Characteristics.

	Rates/100		
Characteristic	*Major depression*	*Minor depression*	*Major and minor depression*
Race			
White (n=458)	20.8	9.4	27.8
Nonwhite (n=53)	13.2	7.5	17.0
Significance	NS[b]	NS	NS
Social class			
I and II (n=65)	21.5	10.8	27.7
III (n=98)	14.3	12.2	25.5
IV (n=225)	24.4	6.7	28.4
V (n=123)	15.6	10.7	23.8
Significance	$p < 0.1$	NS	NS
Currently married			
No (n=136)	23.0	9.6	29.6
Yes (n=375)	18.9	9.1	25.6
Significance	NS	NS	NS
Sex			
Male (n=220)	12.3	5.9	17.4
Female (n=291)	25.8	11.7	33.7
Significance	$p < 0.001$	$p < 0.05$	$p < 0.001$
Age, yr.			
26-45 (n=210)	23.8	12.4	33.3
46-65 (n=190)	19.0	7.9	23.8
$\geq$ 66 (n=111)	14.4	5.4	18.9
Significance	NS	$p < 0.1$	$p < 0.05$
Total (n=511)			
Probable and definite	20.0	9.2	26.7
Definite only	18.0	8.6	24.7

[a]Grief reactions are excluded.
[b]Not significant.

most frequently alcoholism. There were no sociodemographic differences between primary and secondary depression. However, the sample of secondary depressives is quite low.

TABLE 4
Primary and Secondary Depression and Preceding Disorders in Secondary Depression.

	No.	%
Primary depression	88	86
Secondary depression	14	14
Total lifetime major depression	102	100
Preceding disorders in secondary depression		
Schizophrenia	3	21
Phobia	2	14
Alcoholism	6	44
Drug Abuse	2	14
Panic	1	7
TOTAL	14	100

Mania-Hypomania
Bipolar I and II Disorders

There were no current cases of mania or hypomania. The lifetime rates were low, 0.8% for each (table 5). Respondents with both major depression and mania were diagnosed as bipolar I; their lifetime rate was 0.6%. Respondents with major depression and hypomania were diagnosed as bipolar II; their lifetime rate was also 0.6%. Therefore, the total rate for the bipolar disorders was 1.2%. There was a strong relationship between bipolar disorder and upper social class, e.g., the rates of bipolar I and II disorders were 4.6% in social classes I and II combined, 1.0% in class III, 0.95% in class IV, and no cases in class V. These differences were significant at $P < 0.05$. Caution must be exerted, due to the small samples, in interpreting any relationship with risk factors; therefore, the variations in rates by sociodemographic characteristics are not presented here for disorders with low frequency.

Schizo-Affective Disorders

There were no current cases of schizo-affective disorders and the lifetime rates were low, 0.2% for schizo-affective-mania and 0.4% for schizo-affective-depressed (table 5).

TABLE 5
Lifetime Rates of Mania, Hypomania, Bipolar I and II Disorders, and Schizo-Affective Disorders.

	Rates/100	
Disorder	*Probable and definite*	*Definite*
Mania	0.8	0.8
Hypomania	0.8	0.6
Bipolar with mania (bipolar I)	0.6	0.6
Bipolar with hypomania (bipolar II)	0.6	0.6
Total bipolar I and II	1.2	1.2
Schizo-affective disorder		
Manic	0.2	0.2
Depressed	0.4	0.4
TOTAL	0.6	0.6

Grief

Table 6 shows that 10.4% of the respondents (2.7% of the men and 16.2% of the women) had grief reactions during their lifetime. The rates were highest in the lower social classes, men not currently married, and women. Ideally, the denominator for these rates should be only those persons who have experienced the death of a significant other.

Cyclothymic and Depressive Personality Disorders

Table 7 shows that the lifetime rates of cyclothymic personality (0.4%) are low but lifetime rates of depressive personality are considerably higher (4.7%). Of interest is the slightly higher rate of depressive personality in men and in the younger age group.

Multiple Diagnoses

Table 8 shows the high rate of multiple diagnoses. Approximately half of the respondents with a current major depression had one or more other current diagnoses and one or more other past diagnoses. Alcoholism was the most common other diagnosis; this will be explored more fully in future publications.

TABLE 6
Lifetime Rates for Grief Reactions by Sex and Sociodemographic Characteristics.

Characteristic	Rates/100 for grief	Men No.	Men %	Women No.	Women %
Race					
White (n=458)	10.9	201	3.0	256	17.2
Nonwhite (n=53)	5.3	18	0.0	35	8.6
Significance	NS[a]	NS		NS	
Social class					
I and II (n=65)	4.6	28	0.0	37	8.1
III (n=98)	3.1	42	0.0	56	5.4
IV (n=225)	12.9	103	3.9	122	20.5
V (n=123)	14.8	46	4.3	76	21.1
Significance	$p < 0.01$	NS		$p < 0.05$	
Currently married					
No (n=136)	15.6	41	9.8	94	18.1
Yes (n=375)	8.5	178	1.1	197	15.2
Significance	$p < 0.05$	$p < 0.05$		NS	
Sex					
Male (n=220)	2.7	—	—	—	—
Female (n=291)	16.2	—	—	—	—
Significance	$p < 0.001$	—		—	
Age, yr.					
26-45 (n=240)	9.0	78	1.3	132	13.6
46-65 (n=190)	13.2	84	4.8	105	20.0
≥66 (n=111)	8.1	57	1.8	54	14.8
Significance	NS	NS		NS	
Total (n=511)	10.4	219	2.7	291	16.2

[a]Not significant.

Comment

This is, to our knowledge, the first application of Research Diagnostic Criteria to a community sample. There are no directly comparable community data based on similar diagnostic procedures. However, before discussing the substantive findings of these data, their limitations should be emphasized.

TABLE 7
Lifetime Rates of Cyclothymic and Depressive Personality by Sociodemographic Characteristics.

	Rates/100	
Characteristic	*Cyclothymic personality*	*Depressive personality*
Race		
White (n=458)	0.4	5.3
Nonwhite (n=53)	0.0	0.0
Significance	NS[a]	NS
Social class		
I and II (n=65)	0.0	6.2
III (n=98)	0.0	6.1
IV (n=225)	0.9	4.4
V (n=123)	0.0	3.3
Significance	NS	NS
Currently married		
No (n=136)	0.0	5.2
Yes (n=375)	0.5	4.5
Significance	NS	NS
Sex		
Male (n=220)	0.9	5.5
Female (n=291)	0.0	4.1
Significance	NS	NS
Age, yr.		
26-45 (n=210)	0.0	7.1
46-65 (n=190)	0.5	3.7
≥ 66 (n=111)	0.9	1.8
Significance	NS	$p < 0.1$
Total (n=511)		
Probable and definite	0.4	4.7
Definite only	0.2	4.5

[a]Not significant.

Limitations in the Design

The limitations in the design of this present study for the purpose of obtaining the rates of psychiatric disorders should not be underestimated. First, this is a follow-up study. While the sample originally derived from systematic sampling of an urban community in 1967, by 1975 attrition had occurred due to deaths, geographic moves, or refusals to cooperate. Since there are differential mortalities for persons with psychiatric disorders (Winokur et

TABLE 8
Respondents With Additional Diagnoses.

Current diagnosis	% of Respondents: No other current diagnosis	One or more other current diagnoses	One or more other past diagnoses
Major depression (n=22)	54.5	45.5	54.5
Minor depression (n=13)	84.6	15.4	53.8
Major or minor depression (n=35)	65.7	34.3	45.7
Grief (n=1)	100.0	0.0	0.0

Lifetime diagnosis	% of Respondents: No other diagnosis	One other diagnosis	Two other diagnoses	Three or more diagnoses
Major depression (n=102)	51.0	22.5	17.6	8.9
Minor depression (n=47)	51.1	27.7	17.0	4.3
Bipolar disorder (n=6)	50.0	33.3	16.6	0.0
Depressive personality (n=24)	12.5	33.3	33.3	20.8
Cyclothymic personality (n=2)	50.0	0.0	0.0	50.0
Grief (n=53)	45.3	26.4	15.1	13.2

al., 1969), particularly schizophrenia, alcoholism, and bipolar disorders (Babigian and Odoroff, 1969; Tsuang and Woolson, 1977), we can anticipate that subjects with these diagnoses are overrepresented in the sample of subjects who died. Therefore, their more severe disorders are most likely underrepresented in the rates presented here. Also, there was a slight loss of nonwhites and lower-class persons in the reinterviewed sample, which may add to the underrepresentation of schizophrenia and alcoholism.

Due to the original conditions of the sample selection, there is undoubtedly an underrepresentation of persons with the psychiatric disorders requiring institutionalization. In the original sample, persons living in the community were selected, while persons in institutions such as mental hospitals, prisons, etc. were not included. However, respondents who were institutionalized at the time of follow up in 1975 were included in the reinterviewed sample.

Alternately, there could be an overrepresentation of depressives if there were any tendency for depressives not to move out of the area. Finally, while more than 500 persons were interviewed, this sample is small for disorders of low frequency, especially for examining variations in rates by risk factors.

Problems in the Lifetime Prevalence Rate

While there is considerable interest and utility in determining the likelihood of a person getting a disorder during his lifetime, a lifetime prevalence estimate, as presented here, is a poor approximation of this information. Moreover, the other commonly used methods, such as morbid risk rates or life-table analyses, have not solved the problem. Ideally, the only certain way to determine the lifetime expectancy of any disease in a population is to plot the illness experience of a representative cohort over the entire period of risk. This requires a long-term prospective study to determine the incidence of the disorder. A cross-sectional survey is not a substitute because the population studied comprises only the surviving members of each generation. The lifetime prevalence statistic is an effort to capture retrospectively the information from a probability sample of those who are alive.

The lifetime prevalence, morbid risk, or lifetable methods are based on the following assumptions:

1. *Mortality is consistent in the different diagnostic groups.* If mortalities of persons with a history of mental illness are identical with those of persons with no history, then lifetime prevalence at a specific age is solely a function of incidence at earlier ages (Kramer, 1965). If mortalities are not equal, the lifetime prevalence is a function of incidence rates of persons who become mentally ill at a specific age and of the mentally ill who survived to that age and the mortality of persons with no history of mental illness. The assumption of consistent mortality is, of course, unreasonable because we know that persons with a history of mental illness have higher mortalities than those without such a history (Babigian and Odoroff, 1969; Tsuang and Woolson, 1977; Reveley et al., 1977).

2. *There is no cohort effect,* i.e., the lifetime prevalence of a person of a certain age does not reflect a rate of persons born in that generation only. Scientific evidence for a cohort effect is lacking. However, there are suggestions in the clinical literature that depression may be increasing or that certain personality disorders are decreasing.

3. *There is no memory effect.* Persons can recall their recent and past episodes of illness with equal accuracy.

Relationship to Other Community Data

Major Depression

A major finding of this study is that primary major depression is the most common disorder with relatively high current and lifetime prevalence. While these current rates are quite high, they are considerably lower than rates based on depression symptom scales such as Zung, Beck, and Center for Epidemiologic Studies-Depression scales, when applied to community samples. Estimates from studies using symptom scales range from 15% to 20% current point prevalence (Weissman and Myers, 1978).

The range of findings for population studies using diagnostic criteria varies tremendously. Many of these variations may be explained by variation in methodology, particularly in the diagnostic criteria used. In future publications, we intend to report on an examination of our data by varying symptom, severity, and/or duration criteria used in other studies to determine comparability of rates. However, the 4.3% current rate of major depression is close to the rate of 3.8% of neurotic and psychotic depression reported by Helgason in his 1957 study of a cohort of 3,843 persons born between 1895 and 1897 in Iceland and the rate of 3.4% reported by Sorensen and Stromgren in their 1960 study of the total population (6,447) of Samso Island in Denmark (Silverman, 1968). Other surveys, dividing depressive disorders into psychosis and neurosis, report current rates considerably lower for psychosis, usually less than 1%, but higher and more variable for neurosis, less than 1% to 7.2% (Silverman, 1968). We did not make a distinction between psychosis and neurosis, and the rates of major depression would presumably include both.

It should be emphasized that the RDC definition of major or minor depression does not require that the person seek treatment, although functional role impairment is required. If we had used the diagnostic requirement that the person seek treatment for the symptom, then our rates would have been considerably lower.

Bipolar Disorder

The high rates of major depression are in sharp contrast to the rates for bipolar disorders, which were 1.2% when both bipolar I and II disorders were included. While the lower rates for bipolar as contrasted with unipolar disorders are consistent with clinical experience, again there are no comparable data assessing bipolar disorder in the community using criteria similar to the RDC. Manic-depressive disease based on Kraepelin's definition is used most commonly in European and Scandinavian surveys. However, this definition does not require the presence of a manic episode and is, therefore, not comparable to bipolar disorder. In a comprehensive report, Krauthamer and Klerman (1978) have reviewed the diagnostic classification and epidemiology of bipolar disorder. They conclude that 10% to 20% of persons with the diagnosis of manic depression are in fact bipolars. Following this estimate, they conclude that the lifetime prevalence of bipolar disorder is slightly less than 1%, a figure quite close to ours.

Primary-Secondary Depression

The primary-secondary distinction in depression is of recent origin, and the best data derive from clinic studies. We found that secondary depression constituted only 14% of the major depressions in the community, i.e., a rate of about 6:1, primary to secondary. The rate of secondary relative to primary depression is considerably higher in clinic studies, e.g., Robins et al. (1977) found in an emergency room a rate of 1.5:1, primary to secondary depression. The differences between community and clinic studies in rates of secondary depression relative to primary depression suggest that secondary depressives more frequently seek treatment, an observation consistent with the finding in medical clinics that persons with two or more diagnoses have a higher probability of seeking treatment as compared with those with one diagnosis (Weissman et al., 1977). In regard to the type of primary diagnosis among the secondary depressives, we found that alcoholism was the most frequent primary diagnosis among the secondary depressives, accounting for 44% of the secondary depressives. This finding is similar to that of Robins et al. (1977) who also found that 44% of the secondary depressives had alcoholism as their primary diagnosis.

Grief

Grief reactions occurring after a death and meeting the criteria of major depressives are relatively common. We found a lifetime rate of about 10%, which was higher in women than in men, in the lower social class, and in men who were currently unmarried—suggesting, as others have noted, that grief reactions are strongest when there are fewer social supports. The increase in grief reactions in women may have to do with the fact that more women than men are at risk for grief reactions because of longer life span.

Variation with Sociodemographic Characteristics

The associations with sociodemographic risk factors further support the heterogeneity of affective disorders, and the need to examine subtypes separately and to define precisely the prevalence period under scrutiny. Of the sociodemographic factors, two are of the most interest here—social class and sex.

Social Class

The association with risk factors varied considerably by type of affective disorder and by the time period assessed. Current rates of major depression showed no strong relationship to social class, although the rates were higher in the lower social classes whereas lifetime major depression was higher in the upper social classes. Current minor depression was highest in the lower social class, and bipolar disorders were highest in the upper social class. The variability of the relationship of class and disorder is of considerable interest because previous surveys using symptoms scales (Weissman and Myers, 1978) or differentiated measures of impairment as the dependent variable (Dohrenwend, 1975) have consistently found a relationship between lower social class and impairment or symptoms. Our data suggest that this relationship exists for the minor disorders, which is a diagnosis probably related to demoralization, a concept suggested by Jerome Frank, and could be related to less access to health care. The relationship between lower social class and diagnosis also is found in current but not lifetime rates of major depression. This latter finding is possibly explained by the fact that the lower class has poorer access to treatment and, therefore, has longer duration of symptoms, although the actual number of episodes may not differ between classes.

Moreover, our data suggest that the relationship between low social class and psychiatric symptomatology is not consistent across all affective disorders. The relationship of bipolar disorder and higher social class that we found has been suggested by some studies (Malzberg, 1956; Faris and Dunham, 1939), but the association has not been strong or consistent (Klerman and Barrett, 1973).

Sex

The higher rates of affective disorders for women generally found here have been reported by others (Weissman and Klerman, 1977). However, again there were variations. For lifetime rates of major depression, minor depression, and grief, women predominated, but the rates were equal between the sexes for depressive personality.

Conclusion

This survey of a U.S. urban community in 1975-1976 found that nearly 18% of an interviewed sample had a current psychiatric diagnosis and that major depression was the most frequent diagnosis. Contrary to common belief, this study showed that psychiatric diagnoses can be made in the community. Nonpsychiatric raters can be trained to administer structured interviews and to obtain the systematic information necessary for making a diagnosis. Respondent compliance was good. The completion rate was excellent: only 11% of persons contacted refused to cooperate. Interrater reliability was excellent. Similar efforts are now ongoing by Wing et al. (1974) and Brown et al. (1977) and others in England using the Present State Examination.

Although psychiatric disorders were common, they were not ubiquitous. Over 80% of the subjects had no current diagnosis, either probable or definite, including any type of personality disorder, anxiety reaction, or minor depression.

There is considerable heterogeneity within the affective disorders. This heterogeneity exists by time period assessed and by association with sociodemographic risk factors. This heterogeneity certainly adds to the confusion in interpreting findings from existing studies that use as the dependent variable overall rates of impairment independent of diagnosis, depressive symptoms independent of subtypes, or diagnostic categories that are not precisely defined.

Aside from the data presented here, recent rates of discrete psychiatric disorders based on community samples in the United States are not available. Such data are most important scientifically and for health care and planning. Scientifically, these rates and their variation with risk factors can provide clues to etiology. In health care planning, rates of specific disorders are crucial for calculating costs and allocation of resources, a point made strongly in the recent report on the mental health needs of the nation by the President's Commission on Mental Health (1978). The absence of such rates can hinder adequate projections and make it difficult to formulate policy decisions regarding the extent of coverage or manpower needs for mental illness under various health insurance plans.

The data we have presented are imperfect, preliminary, and from a local sample of one community. The results should be accepted with considerable caution and are presented with modesty. While we believe these results demonstrate the feasibility of this approach, before any conclusions are drawn, a replication of this study is required on a different and larger community sample, which would overcome the design problems we have described.

Acknowledgments

This research was supported by Alcohol, Drug Abuse,and Mental Health Administration grants MH25712 and MH28274 from the Center for Epidemiologic Studies, National Institute of Mental Health, Rockville, Maryland.

References

Babigian, H. T. & Odoroff, C. (1969), The mortality experience of a population with psychiatric illness. *Am J Psychiat* 126:470-480.

Brown, G. W., Davidson, S., Harris, T., et al. (1977), Psychiatric disorder in London and North Uist. *Soc Sci Med* 2:367-377.

Dohrenwend, B. P. (1975), Sociocultural and sociopsychological factors in the genesis of mental disorder. *J Health Soc Behav* 16:365-392.

Endicott, J. & Spitzer, R. L. (1977), A diagnostic interview: the schedule for affective disorders and schizophrenia. Read before the annual meeting of the American Psychiatric Association, Toronto.

Faris, R. E. L. & Dunham, H. W. (1939), *Mental Disorders in Urban Areas: An Ecological Study of Schizophrenia and Other Psychoses.* Chicago: University of Chicago Press.

Gurin, G., Veroff, J., & Feld, S. (1960), *Americans View Their Mental Health: A Nationwide Interview Study.* New York: Basic Books, Inc.

Klerman, G. L. & Barrett, J. E. (1973), Clinical and epidemiological aspects of affective disorders. In: *Lithium: Its Role in Psychiatric Research and Treatment,* ed. S. Gershon & B. Shopsin. New York: Plenum Press, pp. 201-232.

Kramer, M. M. (1965), *The Concept of Lifetime Prevalence.* Bethesda, Md.: National Institute of Mental Health.

Krauthamer, C. & Klerman, G. L. (1978), The epidemiology of mania. In: *Mania,* ed. B. Shopsin. New York: Plenum Press.

Leighton, D. C., MacMillan, A. M., Harding, J. S. et al. (1963), *The Character of Danger.* New York: Basic Books, Inc.

MacMillan, A. M. (1957), The health opinion survey: Technique for estimating prevalence of psychoneurotic and related types of disorder in communities. *Psychol Rep* 3:325-329.

Malzberg, B. (1956), Mental disease in relation to economic status. *J Nerv Ment Dis* 123:256.

Myers, J. K., Lindenthal, J. J., & Pepper, M. P. (1971), Life events and psychiatric impairment. *J Nerv Ment Dis* 152:149-157.

Myers, J. K., Lindenthal, J. J., & Pepper, M. P. (1975), Life events, social integration and psychiatric symptomatology. *J Health Soc Behav* 16:421-427.

Myers, J. K., Lindenthal, J. J., & Pepper, M. P., et al. (1972), Life events and mental status: A longitudinal study. *J Health Soc Behav* 13:398-406.

Report to the President from the President's Commission on Mental Health. (1978), Stock No. 040-000-00390-8. Washington, D.C.: U.S. Government Printing Office.

Reveley, M. A., Woodruff, R. A., Robins, L. E., et al. (1977), Evaluation of a screening interview for Briquet's syndrome (hysteria) by the study of medically ill women. *Arch Gen Psychiat* 34:145-149.

Robins, E., Gentry, K., Munoz, R., et al. (1977), A contrast of the three more common illnesses with the ten less common in a study and 18-month follow-up of 314 psychiatric emergency room patients: II. Characteristics of patients with the three more common illnesses. *Arch Gen Psychiat* 34:269-281.

Silverman, C. (1968), *The Epidemiology of Depression*. Baltimore: Johns Hopkins University Press.

Spitzer, R. L., Endicott, J., & Robins, E. (1975), Clinical criteria for psychiatric diagnosis and the DSM-III. *Am J Psychiat* 132:1187-1192.

Spitzer, R. L., Endicott, J., & Robins, E. (1977), Research diagnostic criteria: rationale and reliability. Paper read before the annual meeting of the American Psychiatric Association, Toronto.

Srole, L., Langner, T. S., Michael, S. T., et al. (1962), *Mental Health in the Metropolis: The Midtown Manhattan Study*. New York, McGraw-Hill Book Co., Inc.

Tsuang, M. & Woolson, R. F. (1977), Mortality in patients with schizophrenia, mania, depression and surgical conditions. *Br J Psychiat* 130:162-166.

Weissman, M. M. & Klerman, G. L. (1977), Sex differences and the epidemiology of depression. *Arch Gen Psychiat* 34:98-111.

Weissman, M. M. & Klerman, G. L. (1978), The epidemiology of mental disorders: emerging trends. *Arch Gen Psychiat* 35:705-712.

Weissman, M. M. & Myers, J. K. (1978), Rates and risks of depressive symptoms in a United States urban community. *Acta Psychiat Scand* 57:219-231.

Weissman, M. M., Pottenger, M., Kleber, H. D., et al. (1977), Symptom patterns in primary and secondary depression. *Arch Gen Psychiat* 34:854-862.

Wing, J., Cooper, J. E., & Sartorius, N. (1974), *Measurement and Classification of Psychiatric Symptoms*. New York: Cambridge University Press, pp. 189-228.

Winokur, G., Clayton, P., & Reich, T. (1969), *Manic Depressive Illness*. St. Louis: C. V. Mosby Co., p. 29.

Chapter 9

The Community Mental Health Assessment Survey and the CES-D Scale

LENORE SAWYER RADLOFF
BEN Z. LOCKE

The Community Mental Health Assessment (CMHA) program was initiated in 1969 by staff at the Center for Epidemiologic Studies (CES). The goals of the CMHA program were both methodologic and substantive. The major methodologic purpose was the development and field-testing of an epidemiologic measure of depressive symptomatology, the CES-D Scale. Other methodological issues (which will not be detailed here) included, for example, feasibility of coordinated surveys in two different communities; maximization of response rates; estimation of biases due to various conditions of the interview; feasibility of representative samples over time, to estimate time variations in mental health measures and comparisons with community indicators such as unemployment rates; and feasibility of immediate data processing and reporting procedures. The major substantive purpose was the identification of risk factors associated with depressive symptomatology. Both cross-sectional and reinterview data were collected for this purpose. Other substantive issues included analyses of other mental health-related measures. This chapter describes the two main purposes: the development and evaluation of the measure of depression (the CES-D Scale) and the major substantive findings relating to the epidemiology of depression.

The CMHA program included several related components (see Radloff, 1977 for more complete details). The first survey was carried out in both Washington County, Maryland and Kansas City, Missouri in 1971-73. Work in the two sites was designed and coordinated to be as similar as possible. The first survey used the longest questionnaire (Q1) which included the CES-D Scale, several other standard scales (e.g., from Bradburn, 1969; Lubin, 1967; Langner, 1962; Cantril, 1965; Crowne & Marlowe, 1960), measures of life events, alcohol problems, social functioning, physical illness, use of medications, and sociodemographic information. An individual (aged 18 and over) was randomly selected for interview from each household in the sample. The response rate in Kansas City was about 75%, with a total of

1,173 completed interviews; in Washington County the response rate was about 80%, with 1,673 completed interviews.

Demographic distributions of the samples have been reported by Comstock and Helsing (1976). Those who refused to be interviewed were found to be significantly more likely to have less education and come from smaller households than respondents (Comstock and Helsing, 1973). These and other (unpublished) analyses suggest that the samples probably had some underrepresentation of males and the poorly educated. However, they included respondents with a wide range of demographic characteristics, in numbers adequate for analyses of relationships among variables.

The second survey used a shorter questionnaire (Q2) which included the CES-D Scale. It was done in Washington County only, in 1973-74. The response rate for the Q2 survey was about 75%, with 1,089 completed interviews, and about 22% refusals. Therefore, the obtained sample for Q2 may be slightly less representative than that of the Washington County Q1 survey.

In 1973-74, each respondent to Q2 was asked to fill out and mail back one retest on the CES-D Scale either two, four, six, or eight weeks after the original interview. A total of 419 mailbacks was received (about 56% response rate). The CES-D was also included in a reinterview (Q3) of samples of the original respondents to Q1 and Q2. In Kansas City, in 1973, 343 respondents (78% of those attempted) were reinterviewed about 12 months after the original interview. In 1973-74, in Washington County, 1,209 respondents (about 79% of those attempted) were reinterviewed once—either three, six, or twelve months after the original interview.

The CES-D Scale

The Center for Epidemiologic Studies Depression Scale (CES-D Scale) was developed to be appropriate for use in studies of the epidemiology of depressive symptomatology in the general population. It was not intended or expected to discriminate among subtypes of depression (e.g., endogenous vs. reactive; bipolar vs. unipolar) nor to distinguish primary depressive disorders from secondary depression, (depressive symptomatology accompanying other primary diagnoses). It was, however, intended and expected to identify not only the presence but also the severity (number of symptoms weighted by frequency/duration) of depressive symptomatology. Choice of items was based on published item validity data and on coverage of depressed mood, feelings of guilt and worthlessness, feelings of helplessness and hopelessness, psychomotor retardation, loss of appetite, and sleep disturbance. Four items were worded in the positive direction to break tendencies toward response set as well as to assess positive affect (or its absence). The scale was designed to reflect current state and to be responsive to changes in state, by asking how often the symptoms occurred during the past week. Each response was scored from zero to three on a scale of frequency of occurrence of the symptom during the past week. The scoring of positive items is reversed, with less frequent scoring higher. The possible range of scores is zero to 60, with the higher scores indicating the presence of more symptomatology (see table 1).

TABLE 1
CES-D Scale.

Instructions For Questions: Below is a list of the ways you might have felt or behaved. Please tell me how often you have felt this way during the past week.

HAND CARD A.

Rarely or none of the time (less than 1 day)
Some or a little of the time (1-2 days)
Occasionally or a moderate amount of time (3-4 days)
Most or all of the time (5-7 days)

During the past week:

1. I was bothered by things that usually don't bother me.
2. I did not feel like eating; my appetite was poor.
3. I felt that I could not shake off the blues even with help from my family or friends.
4. I felt that I was just as good as other people.
5. I had trouble keeping my mind on what I was doing.
6. I felt depressed.
7. I felt that everything I did was an effort.
8. I felt hopeful about the future.
9. I thought my life had been a failure.
10. I felt fearful.
11. My sleep was restless.
12. I was happy.
13. I talked less than usual.
14. I felt lonely.
15. People were unfriendly.
16. I enjoyed life.
17. I had crying spells.
18. I felt sad.
19. I felt that people dislike me.
20. I could not get "going."

The first field test of the CES-D Scale was in the CMHA surveys. The scale was found to be acceptable and understandable to a wide range of general population respondents. The average scores for the full samples in the two sites ranged from 7.80 to 9.92, with standard deviations between 7.50 and 9.31. The distributions in these samples had large positive skews (about 1.5). A cutoff score of 16 and above was approximately the 80th percentile of the Q1 sample. Very similar results were found in a national sample by the National Center for Health Statistics, Health and Nutrition Examination Survey (NCHS-HANES). For example, the average CES-D Score was 8.7, with a standard deviation of 8.4 (NCHS, 1980).

Psychometric properties of the scale derived from the CMHA surveys have been described in detail by Radloff (1977). The properties were replicated on three separate equivalent samples from the CMHA Survey (Q1, whites; Q2, whites; Q3, whites) and on age, sex, and race subgroups. High levels of internal consistency were found in all groups (coefficients alpha about 0.85; split-halves correlations corrected for attenuation about 0.87). Test-retest correlations were considerably lower, as would be expected if the scale is sensitive to current depressive state.

The pattern of correlations of the scale with other mental health measures in the CMHA interview gave reasonable evidence of discriminant validity. For example, the CES-D correlated about 0.60 with the Bradburn Negative Affect Scale, about -0.20 with the Bradburn Positive Affect Scale, about 0.50 with the Langner 22-item Scale, and about 0.30 with disability days. The average CES-D scores were considerably and significantly higher for those who answered "yes" to the question, "Did you have an emotional problem for which you felt you needed help?" (x about 18 for "yes" vs. about 8 for "no"). Those who reported certain life events losses had significantly higher than average CES-D scores.

Factor analysis of the scale revealed a strong depressed affect factor, a separate positive affect favor, a somatic/vegetative factor and a weak fourth factor mainly weighted with the two interpersonal items (dislike and unfriendly). However, there was some overlap among factors as would be expected from the very high internal consistency of the scale as a whole.

The CMHA study demonstrated acceptability and internal consistency across age and sex subgroups and for Blacks and Whites. Roberts (1980) found satisfactory internal consistency and also similar factor structure in groups of Anglos, Blacks and Mexican-Americans in Alameda County, California. He also found that a Spanish translation used for part of the Spanish-speaking sample had similar properties. Other foreign language versions of the scale have also been developed.

The CMHA and Roberts results were based on studies using lay interviewers. Some studies using the scale as self-administered have found somewhat higher rates of unusable or questionable data due to errors, especially involving the four positively worded items. The use of the scale in telephone interviews has been tested and found equivalent to the personal interview method (Aneshensel et al., 1982).

A small clinical validity study using the CES-D in psychiatric inpatients with a variety of diagnoses (N=70) has been reported by Craig and Van Natta (1976a, 1976b). The average CES-D score for the patients was about 24 (compared with the general population average of about 9; $p < 0.01$). The CES-D scores correlated 0.56 with severity of depression as rated by the nurse-clinician most familiar with the patient.

A larger clinical validity study has been reported by Weissman, Sholomskas, et al. (1977). A carefully diagnosed group of acutely depressed outpatients plus four other groups (treated depressives, drug methadone maintenance patients, alcoholics and schizophrenics) were assessed with a variety of self-report and clinician rating scales. The correlations of the CES-D with the SCL-90 (Derogatis et al., 1973) depression subscale ranged in the five groups from 0.73 to 0.89; with the Hamilton clinician rating

(Hamilton, 1960) 0.49-0.85; with the Raskin clinician rating (Raskin, et al., 1969), 0.28-0.79. The low correlations with the Hamilton and Raskin were in the acutely depressed group, which was selected partly on the basis of Raskin scores above 6; this truncation of the range of clinician ratings makes a high correlation with other depression measures unlikely. In the treated depressed group, with a larger range of clinician rating scores, the correlations were higher: 0.65 with the Hamilton and 0.64 with the Raskin. The average CES-D scores were substantially higher for the acute depressed group (x = 38.10) than for the other groups (ranging from alcoholics, x = 23, to schizophrenics, x = 13). The three groups with diagnoses other than depression had average CES-D scores higher than the general population. This is consistent with the findings of Weissman, Pottenger, et al. (1977): 59% of the alcoholic group, 32% of the Methadone maintenance group, and 28% of the schizophrenics were diagnosed as having a depressive disorder secondary to their primary diagnosis.

In a substudy, Weissman et al. (1975a) found that in 35 depressed patients, the average scores went down from 39.11 to 20.91, reflecting improvement over the course of four weeks of treatment with antidepressant medication and supportive psychotherapy. In 25 depressed outpatients, at intake (with attenuated range), the CES-D correlated 0.72 with the Zung Self-Rating Depression Scale and 0.52 with the Beck Depression Inventory; at termination of treatment (with larger range), the CES-D correlated 0.90 with the Zung and 0.81 with the Beck (Weismann et al., 1975b).

Husaini and Neff (1980) reported a validation study comparing a rural general population sample (n=713) with a sample of rural mental health clinic outpatients (n=200 with a variety of diagnoses and levels of problem severity). They found that the CES-D discriminated well between the general population (x = 6.88) and the patient sample (x = 27.01). Within the patient sample, there was a significant overall difference in average CES-D scores among diagnostic groups (marital maladjustment highest, x = 35.24; alcoholics lowest, x = 19.68). There were also significantly higher CES-D scores for those rated by clinicians as presenting with more severe problems, for those tested at intake rather than after some treatment, and for those receiving antidepressant medications. Cutoff scores on the CES-D were evaluated according to their ability to discriminate depressed patients from other patients, taking problem severity into account. These cutoffs were then tested for their ability to discriminate within the community sample between those who reported emotional problems and/or felt a need for help. The authors suggest a CES-D score of 17 and over be used to designate "possible" cases, with a score of 23 and over used for "probable" cases. In most studies, a score of 16 and over has been used as a cutoff, because it allows comparison with findings from the CMHA surveys.

Hankin and Locke (1982) reported on a study using the CES-D Scale in a prepaid group practice medical setting. Patients filled in the CES-D while waiting to see a health care provider; the provider rated the patient on depressed mood after seeing the patient (but without seeing the CES-D Scale results). Twenty-one percent of the patients scored 16 and above on the CES-D Scale, which is very similar to the rate in the CMHA survey. However, the providers judged a very small number of patients as depressed.

The authors state that the CES-D Scale would be a useful screening instrument in general medical settings, to alert health care providers to the presence of significant depressive symptomatology so that appropriate action can be taken.

In a community survey in New Haven, Myers and Weissman (1980) compared the CES-D Scale with Research Diagnostic Criterion (RDC) diagnosis based on the Schedule for Affective Disorders and Schizophrenia (SADS) structured diagnostic interview (Spitzer, et al., 1978; Endicott & Spitzer, 1978). The study, done in 1975-76, reinterviewed, for the second time, about 55% (N=515) of a sample originally interviewed in 1967. CES-D Scale data were available for 482 of the respondents. The average CES-D Score for this sample was lower than that found in the CMHA surveys. Less than 10% of the sample scored at or above the 80th percentile cutoff of 16. Using the SADS-RDC diagnosis of current major depression as criterion gave a false positive rate of 6.1% and a false negative rate of 36.4% for the CES-D Scale (with the cutoff of 16). Very similar findings have been reported by Roberts and Vernon (1983) from a 1978-79 follow-up of a sample originally studied in 1974-75. The study was done in Alameda County, California and included Anglos, Blacks and Chicanos. The CES-D was included in an interview given by trained lay interviewers; the SADS was administered 1-2 weeks later by trained clinicians. The overall level of the CES-D scores was fairly similar to the CMHA study with 17% scoring at or above 16. The CES-D cutoff score of 16 gave a false positive rate of 16.6% and false negative rate of 40% for current major depression on the SADS-RDC.

In a case-by-case analysis of the false positives and negatives from the New Haven study, Boyd et al. (1982) found that many of the discrepancies could be explained. Of the eight false negatives (RDC major depression but CES-D score under 16), three were noted by the interviewers as having serious difficulty completing the CES-D because of its self-administered format. Four were noted as having a tendency to deny symptoms; even during the SADS, probing was necessary to elicit positive responses. One case was explainable only by the comment "seems to accept her current depression as transient episode and is sure she will get better." Of the 28 false positives (above 16 on CES-D but not major depression on RDC), 15 (36%) had depressive symptoms on the SADS interview but did not meet RDC criteria for major depression either because of too few symptoms, too short a duration, absence of functional impairment, or exclusion criteria such as bereavement or medical illness. Five respondents (12% of the false positives) seemed to be deniers on the SADS interview, since the interviewer noted an impression of depression which agreed with the CES-D results rather than the SADS results. Seven respondents (17%) were not depressed according to the SADS or interviewer observation but did have other RDC diagnoses. In summary, 81% of those above cutoff on the CES-D had some other evidence of depressive symptoms (though not necessarily major depression). Another 17% had other disorders which might have led to the high CES-D scores. Only one respondent had a high CES-D with no other evidence of problems.

These results help to evaluate the CES-D as a screening measure. If the purpose of screening is to refer individuals for further diagnosis, then some false positives are acceptable, since they will be corrected in the second stage. Furthermore, Boyd's analyses suggest that most of the high CES-D scores do reflect problems of some sort. The false negatives would present a more serious problem in screening. Boyd's finding that some respondents had trouble with the self-administered version would suggest that administration by interviewers should reduce the false negatives. However, the Roberts study, with interviewer administration, had equally high false negative rates. The Roberts study, however, did have a one to two-week interval between the CES-D and the SADS. Depression may have developed or worsened during this interval for some but not all of the false negatives. A more likely explanation is that there is a core of people who will deny symptoms, especially on a structured self-report scale on which the interviewer is not free to probe. It is possible—but yet to be verified—that these are people who perceive their symptoms as transient or not significant and who would resist treatment if it were offered. If this is the case, then their loss in screening might be acceptable. For research purposes, however, they would be an interesting group to study.

Substantive Findings on the CES-D Scale from the CMHA Survey

Comstock & Helsing (1976) reported the relationship of high scores (16 and above) on the CES-D to the standard demographic variables assessed in the CMHA survey, separately for Kansas City Blacks, Kansas City Whites and Washington County Whites. They used binary multiple regression, so the relationship reported for each variable has been adjusted for all the other variables. Variables which did not relate to depression and were therefore omitted from the regression were: relationship to household head, size of household, and urban-rural subdivisions of Washington County. For the Kansas City Blacks, lower adjusted rates of high CES-D scores were associated with older age, being currently employed, being married, and higher household income. For both Kansas City and Washington County Whites, lower adjusted rates of depression were associated with older age, being currently employed, male sex, and higher education. In all three groups, the relationship of adjusted rates of high CES-D scores to age was strong and monotonic with highest rates at age 18-24. Eaton & Kessler (1981) replicated these analyses on the national data of the NCHS-HANES, and found very similar results.

Radloff has reported the relationship of CES-D scores to sex and other risk factors. The sex-marital status interaction noted by Gove (1972) was partially confirmed in the CMHA data: women had higher average CES-D scores than men among the married, the divorced/separated, and the never married who were not heads of households; men had higher scores among the widowed and the never-married heads-of-household. Comstock and Helsing also noted this interaction in rates of high scores. Adjustments for current employment, age, education, income, presence and age of children, and physical illness did not eliminate this pattern (Radloff, 1975; Radloff, 1980).

TABLE 2
Percentage of Population with CES-D Scores of 16 or More by Selected Characteristics Among Kansas City Blacks and Whites and Washington County Whites.[a]

	Crude percentages			*Adjusted percentages*[b]		
	Kansas City		*Washington County*	*Kansas City*		*Washington County*
Characteristic	*Blacks*	*Whites*	*Whites*	*Blacks*	*Whites*	*Whites*
Total	26.4	19.8	17.0	17.6	20.1	17.0
Sex						
Male	22.2	15.7	11.9	18.6	17.4	13.6
Female	29.6	22.4	20.7	16.9	22.1	19.5
Age						
18-24	39.6	27.9	29.0	31.1	30.6	31.6
25-44	25.4	20.7	17.4	21.7	24.3	20.8
45-64	22.2	15.5	14.7	15.2	16.8	14.7
65+	25.6	18.1	12.3	3.9	10.3	3.0
Marital Status						
Single	45.2	22.0	20.4	37.9	22.6	15.4
Married	16.0	18.1	14.7	11.3	18.8	15.7
Widowed	34.0	22.8	19.4	28.8	23.6	19.9
Other	35.8	24.4	30.1	29.6	23.5	26.8
Years of Schooling						
0-6[c]	25.0	20.0	25.2	14.9	21.2	27.6
7-11	29.6	26.7	18.8	19.1	25.8	18.9
12	25.0	20.6	16.9	15.7	19.0	14.9
13+	21.7	14.3	11.7	19.0	12.7	13.5
Employment status						
Working	22.4	17.1	14.4	12.3	17.8	15.1
Housewife	29.4	21.7	21.3	21.4	20.8	18.1
Retired or student	30.0	22.0	16.8	28.3	26.0	21.3
Other	40.5	28.8	28.1	30.1	28.5	21.8
Household income (in $1000)						
0-3	39.0	29.0	23.4	32.4	26.5	21.9
4-7	31.5	20.1	18.5	25.6	19.6	16.9
8-11	17.4	17.6	17.2	17.7	17.8	16.4
12-15	8.7	21.1	14.2	10.9	22.7	16.3
16+	6.7	15.9	8.5	11.3	19.5	12.3
Not stated	17.6	11.1	21.2	-2.3	11.1	18.8

[a]Reprinted with permission from G. W. Comstock & K. J. Helsing, "Symptoms of Depression in Two Communities," *Psychol Med* (1976):551-563. Cambridge University Press.

[b]The percentages for each characteristic have been adjusted for the effects of all the other characteristics in this table by a method of binary multiple regression (Feldstein, 1966).

[c]Includes a few persons with years of schooling not stated.

Risk factors were examined for their relationship to CES-D scores separately for men and women (Radloff and Rae, 1981) and for men and women classified by marital and household status (Radloff and Rae, 1979). With the notable exception of marital status, the risk factors related to depression similarly for men and women. There was some evidence of stronger relationships for the women, however, so that men and women were more similar on CES-D scores at low levels of risk, but diverged, with women scoring higher, at high levels of risk (Radloff and Rae, 1981). The strongest and most consistent risk factors, significant in multiple regression for both sexes, were young age, current illness, recent illness, marital losses (past year), other life events losses (past year), excessive sleeping, and lack of leisure activities.

High CES-D scores were significantly related to life events scored in life change units (LCU) for the overall CMHA sample (Markush and Favero, 1974). There was considerable but unpatterned variation in the strength of this relationship across subgroups of site (Kansas City and Washington County), race, sex, age and education. Analyses of the longitudinal relationship of life events and CES-D scores were possible, using the reinterview subsample of respondents (Q3). Hornstra and Klassen (1977) reported that those who reported high depression or high life events at the first interview were those most likely to report high depression or high life events (respectively) at the reinterview (high is defined as at and above the 80th percentile). Radloff (1977) found that negative life events and CES-D scores were related concurrently at both first and second interview. Overall, the average CES-D scores were lower at the second interview, except for the group reporting no negative life events at first interview but at least one at second interview. Those who reported negative events at only the first interview showed a large decrease in CES-D scores; those reporting negative events at both interviews showed a similarly large decrease, but their average CES-D scores were higher than the other groups at both interviews (table 3).

High CES-D scores were found to be consistently related to reported disability days in the past week, in multiple regression adjusting for age, sex, marital status, education, employment, income and alcohol problems (Craig and Van Natta, 1983). CES-D scores were not related to treatment for the disabling condition, but among whites were negatively related to reported current improvement of the condition (i.e., less depression if the condition was currently improved). Among women, those reporting specific causes (illness or injury) of the disability had a lower rate of high CES-D scores than those reporting nonspecific causes; this was not the case with the male respondents. High scores on the CES-D Scale were also found to be associated with use of multiple medications (Craig and Van Natta, 1978). Among women, high scores were associated with the use of minor tranquilizers and sedatives. Although high CES-D scores were found to be related to current or recent past physical illness, they do not seem to predict subsequent serious illness (Goldberg, et al., 1979). Respondents who died or were hospitalized during the interval between the first (Q1 or Q2) and second (Q3) interviews were not significantly different from matched controls on the first interview CES-D scores nor on four other mental health measures.

TABLE 3
CES-D Average Scores By Life Events Losses Reported at Each Interview.[a]

Life events loss reported at		*No.*	*X*[b]
First interview:	No	608	7.40
Second interview:	No		6.71
First interview:	Yes	362	9.54
Second interview:	No		7.55
First interview:	No	270	8.25
Second interview:	Yes		8.92
First interview:	Yes	302	11.66
Second interview:	Yes		9.80

[a]Reprinted in part with permission from L. S. Radloff, "The CES-D Scale: A Self-Report Depression Scale for Research in the General Population," *App Psychol Meas* 1.3(1977):385-401. Copyright© West Publishing Company.

[b]Overall significance of difference between groups in change scores: $p < 0.01$ in one-way analysis of variance and in one-way analysis of covariance, with score at time 1 as covariate.

Summary

The CES-D scale was developed by the Center for Epidemiologic Studies of the National Institute of Mental Health and tested as a measure of depressive symptomatology for use in studies of the general population. The Community Mental Health Assessment Survey which field tested the CES-D contributed psychometric information on the scale and also produced useful epidemiologic information on the relationship of the scale to other variables. Other investigators have also reported reliability and validity data. The results support the use of the scale in epidemiologic research, in needs assessment studies conducted by or for health planners, and as a screening measure. The only moderate concordance with psychiatric diagnosis should, however, be noted. The scale has been or is currently being used in these ways. The use of the scale in a variety of settings and populations by different investigators with a variety of hypotheses will contribute substantially to normative data and construct validation of the scale. At the same time, the use of the same measure in a variety of studies will facilitate the accumulation of knowledge about the epidemiology and eventually the etiology of depression.

References

Aneshensel, C. S., Frerichs, R. R., Clark, V. A. & Yokopenic, P. A. (1982), Measuring depression in the community: A comparison of telephone and personal interviews. *Public Opinion Quarterly*, 46:110-121.

Boyd, J. H., Weissman, M. M., Thompson, W. D. & Myers, J. K. (1982), Screening for depression in a community sample. *Arch Gen Psychiatr* 39:1195-1200.

Bradburn, N. M. (1969), *The Structure of Psychological Well Being*. Chicago: Aldine.

Cantril, H. (1965), *The Pattern of Human Concern*. New Brunswick: Rutgers University Press.

Comstock, G. W. & Helsing, K. J. (1973), Characteristics of respondents and non-respondents to a questionnaire for estimating community mood. *Am J Epidemiol* 97:233-239.

Comstock, G. W. & Helsing, K. J. (1976), Symptoms of depression in two communities. *Psychol Med* 6:551-563.

Craig, T. J. & Van Natta, P. A. (1976a), Presence and persistence of depressive symptoms in patient and community populations. *Am J Psychiatr* 133:1426-1429.

Craig, T. J. & Van Natta, P. A. (1976b), Recognition of depressed affect in hospitalized psychiatric patients: Staff and patient perceptions. *Dis Nerv Syst* 37:561-566.

Craig, T. J. & Van Natta, P. A. (1978), Current medication use and symptoms of depression in a general population. *Am J Psychiatr* 135:1036-1039.

Craig, T. J. & Van Natta, P. A. (1978), Current medication use and symptoms of depression in a general population. *Am J Psychiatr* 135:1036-1039.

Craig, T. J. & Van Natta, P. A. (1983), Disability and depressive symptoms in two communities. *Am J Psychiatr* 140:598-600.

Crowne, D. P. & Marlowe, D. (1960), A new scale of social desirability independent of psychopathology. *J Consult Psychol* 24:349-354.

Derogatis, L. R., Lipman, R. S., & Covi, L. (1973), SCL-90: An outpatient psychiatric scale: Preliminary report. *Psychopharmacol Bull* 9:13-27.

Eaton, W. W. & Kessler, L. G. (1981), Rates of symptoms of depression in a national sample. *Am J Epidemiol* 114:528-537.

Endicott, J. & Spitzer, R. L. (1978), A diagnostic interview: The schedule for affective disorders and schizophrenia. *Arch Gen Psychiatr* 35:837-844.

Goldberg, E. L., Comstock, G. W. & Hornstra, R. K. (1979), Depressed mood and subsequent physical illness. *Am J Psychiatr* 136:530-534.

Gove, W. (1972), The relationship between sex roles, marital status, and mental illness. *Soc Forces* 51:34-44.

Hamilton, M. (1960), A rating scale for depression. *J Neurol Neurosurg Psychiatr* 23:56-62.

Hankin, J. R. & Locke, B. Z. (1982), The persistence of depressive symptomatology among prepaid group practice enrollees: An exploratory study. *Am J Pub Health*, 72:1000-1006.

Hornstra, R. K. & Klassen, D. (1977), The course of depression. *Compr Psychiatr* 18:119-125.

Husaini, B. A., Neff, J. A., Harrington, J. B., Hughes, M. D., & Stone, R. H. (1980), Depression in rural communities: Validating the CES-D Scale. *J Community Psychol* 8:20-27.

Langner, T. S. (1962), A twenty-two item screening score of psychiatric symptoms indicating impairment. *J Health Hum Behav* 3:269-276.

Lubin, B. (1967), *Manual for the Depression Adjective Lists.* San Diego: Educational and Industrial Testing Service.

Markush, R. E. & Favero, R. V. (1974), Epidemiologic assessment of stressful life events, depressed mood, and psychophysiological symptoms: A preliminary report. *Stressful Life Events: Their Nature and Effects,* eds. B. S. Dohrenwend & B. P. Dohrenwend. New York: Wiley & Sons.

Myers, J. K. & Weissman, M. M. (1980), Use of a self-report symptom scale to detect depression in a community sample. *Am J Psychiatr* 137:1081-1084.

National Center for Health Statistics. (1980), Basic data on depressive symptomatology: United States, 1974-75, by R. B. Sayetta & D. P. Johnson. Vital and Health Statistics. Series 11-No. 216. DHEW Pub No.(PHS) 80-1666. Public Health Service. Washington, D.C.: Government Printing Office.

Radloff, L. S. (1975), Sex differences in depression: The effects of occupation and marital status. *Sex Roles* 3:249-265.

Radloff, L. S. (1977), The CES-D Scale: A self-report depression scale for research in the general population. *App Psychol Meas* 3:385-401.

Radloff, L. S. (1980), Risk factors for depression: What do we learn from them? *Mental Health of Women: Fact & Fiction,* eds. D. Belle & S. Salasin, NY: Academic Press.

Radloff, L. S. & Rae, D. S. (1979), Susceptibility and precipitating factors in depression: Sex differences and similarities. *J Abnorm Psychol* 88:174-181.

Radloff, L. S. & Rae, D. S. (1981), Components of the sex difference in depression. *Research in Community and Mental Health,* Vol. III, ed. R. G. Simmons, Greenwich, CT: JAI.

Raskin, A., Schulterbrandt, J., Reatig, N. & McKeon, J. (1969), Replication of factors of psychopathology in interview, ward behavior, and self-report ratings of hospitalized depressives. *J Nerv Ment Dis* 148:87-96.

Roberts, R. E. (1980), Reliability of the CES-D scale in different ethnic contexts. *Psychiatr Res* 2:125-134.

Roberts, R. E. & Vernon, S. W. (1983), The center for epidemiologic studies depression scale: Its use in a community sample. *Am J Psychiatr* 140:41-46.

Spitzer, R. L., Endicott, J. & Robins, E. (1978), Research diagnostic criteria: Rationale and reliability. *Arch Gen Psychiatr* 35:773-782.

Weissman, M. M., Pottenger, M., Kleber, H., Ruben, H. L. & Williams, D. (1977), Symptom patterns in primary and secondary depression: A comparison of primary depressives with depressed opiate addicts, alcoholics, and schizophrenics. *Arch Gen Psychiatr* 34:854-862.

Weissman, M. M., Prusoff, B. A. & Newberry, P. (1975a), Comparison of the CES-D with standardized depression rating scales at three points in time. Technical Report, Yale University, Contract ASH 74-166, National Institute of Mental Health.

Weissman, M. M., Prusoff, B. A. & Newberry, P. (1975b), Comparison of CES-D, Zung Self Rating Depression Scale and Beck Depression Inventory. Progress report, Contract 42-74-83, National Institute of Mental Health.

Weissman, M. M., Sholomskas, D., Pottenger, M., Prusoff, B. A. & Locke, B. Z. (1977), Assessing depressive symptoms in five psychiatric populations: A validation study. *Am J Epidemiol* 106:203-214.

Chapter 10

An Epidemiologic Assessment of Mental Health Problems in the Southeastern United States

GEORGE J. WARHEIT
ROGER A. BELL
JOHN J. SCHWAB
JOANNE M. BUHL

This paper reports findings from a number of independent but interrelated research projects designed to establish the prevalence of mental health problems in the general population. Additional objectives of the research included the use of these prevalence rates to identify the differential need for and utilization of mental health services among various social and demographic groups. In keeping with the objectives of this monograph, this paper presents findings only from the prevalence phase of the projects. All research was conducted in the southeastern United States.

Background

The data reported took approximately seven years to collect. During this period, a series of socioanthropological field studies, a rates-under-treatment study, and six separate epidemiologic field surveys were conducted. The communities that served as research sites included open country areas, scattered rural settlements, small villages, moderately sized cities, and Standard Metropolitan Statistical Areas (SMSAs). The first community studied served as the model for the later research. This county was typical of many in the region; it was changing from a stable, traditionally oriented, rural, agricultural community to one with a rapidly expanding economic base; shifting from a rural to an urban dominated power structure; and experiencing racial tensions and institutional transitions. In many ways, it exhibited most of the changes taking place in the southeastern United States as described by McKinney and Bourque in their work on the incorporation of the region into the wider national economy (1971). (see also Schwab et al., 1979.)

Design of the Model Study

The research design of the model study contained three major components: *(a)* a socioanthropologic one, *(b)* a rates-under-treatment one, and *(c)* an epidemiologic prevalence one. And, although the findings are presented only for the epidemiologic component, brief descriptions of the other two are presented since they help put the total project in perspective.

Socioanthropological Field Study

The socioanthropologic phase of the research grew out of our experience which suggested that many psychiatric symptoms and syndromes have both a sociocultural context and content. Hence, the anthropological field study had as a primary function the identification of the social and cultural factors associated with the development, definition and treatment of persons who manifested aberrant thoughts, behaviors, or other forms of social deviance. The data obtained during this phase also included information on health-seeking behaviors; health providers, particularly for mental health problems; and description summaries of the community's geographic and land use patterns, history, local norms, social participation, economic bases, support networks, political structures, educational facilities and programs, racial and other attitudes and behaviors, recreational practices, religious beliefs, and kinship patterns.

Once analyzed, the findings constituted a general descriptive background of the community and its people; they were also useful in preparing the interview schedule, and they provided a framework for the analysis and interpretation of the data secured as part of the rates-under-treatment and epidemiologic phases of the research.

The anthropological field work, which took 12 months to complete, supplied information on every "community" in the county. Some of these had clearly demarcated political, geographic, and social boundaries; others were communities largely in the psychological sense in that they consisted primarily of persons who shared a common identification with one another and with the geographic area in which they lived.

Rates-Under-Treatment

The second phase of the initial project consisted of rates-under-treatment studies. These were designed to address the following questions: *(a)* who in the various communities are being treated in hospital and agency settings; *(b)* for what conditions are they being treated; *(c)* what are the rates of utilization for differing social, demographic and geographic groups; and *(d)* what services are being provided? Answers to these questions were sought for two primary reasons. First, it was recognized that treatment rates constitute one method of estimating the prevalence of differing psychiatric disorders and, implicitly, the need for mental health services. And, it was also known from earlier research that many persons treated in the general hospitals and clinics for physical health problems were treated concomitantly for mental health ones as well. It was anticipated that the hospital and agency data would provide information regarding the prevalence of mental health problems and use patterns that could not be gained from the household surveys alone. This proved to be true.

The data necessary to complete this component were secured from a 10% sample of the medical records of all patients treated in hospitals during the one-year period prior to the commencement of the project. No data were obtained on females admitted for childbirth unless there were specific psychiatric aspects to their hospitalization. In addition to this sampling of general medical records, a total enumeration was made of the records of all patients and clients who had received treatment in public hospitals, clinics, and/or other agencies for mental health related problems. Altogether, data were secured on approximately 2,500 adults who had used physical or mental health services during a one-year period. This phase of the research took eight months to complete.

The Epidemiologic Field Surveys

The data from the socioanthropological and rates-under-treatment studies were informative in their own right; moreover, they constituted an excellent base for conducting the cross-sectional field surveys designed to establish the prevalence rates of mental health problems among the general population. This phase of the research was specifically begun with the construction of an interview schedule. It ultimately consisted of 317 individual items that obtained approximately 800 pieces of information on each respondent. The instrument was constructed so its components were dynamically interrelated, that is, a conscious effort was made to give the schedule a systemic, active interrelatedness. This conscious effort reflects two basic theoretical assumptions: one, individuals are in a state of continuous adaptation to their internal, interpersonal, social, and cultural environments; and, two, the processes of adaptation are made more complex and stressful in rapidly changing social situations. To secure the data needed to test these and other assumptions, the following information was obtained by means of the field surveys.

1. Social and demographic factors.
2. Occupational and work pattern histories.
3. Marital histories on both the respondent and his/her family of orientation.
4. Patterns of social interaction between the respondents, their immediate and extended family systems, and friendship networks.
5. Religious belief and practices and community involvement through both formal and informal organizations.

6. The perception of and attitudes toward social change.
7. A comprehensive physical health inventory that included past and/or present illnesses, operations, major accidents, hospitalizations, and medications taken in the past or present.
8. An extensive physical health symptoms review.
9. A comprehensive mental health inventory consisting of approximately 100 different items related to a broad spectrum of psychiatric symptoms, syndromes, and related dysfunctions including drug and alcohol use.
10. A series of life satisfaction scales dealing with family, work, and community.
11. A health services utilization inventory that related patterns of past or present health care along with sources of care.
12. The final section included a modified version of the Cantril Self-Anchoring-Striving Satisfaction Scale (1965) and an anomie scale.

As a composite, these items secured data on each respondent's mental and physical health, coping resources, social functioning, interpersonal well-being, and ability to achieve satisfaction from daily life.

Theoretical Assumptions and Guidelines

The working hypotheses that guided the research included three basic assumptions: *(a)* psychiatric symptoms and related dysfunctions are not randomly distributed in a population but rather are clustered among certain social and demographic subpopulations; *(b)* differential symptom and dysfunction levels are associated with the number and kinds of environmental stressors experienced by varying social and demographic groups; and, *(c)* differing groups do not have the same access to or utilization of coping resources. In short, when psychiatric scale scores are found to be high for subpopulations which share a particular quality, e.g., age, race, sex, marital status, and/or socioeconomic status, we hypothesize that these elevated scores are related to the group's degree of vulnerability to life stressors and/or its access to and utilization of coping resources. Logically, the items included in the schedule were intended to elicit information by which these assumptions could be tested.

This model is, of course, a social one and as such is incomplete when viewed from epidemiologic and etiologic perspectives. We were aware of these limitations as the study was designed but decided, nonetheless, to focus primarily on the relationships between mental health problems and social factors for two reasons. First, we believed it was necessary to develop a number of symptoms and dysfunction scales that could be analyzed using statistical normative techniques. We envisaged that the results of these analyses could be used to identify the varying kinds and levels of need for mental health services among differing social and demographic groups. Second, we believed that etiologic assumptions involving genetic, biochemical and/or other biologically oriented models were all but impossible to test in field settings given the theoretical and methodological problems associated with their conceptualization and design. In contrast, the development of the field of psychiatric epidemiology did permit at least some testing of etiologic issues as they related to social structural and psychosocial variables.

As a consequence of these assumptions and beliefs and in keeping with our goal to identify as completely as possible those in the general population with mental health problems amenable to treatment in community based settings, we designed a cross-sectional survey that would yield the most reliable and valid data obtainable given the theoretical and methodological limitations of the field.

Sampling Procedures

The procedures employed in the initial project and all subsequent ones permitted the construction of a sampling frame from which a multi-staged probability sample could be drawn. The enumeration of households was made possible from electrical utility lists. This method was chosen after extensive efforts to identify households by postal addresses, telephone and city directories, voter registration lists, and other sources proved inadequate. It was found that over 98% of all households in the communities researched were serviced by an electrical utility, and this near universal pattern permitted a convenient and efficient population frame from which to select a probability sample of households. Once a household was identified, the adult to be interviewed was selected by a multistage method developed by Kish (1965). This procedure proved, upon close examination, to be extremely accurate. Analysis of census reports indicated that the social and demographic characteristics of the samples were strikingly similar to those of the populations from which they were selected.

Approximately 85% of all individuals contacted were successfully interviewed. The major sources of nonresponse consisted of the following: refusals, 8%; respondents not found at home after a minimum of 4 visits, 4.5%; addresses not located, 1.2%; and respondents too ill to be interviewed, 1.3%. This paper presents data on 4,202 of these respondents.

Mental Health Problems

The research design called for the identification of mental health problems using psychiatric symptom and dysfunction scales. The 110 items on which these scales are based were drawn from the epidemiologic literature and from clinical experience. Scale development began with a factor analysis which isolated subsets of items from within the larger pool. Once identified, these subsets were refined further using principal components analysis and the following measures were constructed: a depression scale, an anxiety scale, a general psychopathology scale, a cognitive impairment scale, a phobia scale, and a psychosocial dysfunction scale. Each scale was tested for reliability by means of Cronbach's Alpha using the method developed by Bohrnstedt (1969). All scales were found to have coefficients of reliability above 0.80. For purposes of this paper, findings based on three of these scales are presented. These are depression, anxiety, and psychosocial dysfunction. These were selected because depression and anxiety are the symptoms most commonly reported in the field studies of psychiatric epidemiology. The psychosocial dysfunction scores are reported because this scale taps the behavioral consequences of psychiatric symptomatology rather than symptoms alone, and our analysis has shown it to be less influenced by socioeconomic factors than any of the other measures included in the research.

All of the scales were also tested extensively for criterion validity. These tests included judgments by three psychiatrists who were asked to rate the impairment levels of 322 field survey respondents and 107 known psychiatric patients; both groups were interviewed as part of a pilot study. Fifty of the patients were being treated in private settings; 57 were from hospital inpatient and outpatient units. The rating protocols, which were the same for the community and patient samples, included social and demographic data and information regarding physical health, mental health, and social functioning. The responses to symptom and dysfunction items were included in the protocols, but the raters were not given scale score distributions or other information that would contaminate their judgments. These impairment estimates, which were made independently and blind, rated all community respondents and patients along a continuum from no impairment to incapacitation. Overall, the raters significantly agreed on the levels of impairment for both the patient and nonpatient groups. When scores were compared, it was found that those of the patients and those from the community sample rated as having some level of impairment were significantly higher than those of the community sample rated as nonimpaired.

Other tests to determine the construct validity of the scales included the comparisons of scale scores for community respondents identified as being at psychiatric risk with those of 237 inpatients being treated in community mental health centers in the counties where the research was being conducted. These patients were interviewed as quickly after admission as medically possible, usually within five days. The interview schedule included the scales developed as part of the field surveys. The patient data were reviewed by judges (which included research psychiatrists), and individuals were placed into categories on the basis of their symptoms, past medical histories, admission and treatment diagnoses, and the psychotropic drugs being prescribed for them. Three groups were established: psychotic, neurotic, and other. The "other" group consisted of patients who did not clearly fit into the psychotic or neurotic categories. Retarded patients and those being treated for substance abuse or organic brain syndromes were excluded from the sample.

Risk categories for the field survey sample were established by enumerating the number of events, conditions, and characteristics they reported that are known from epidemiologic and clinical research to predispose persons to mental health problems. Ten risk factors were used. These included recent life events such as separation or divorce, prior diagnosed physical or mental health problems, occupational disability, and self-assessment of physical and mental health. Survey respondents were placed into one of four groups based on the number of risk factors they reported. Their symptom/dysfunction scale scores were then compared to those of the various patient groups. The results of these comparisons are shown in table 1.

TABLE 1
Scale Score Means For General Population Risk Groups and Psychiatric Inpatients: Depression, Anxiety, and Psychosocial Dysfunction.

Risk groups or patients	*Mean depression*	*Mean anxiety*	*Mean psychosocial dysfunction*
Risk groups			
0 Risk factors[a]	12.3	3.2	0.8
1-2 Risk factors[a]	16.9	5.7	2.4
3-4 Risk factors[b]	26.6	12.7	7.1
5-8 Risk factors[c]	34.0	20.0	14.4
Patients			
Psychotic patients	26.4	16.5	12.5
Neurotic patients	38.6	19.9	15.4
Other patients	30.9	18.1	12.9

[a]The differences between the no risk and 1-2 risk group scores were significantly different from one another.

[b]The 3-4 risk group scores were significantly higher than those of either the none or 1-2 risk groups. The scores of this group were not significantly different from those of the psychiatric patients on the depression scale. They were, however, significantly lower than all other patient scores on the three scales.

[c]The 5-8 risk factor group had scores significantly higher than those of the other general population risk groups and were not significantly different from those of the patient groups on the various scales.

The scores of the patients were significantly higher than those of the general population low risk groups. Neurotic patients had the highest scores on two of the three scales being reported. Those in the field survey sample with five to eight risk factors had the highest anxiety scores, and also the second highest scores on the other two scales. A more detailed description of these and other tests for reliability and validity is found in Kuldau, Warheit and Holzer (1977), Schwab et al. (1979), and Warheit et al. (1980).

On the basis of these extensive procedures, it was concluded that the scales developed to measure the prevalence of mental health problems in the various populations were both reliable and valid.

Findings

While the data obtained in these field surveys could not be used to classify respondents accurately into various diagnostic categories such as those found in the DSM (1968), the project was designed to assess the prevalence of mental health problems by means of scale score distributions. The analysis of scores for differing social and demographic groups is presented in two ways. First, the means and standard deviations are reported for age, sex, race, marital status, and socioeconomic status (SES) groups, then the results of stepwise multiple regression analyses are outlined. Socioeconomic status is an index that represents a composite average of scores on income, years of education, and occupational status. For our purposes, respondents were placed in quintile groups on the basis of their scores. The procedures for establishing the index are found in Nam et al. (1975) and a U.S. Bureau of the Census publication (1967).

Tables 2-4 present the mean scale score distributions, standard deviations, t-tests and analysis of variance for the social and demographic subgroups.

Depression Scale Scores

The depression scale consists of 18 items. The possible score ranges are 0 to 72. The Cronbach's alpha was 0.84. The depression scale scores are found in table 2. Of the total sample, 15.9% had scores 1 or more standard deviations above the mean. The percentage scoring 1-2 standard deviations above the mean was 10.3%, and 5.6% scored 2 or more standard deviations above the mean. Blacks, females, the poor, the separated, the widowed, and the divorced had significantly higher scores than their counterparts ($p < 0.001$). The score distributions for age groups were highest for those aged 40-59. Although the scores were significantly different ($p < 0.05$) for age categories, there is no consistent pattern. The separated had the largest percentage of persons 2 or more standard deviations above the mean (20.0%), followed by those in the lowest SES quintile (17.1%). Whites, males, and those in the two highest SES quintiles had the lowest scores. For example, only 1.3% of those in the highest SES groups had scores 2 or more standard deviations above the sample mean.

Anxiety Scale Scores

The anxiety scale contains 12 items with a score range of 0 to 48. The Cronbach's alpha was 0.82. The findings are presented in table 3. The mean score for the entire sample was 6.1; a total of 14.6% had scores 1 or more standard deviations above this mean. Of this total, 8.4% had scores 1-2 standard deviations above the mean and 6.2% had scores 2 or more standard deviations higher than the mean. Again, blacks, females, the more aged, those in the lowest SES groups, and the separated, widowed, and divorced had the highest scores. All differences were significant at the $p < 0.001$ level. Whites, males, those under 40 years of age, the highest SES groups, the single, and the married had the lowest percentages of persons with scores above the normal range.

TABLE 2
Depression Scale Scores by Race, Sex, Age, SES, and Marital Status.

Characteristic	*No.*	*Mean*[a]	*Significance level*	*% 1-2 S.D.*	*% 2 or more S.D.*	*Total % 1 S.D. above mean*
Total	4202	14.28	—	10.3	5.6	15.9
Race						
White	3469	13.61	t=10.17[b]	9.1	4.8	13.9
Black	707	17.59		16.5	9.5	26.0
Sex						
Male	1807	12.51	t=10.58[b]	7.5	3.4	10.9
Female	2395	15.63		12.4	7.2	19.6
Age						
< 20	197	15.78		9.1	6.1	15.2
20-29	907	14.24	ANOVA	8.5	3.7	12.2
30-39	631	13.99	F=2.53[c]	10.8	4.4	15.2
40-49	639	14.58	df=6,4187	11.9	6.6	18.5
50-59	621	15.02	R=0.0281	12.1	7.4	19.5
60-69	624	13.92		9.9	6.4	16.3
70 +	575	13.43		9.7	5.7	15.4
SES						
1. 0-19	432	19.47		18.1	17.1	35.2
2. 20-39	798	16.59	ANOVA	15.1	8.8	23.9
3. 40-59	933	14.54	F=73.02[b]	9.8	6.1	15.9
4. 60-79	1246	12.29	df=4,4194	7.7	1.9	9.6
5. 80-99	790	11.96	R=0.2469	5.9	1.3	7.2
Marital status						
Single	527	15.54		9.9	5.1	15.0
Married	2765	13.07	ANOVA	8.5	4.0	12.5
Widowed	535	16.25	F=45.81[b]	15.5	8.6	24.1
Separated	130	22.15	df=4,4178	23.1	20.0	43.1
Divorced	226	16.41	R=0.1085	12.8	9.3	22.1

[a]The standard deviation for the entire sample was 9.6.
[b]$p < 0.005$
[c]$p < 0.05$

The Psychosocial Dysfunction Scale Scores

The psychosocial dysfunction scale consists of 11 items with possible scores ranging from 0 to 44. The Cronbach's alpha was 0.88. As shown in table 4, the mean for the total sample was 1.92 with 11.7% having scores 1 or

TABLE 3
Anxiety Scale Scores by Race, Sex, Age, SES, and Marital Status.

Characteristic	*No.*	*Mean*[a]	*Significance level*	*% 1-2 S.D.*	*% 2 or more S.D.*	*Total % 1 S.D. above mean*
Total	4002	6.11	—	8.4	6.2	14.6
Race						
White	3469	5.77	t=7.25[b]	7.5	5.6	13.1
Black	707	7.86		13.2	9.5	22.7
Sex						
Male	1807	5.20	t=7.36[b]	5.5	5.4	10.9
Female	2395	6.80		10.6	6.8	17.4
Age						
< 20	197	4.75		4.1	2.0	6.1
20-29	907	4.82	ANOVA	6.1	2.2	8.3
30-39	631	5.14	F=19.74[b]	7.6	3.5	11.1
40-49	639	5.81	df=6,4187	8.3	5.2	13.5
50-59	621	6.89	R=0.1625	10.0	9.0	19.0
60-69	624	7.05		9.1	9.8	18.9
70 +	575	8.09		12.0	11.3	23.3
SES						
1. 0-19	432	12.09		23.4	19.4	42.8
2. 20-39	798	7.71	ANOVA	9.6	10.4	20.0
3. 40-59	933	5.96	F=139.95[b]	8.2	5.9	14.1
4. 60-79	1246	4.46	df=4,4194	5.4	2.5	7.9
5. 80-99	790	3.98	R=−0.3199	3.7	1.1	4.8
Marital status						
Single	527	4.96		5.9	2.5	8.4
Married	2765	5.64	ANOVA	7.7	5.2	12.9
Widowed	535	8.32	F=30.14[b]	11.2	12.3	23.5
Separated	130	9.84	df=4,4178	16.2	14.6	30.8
Divorced	226	6.63	R=0.1184	10.6	7.1	17.7

[a]The standard deviation for the entire sample was 6.1.
[b]$p < 0.005$

more standard deviations above the mean. About 6.5% of the sample had scores 1-2 standard deviations above the mean and 5.2% had scores 2 or more standard deviations above the mean. The total percentage of respondents with scores above the mean, (11.7%) was lower on this measure than those reported for the three symptom scales. This is due to the smaller number in the 1-2 standard deviation group. As in the case of the symptom

TABLE 4
Psychosocial Dysfunction Scale Scores by Race, Sex, Age, SES, and Marital Status.

Characteristic	*No.*	*Mean*[a]	*Significance level*	*% 1-2 S.D.*	*% 2 or more S.D.*	*Total % 1 S.D. above mean*
Total	4202	1.92	—	6.5	5.2	11.7
Race						
White	3469	1.81	t=3.81[b]	6.4	4.6	11.0
Black	707	2.49		7.1	8.1	15.2
Sex						
Male	1807	1.38	t=7.14[b]	4.9	3.3	8.2
Female	2395	2.33		7.6	6.6	14.2
Age						
< 20	197	2.21		7.1	5.6	12.7
20-29	907	2.30	ANOVA	8.7	6.4	15.1
30-39	631	2.08	F=5.72[b]	5.9	6.2	12.1
40-49	639	2.20	df=6,4187	5.2	6.3	11.5
50-59	621	1.95	R=−0.0819	6.1	5.2	11.3
60-69	624	1.51		6.6	3.4	10.0
70 +	575	1.17		5.2	2.8	8.0
SES						
1. 0-19	432	2.62		8.8	8.1	16.9
2. 20-39	798	2.34	ANOVA	6.6	7.1	13.7
3. 40-59	933	1.98	F=7.89[b]	7.0	5.7	12.7
4. 60-79	1246	1.57	df=4,4194	5.9	3.6	9.5
5. 80-99	790	1.60	R=0.0823	5.2	3.4	8.6
Marital status						
Single	527	2.31		8.7	5.7	14.4
Married	2765	1.66	ANOVA	5.7	4.2	9.9
Widowed	535	1.84	F=19.61[b]	6.7	4.7	11.4
Separated	130	4.76	df=4,4178	10.0	19.2	29.2
Divorced	226	2.65	R=0.0605	7.5	8.4	15.9

[a]The standard deviation for the entire sample was 1.9.
[b]$p < 0.005$

scales, blacks, females, and those in the lowest SES groups had significantly higher scores than whites, males, and those in the upper SES quintiles ($p < 0.001$). The distribution of scores among age and marital status groups are significantly different ($p < 0.001$) but the patterns are unlike those found for the symptom measures.

When controlled for age, the lowest scores were found among the older age groups, particularly for those 60 and over. Another variation from the symptom scales is found among marital status groups. The separated and divorced had the highest scores, but the widowed had lower scores than the single. Importantly, the variations between SES quintiles are far less pronounced than they are for the other measures.

The uncontrolled scale score findings present a generally consistent configuration: blacks, females, the aged, those in the lower SES quintiles, and those with disrupted marital status, especially the separated, had significantly higher scores than their alter groups. There are variations, but a pronounced general pattern is in evidence.

Multiple Regression Analysis

The scale scores for various social and demographic groups were also analyzed by means of stepwise multiple regression equations. The results are reported in tables 5-7.

Depression Scale Scores

The analysis of depression scores is presented in table 5. Again, all variables were significant at the $p < 0.01$ level. SES, being female, old age, and separation were the best predictors of higher scores. A total of 11.2% of the variance was explained. Of this total, 4.3% was unique to SES; 4.6% was attributable to the non-SES variables combined and 2.3% was shared by all variables in the equation.

Anxiety Scale Scores

The regression results for the anxiety scale are reported in table 6. SES, sex, age, and being separated were significant variables in the equation ($p < 0.01$). The total variance explained was 11.8%. Of this amount, 6.2% was unique to SES; 1.1% was unique to the other social and demographic variables combined, and 4.5% was shared by all variables.

Psychosocial Dysfunction Scale Scores

The findings related to the psychosocial dysfunction scale are shown in table 7. All variables but widowed and black were significant ($p < 0.01$). However, it is important to observe that age, being separated and female entered the equation before SES, a departure from the patterns observed for the symptoms scales. And, although the overall equation was significant ($p < 0.01$), the F was much smaller than it was for the symptom scales. In addition, the total variance explained was markedly lower, only 4.3%. When the variables were tested for interrelationships, it was found that SES uniquely accounted for only 0.7% of the explained variance. The other 6 variables accounted for 3.5% of the explained variance and 0.1% was shared by SES and the other social and demographic variables. It is evident that

TABLE 5
Prediction of Depression Scale Scores From Race, Sex, Socioeconomic Status, Age, and Marital Status.

	Regression Coefficients				
Variable[a]	*B*	*Standardized beta*	*Std. error B*	*F*	*Significance*
SES	−0.09644	−0.24716	0.00672	205.742	$p < 0.01$
Female	2.09075	0.10788	0.29260	51.056	$p < 0.01$
Age	−0.07366	−0.14405	0.00873	71.258	$p < 0.01$
Separated	5.52907	0.09951	0.84028	43.297	$p < 0.01$
Widowed	1.98535	0.06887	0.48370	16.847	$p < 0.01$
Divorced	2.19986	0.05178	0.62481	12.396	$p < 0.01$
Black	0.72166	0.02810	0.41696	2.996	$p < 0.01$
(Constant)	21.14216				

	Analysis of Variance			
	df	*Sum of squares*	*Mean square*	*F*
Regression	*7.*	*43296.90532*	*6185.27219*	*75.05*
Residual	*4183.*	*342666.90762*	*81.91894*	

Multiple R	0.33493
R-square	0.11218
Standard error	9.05091

[a]Uncollapsed scores were used for Age and SES.
Black, Female, Separated, Widowed, and Divorced are dichotomies scored 0=No, 1=Yes.

the dysfunction scale is tapping qualities not included in the symptom scales. We believe these qualities may be related to psychiatric syndromes, the nature of which cannot be derived from the available data.

Comment

The findings are generally consistent with those reported in the literature on psychiatric epidemiology (cf. Dohrenwend and Dohrenwend, 1974, 1975; Warheit et al., 1975). Uncontrolled, the data indicate that the poor, blacks, the separated, divorced or widowed, and the elderly usually had the highest symptom and dysfunction scores. The single had the lowest scores on the depression and psychosocial dysfunction measures. The separated had the highest scores among marital status groups on all three scales. The data on

TABLE 6
Prediction of Anxiety Scale Scores From Race, Sex, Socioeconomic Status, Age, and Marital Status.

	Regression Coefficients				
Variable[a]	***B***	***Standardized beta***	***Std. error B***	***F***	***Significance***
SES	−0.08409	−0.29416	0.00491	293.221	$p < 0.01$
Female	0.85698	0.06035	0.21373	16.078	$p < 0.01$
Age	0.01963	0.05241	0.00637	9.490	$p < 0.01$
Separated	2.28524	0.05614	0.61376	13.863	$p < 0.01$
Widowed	0.45083	0.02135	0.35331	1.628	NS[b]
Black	−0.35345	−0.01878	0.30456	1.347	NS
Divorced	0.39689	0.01275	0.45638	0.756	NS
(Constant)	9.26099				

	Analysis Of Variance			
	df	***Sum of squares***	***Mean square***	***F***
Regression	7.	24364.25017	3480.60717	79.63
Residual	4183.	182819.65582		

Multiple R	0.34292
R-square	0.11760
Standard error	6.61101

[a]Uncollapsed scores were used for Age and SES.
Black, Female, Separated, Widowed, and Divorced are dichotomies scored 0=No, 1=Yes.
[b]Not significant.

age are less patterned. Although those 50 years of age and older did not always have the highest mean scores on the two symptom scales, they did have the greatest percentage of persons scoring 1 or more standard deviations above the mean. For the dysfunction scale, however, those under 30 had the highest mean scores and also the largest percentage in the 1 or more standard deviations above the mean categories.

The most significant relationships between the social and demographic variables and high scores were found for SES. Those in the lowest SES quintile had the largest percentage of respondents scoring 1 or more standard deviations above the mean on the two symptom scales: depression, 35.2%; anxiety, 42.8%. The only scale on which they did not have the largest percentage in the 1 or more standard deviation range was psychosocial dysfunction; the separated had the largest number, 20.2% followed by the lowest SES quintile, 16.9%.

TABLE 7
Prediction of Psychosocial Dysfunction Scale Scores From Race, Sex, Socioeconomic Status, Age, and Marital Status.

	Regression Coefficients				
Variable[a]	*B*	*Standardized beta*	*Std. error B*	*F*	*Significance*
Separated	2.44626	0.09743	0.39417	38.516	$p < 0.01$
Female	0.79270	0.09051	0.13726	33.354	p 0.01
Age	−0.03076	−0.13311	0.00409	56.478	$p < 0.01$
SES	−0.01785	−0.10124	0.00315	32.038	$p < 0.01$
Divorced	0.74091	0.03859	0.29309	6.390	$p < 0.01$
Widowed	0.02293	0.01760	0.22690	1.021	NS[b]
Black	−0.06042	−0.00521	0.19559	0.095	NS
(Constant)	3.73862				

	Analysis of Variance			
	df	*Sum of squares*	*Mean square*	*F*
Regression	7.	3422.79376	488.97054	27.13
Residual	4183.	75402.15828	18.02586	

Multiple R	0.20838
R-square	0.04342
Standard error	4.24569

[a]Uncollapsed scores were used for Age and SES.
Black, Female, Separated, Widowed, and Divorced are dichotomies scored 0=No, 1=Yes.
[b]Not significant.

Multiple regression analyses also indicated that low SES was, by far, the best predictor of high symptom scores and accounted for the greatest percentages of explained variance. It was also a significant variable in the dysfunction equation but entered fourth and explained little of the variance. In short, the data show that low SES is a better predictor of symptoms than of dysfunction. Although the findings are tentative, they suggest that high symptom scores are more related to factors associated with social stress than are high dysfunction scores. At the same time, it appears that the dysfunction scale more likely identifies the signs of a psychiatric syndrome. The evidence for this conjecture comes from three sources: *(a)* the very large dysfunction scale score differences between the patient and the low risk non-patient groups (table 1); *(b)* the smaller amount of variance explained by the social and demographic variables included in the regression analysis presented in table 7; and *(c)* other data in our file that show that 4.0% of those scoring 1-2 standard deviations above the mean on this measure had been psychiatric inpatients at some time during the three years prior to their being interviewed and that 6.5% of those scoring 2 or more standard deviations high had been psychiatric inpatients. By contrast those scoring above the mean on the symptom scales reported significantly lower rates of psychiatric hospitalization (Warheit et al., 1980).

Two competing hypotheses regarding the relationships between low SES and high rates of mental disorder have been posited by the Dohrenwends (1969). These are social causality and social selection. We have used our data to test these hypotheses employing the design they proposed. Regrettably, the findings were ambiguous and inconclusive. After exhaustive analysis, we have concluded that although there are unmistakably high interrelationships between low SES and mental health problems it is not possible to make causal statements about them except, as noted above, to suggest that low SES is probably more related to symptoms than syndromes.

Females had significantly higher scores than males on all scales and the variable "female" was significant in all three regression analyses. It entered the equations second in each instance. This finding is almost universally reported in the literature and although several competing hypotheses have been put forth to explain the phenomenon (e.g., response biases related to social desirability, role conflict, and/or biological predispositions), these cannot be addressed by our data. Earlier analysis of the data reported elsewhere (Warheit et al., 1976) does suggest, however, that the higher scores among females are not significantly related to being married. Other data suggest that being married is a significant coping resource for those experiencing stressful life events (Warheit, 1979; Bell et al., 1982).

The data on race, when uncontrolled for other factors, indicate that blacks had higher scores than whites on all scales. However, when analyzed in regression equations, the variable "black" was not significant for anxiety or psychosocial dysfunction and it was only marginally significant for the depression scale. The findings on the depression scale probably reflect the high rates of physical health problems reported by blacks. Other analysis indicates that these measures are especially influenced by the presence of physical health problems (Schwab et al., 1979). Further, the variable "black" accounted for less than 1.0% of the explained unique variance for any of the three scales analyzed. In short, the data do not suggest a patterned, independent relationship between race and high scale scores when age, sex, and socioeconomic status are controlled simultaneously.

Being separated was the most consistent predictor of high scores among marital status variables. It was significant in all three equations entering first for psychosocial dysfunction. The variable "widowed" was significant for the depression scores although it contributed a very small amount to the total explained variance. It was not significant for anxiety or psychosocial dysfunction. Divorce, while explaining little unique variance, was significant in all regression equations except for the anxiety scale. The statuses "single" and "married" were not significant variables in any of the equations.

The findings show that the symptom and dysfunction scales employed in this research effectively identified the subpopulations at greatest risk for mental health problems. Moreover, the results tend to corroborate the social model that guided the research, i.e., it was found that those in disadvantaged social statuses, be they achieved or ascribed, had the highest scale scores. At the same time, it is important to note that the amount of variance explained by the social and demographic variables was relatively small, ranging from 4.3% for the psychosocial dysfunction measure to 11.7% for the anxiety scale. This low amount of variance explained suggests that other factors, including personality dimensions, social psychological variables such as self-esteem, and biological processes, are playing an important but unidentified role in the development of psychiatric symptomatology and dysfunction.

Finally, the methodologies employed in our research, while of value for general epidemiologic screening, are limited in their ability to distinguish among the heterogeneous symptoms and syndromes that comprise psychiatric disorders. In the United States, however, a number of large epidemiologic field surveys are being conducted which include instruments especially designed to determine the prevalence of specific psychiatric disorders among the general population. If these efforts are successful, and there is no reason to believe they will not be, the field of psychiatric epidemiology will have made a significant step forward. These endeavors may not bring us any closer to understanding the causes of psychiatric disorders and neither will we, in all probability, be able to definitively identify the dynamic interplay of social-structural, psychological, and biological factors as they influence the onset and course of mental illness. The precise identification and enumeration of disorders can, however, provide a sound descriptive base from which further research efforts of a verificational nature can be launched.

References

American Psychiatric Association (1968), *DSM-II: Diagnostic and Statistical Manual of Mental Disorders.* Washington, D.C.: American Psychiatric Association.

Bell, R. A., LeRoy, J. B. & Stephenson, J.J. (1982), Evaluating the mediating effects of social support upon life events and depressive symptomatology. *J Commun Psychol* 10:325-340.

Bohrnstedt, G.W. (1969), Observations on the measurement of change. *Sociological Methodology,* ed. E.F. Borgatta & G.W. Bohrnstedt. San Francisco: Jossey-Bass.

Cantril, H. (1965), *The Pattern of Human Concerns.* New Brunswick, N.J.: Rutgers University Press.

Dohrenwend, B.P. (1975), Sociocultural and socio-psychological factors in the genesis of mental disorders. *J Health Soc Behav* 16(4):365-392.

Dohrenwend, B.P. & Dohrenwend, B.S. (1974), Social and cultural influences on psychopathology. *Ann Rev Psychol* 25:417-452.

Dohrenwend, B.P. & Dohrenwend, B.S. (1969), *Social Status and Psychological Disorder.* New York: John Wiley.

Kish, L.A. (1965), *Survey Sampling.* New York: John Wiley and Sons.

Kuldau, J.M., Warheit, G.J. & Holzer, C.E. (1977), Health opinion survey valid for needs assessment. Presented at the annual meeting of the National Council for Community Mental Health Centers in Atlanta, Georgia.

McKinney, J. & Bourque, L. (1971), The changing South: National incorporation of a region. *Am Sociol Rev* 36:399-412.

Nam, C.B., LaRocque, J., Powers, M.G. & Holmberg, J. (1975), Occupational status scores: Stability and change. *Proc Am Statist Assoc,* pp. 570-575.

Schwab, J.J., Bell, R.A., Warheit, G.J. & Schwab, R.B. (1979), *Social Order and Mental Health,* New York: Brunner/Mazel.

U.S. Bureau of the Census (1967), *U.S. Census of Population: 1960, Subject Reports, Socioeconomic Status,* Final Report PC(2)-5C. Washington, D.C.: U.S. Government Printing Office.

Warheit, G.J. (1979), Life events, coping, stress, and depressive symptomatology. *Am J Psychiatr* 136:502-507.

Warheit, G.J., Holzer, C.E., Bell, R.A. & Arey, S.A. (1976), Sex, marital status and mental health: A reappraisal. *Social Forces* 55:459-470.

Warheit, G.J., Holzer, C.E., Robbins, L. & Buhl, J.M. (1980), *Planning for Mental Health Services: Needs Assessment Approaches.* Rockville, MD: National Institute of Mental Health.

Warheit, G.J., Robbins, L., Swanson, E., McGinnis, N.H. & Schwab, J.J. (1975), *A Review of Selected Research on the Relationship of Sociodemographic Factors to Mental Disorders and Treatment Outcomes: 1968-1974.* Rockville, MD: National Institute of Mental Health.

Chapter 11

The NIMH Epidemiologic Catchment Area Program

WILLIAM W. EATON
DARREL A. REGIER
BEN Z. LOCKE
CARL A. TAUBE

The Epidemiologic Catchment Area (ECA) Program is a developmental series of epidemiologic research studies performed by independent research teams in collaboration with the Division of Biometry and Epidemiology of the National Institute of Mental Health (NIMH). The broad aims of the Program are the historical goals of psychiatric epidemiology: to estimate the incidence and prevalence of mental disorders; to search for etiologic clues; and to aid in the planning of health care services and programs. New substantive developments in the field have emphasized the need for specific types of data collection, and methodologies for carrying out psychiatric epidemiologic studies have improved remarkably over the last decade. The ECA studies have built on these developments and methodological studies to provide a framework for a new generation of epidemiologic and health services research in psychiatry.

Although the ECA Program retains the historical goals of psychiatric epidemiology, the methodologies involved are not in general use. In this paper we discuss five methodologic aspects of the ECA Program that together form the basic research design: the emphasis on specific diagnoses; the integration of community surveys with institutional surveys; the collection of prevalence as well as incidence data; the systematic linkage of service utilization data with other epidemiologic variables; and the multisite comparative-collaborative aspect. None of these aspects is totally new to the field, but they have never been combined in this way, and we therefore believe that data from the ECA Program may address these historical goals in an innovative fashion.

Specific Mental Disorders

One difference between the ECA Program and many other recent epidemiologic studies is that it focuses on specific mental disorders instead of global impairment ratings. Up until the early 1950s, the dominant conceptual framework for psychiatric epidemiology was the medical model, even though social scientists and epidemiologists had been collaborating extensively during and before World War II. For example, specific medical diagnoses were used as dependent variables in most epidemiologic studies up to and including the New Haven study (Hollingshead and Redlich, 1958). But after the war social survey research was established as a practical, accepted technology through the development of multiple-item scaling, accurate and usable survey sampling, and standardized interviewer training, to name just a few methodologies. Social science researchers also became more aware of the need for assessing the reliability and validity of measurement in all their research, and in psychiatric epidemiology it became clear that psychiatric diagnoses could not be made with acceptable reliability and validity using survey technology, or some would say, in standard clinical practice. Therefore, the field of psychiatric epidemiology switched from specific diagnoses to global scales. This trend began with the Midtown study (Langner and Michael, 1963) and has continued to the present, with a few exceptions. The trend toward global mental health ratings satisfied the need of psychiatric epidemiologists to accommodate survey technology, but was in opposition to many changes in the area of psychiatric classification. Increasingly available social epidemiologic evidence suggested that different types of mental disorders were differentially related to demographic variables like sex, social class, and area of residence, (Dohrenwend, 1975). There also began to be genetic evidence suggesting that for the different specific diagnoses the degrees of inheritance were different (Weissman and Klerman, 1978). And new drugs were discovered that had beneficial effects for specific diagnoses and not for others (Berger, 1978). In the areas of classification and diagnosis, operational criteria for diagnoses were developed, along with standardized interview questionnaires and standardized interviewer training techniques, to improve the reliability of diagnosis (Helzer et al., 1977; Endicott and Spitzer, 1978).

The most important change in the ECA Program has been to focus on specific mental disorders without giving up the interest in rigorous survey methodology. The vehicle to accomplish this end is the NIMH Diagnostic Interview Schedule (DIS), which focuses on specific disorders and takes advantage of the recently developed capabilities in diagnostic assessment (Robins et al., 1979). It converts for the first time the methodology of clinical assessment to that of field surveys. The implications of this development for the field of psychiatric epidemiology are rather broad: the conversion not only ties the field into diagnostic categories on which much laboratory and clinical research is being done (thus aiding in the search for etiologic clues), it also ties the field into diagnostic categories used in clinical practice (thus aiding in the planning of mental health facilities).

Part of the ECA Program includes tests of the agreement of the DIS results with other standards of diagnosis. To represent all the diagnoses provided by the DIS, the subjects in the first such study (Robins et al., 1979) were selected according to prior knowledge of their psychiatric condition. The interviewers, however, were not aware of the prior diagnosis or of the diagnosis made by a second interviewer. If the two interviewers had had equivalent training, this study would be simply of the reliability of the DIS. However, one of the basic innovations of the DIS is the superimposition of clinical assessment on survey methodology, and this study is designed to test that crossover by having one of the interviewers be a trained clinical psychiatrist and the other the kind of interviewer generally found in survey organizations, that is a person with no clinical training. The high interrater agreement that was found gave both good evidence of reliability and evidence that lay interviewers can use the DIS as well as psychiatrists. If the DIS in the hands of a clinical psychiatrist is the criterion, then this study is of criterion validity.

Even if the DIS were found to be valid in a clinical setting, one would need to address the question of its agreement with other methods of reaching a diagnosis both in the general population, where the frequency of disorder is low, and under household survey conditions, where the setting is less predictable. A second type of study addresses this need: within three weeks of the survey interviews conducted as part of the ECA Program, a subsample of people are interviewed by a psychiatrist using a criterion instrument. An attempt is made to generate diagnostic heterogeneity by recommending for follow-up a sample of persons with no disorder according to the DIS interviews and a sample with each of the major disorders. The comparison instrument to be used differs at the different sites of research. At one site it is the Schedule for Affective Disorders and Schizophrenia, used by a highly trained clinician. At a second site it is the DIS itself in combination with a standardized clinical assessment based on the third revision of the Diagnostic and Statistical Manual of the American Psychiatric Association (DSM-III); at a third site it is a clinical interview built around the Present State Examination, a structured psychiatric interview widely used around the world, and modified to make DSM-III diagnoses.

The requirement for data on specific disorders necessitates a larger sample size than has been common in psychiatric epidemiologic studies. The sample size for the general population surveys at each site in the ECA Program is set at 4,000 households. If one member of each household is interviewed and we allow for a 75% response rate, the yield will be an estimated 3,000 respondents in the general population. The relatively new emphasis on specific mental disorders requires much larger samples than research conducted on global impairment ratings, because of the rarity of the specific disorders. Ten to 20 percent will have any specific disorder, and for many disorders the point prevalence may be closer to 1% (Weissman et al., 1978). These low frequencies mean that even with a large sample, the yield in cases of disorders is relatively small.

Meeting the goals of the ECA Program entails tasks of estimation (of incidence and prevalence) and analysis (of etiologic factors and of factors affecting service utilization). We have projected what the 95% confidence intervals for prevalence will be for the total sample and for subsamples broken down by age, sex, and socioeconomic status in respect to specific disorders having a true population prevalence of 5% and 1%. For the total sample the interval is about 4%-6% for a disorder with 5% prevalence, and about 0.6%-1.4% for a disorder with 1% prevalence. When the sample is broken down into subcategories considerable precision is lost. The interval is adequate for one-way breakdowns by the three demographic variables just mentioned, but is unacceptable for multivariable analysis of the rare disorders. In terms of the power to analyze and test specific hypotheses the sample from one site is barely of adequate size, and for specific disorders it permits the testing of only the very simplest and strongest hypotheses (concerning either etiology or health services research). When broader groups of specific mental disorders are considered (for example, affective disorders, all mental disorders, or such variables as the total symptom counts) the power for this size sample is much greater.

Community and Institution Surveys

A second aspect of the methodology implemented by the ECA Program is the integration of data from community surveys with data from treatment institutions. The epidemiologist is nearly always faced with this choice of treatment institutions versus community surveys for casefinding; use of both methods simultaneously is rare and rarer still is the rigorous integration of the two methods. The aim in the ECA Program is to study the total true prevalence of disorders, that is, the prevalence without regard to treatment status.

One result of the growth in the social sciences after the war was the realization that many people with bona fide mental disorders never ended up in a treatment setting. The implication was drawn that epidemiologic data based on admission to treatment were of dubious value for etiologic research and for rational planning of facilities. Epidemiologists and social scientists became aware fairly early of this flaw inherent in treatment data, and both groups began to study in detail the processes by which people with personal problems found their way into the psychiatric treatment system (Kitsuse and Cicourel, 1963; Scheff, 1966; Kadushin, 1969). Later on it became apparent that the majority of people treated for psychiatric problems were treated in the general health care sector, not in the psychiatric sector (Locke and Gardner, 1969; Regier et al., 1978). The fact that data on psychiatric problems were not routinely collected in general health care facilities only emphasized the difficulty of studying the total true prevalence of mental disorders.

This problem of total true prevalence is confounded with that of case identification, discussed above. In early studies through the one by Hollingshead and Redlich (1963), treatment agencies were used to find cases, and since treatment agencies routinely make a diagnosis, these studies had data on specific disorders. The dissatisfaction with data on treated cases was one reason for shifting to field surveys, but this shift entailed a loss of data on specific mental disorders. Some researchers decided to completely ignore psychiatric epidemiologic research that relied on studies of treated cases as did the Dohrenwends' classic review (1969). If, in examining the body of research from community studies, one attempts to look at community prevalence data for specific diagnoses instead of the more global "psychological disorder," the number of available studies drops sharply.

The degree to which persons with psychiatric disorders are treated varies by specific diagnosis. After an intensive search for schizophrenic cases in Detroit, Dunham (1965) concluded that "virtually all schizophrenics are eventually hospitalized." In a study in rural Sweden, 12 psychotics were located through a combination of casefinding techniques; all 12 had been seen by a physician, and 11 by a psychiatrist (Hagnell, 1966). These lamentably scanty data suggest that most psychotics end up in some sort of psychiatric treatment, although there are exceptions in some rural societies or premodern societies such as the Hutterites (Eaton and Weil, 1953). For nonpsychotic disorders, the proportion treated is likely to be much lower. Data from treatment institutions probably include a higher proportion of the total population of schizophrenics than do community data. However, since the majority of depressive disorders are probably not treated, community data are more accurate for this diagnosis.

The upshot of these considerations is that data solely from community surveys are also inaccurate because they miss people with severe mental disorders who are in treatment. Thus one requirement of the ECA Program has been the integration of community surveys with surveys of treatment institutions.

There is considerable variation in rates of mental disorder from research studies in different areas, and part of this variation results from the fact that psychiatrically disordered persons select themselves into certain areas (Kantor, 1965). Some of this selection process is related to the presence of institutions in given areas. For example, differences in rates of mental disorder between urban and rural areas probably result largely from the greater availability of facilities in the urban areas. In comparing results from two research studies (or two ECA sites), one would prefer if the greater availability of facilities in one area made no difference: in a broad sense, this sort of difference is measurement error. Paying careful attention to the definition of residence can minimize this source of error. We do this by establishing mutually exclusive and exhaustive definitions of residence in which subjects will be picked up in one, and only one, of the two types of surveys (institutional and general population), and in which their geographic area of residence will be unambiguously established.

In the ECA Program the sites for research are areas that were previously designated Community Mental Health Center (CMHC) Catchment Areas, from which the name of the Program itself comes. These are geographic areas with populations of 75,000-250,000. However, since the Program requires an area with minimum population size of 200,000 to ensure a large enough population base for the sample survey, in some cases CMHC catchment areas must be combined to form the basic geographic unit of study. These catchment areas (and combinations thereof) were chosen because they are the best geographic units for assessing the supply of mental health resources (Regier, 1978). The ECA research will contribute to assessment of demand for these resources using the same geographic units (for those sites involved). This potential linkup of supply and demand for a given area is an important benefit of the ECA Program.

We have specific rules for determining when a person is considered a resident of the CMHC area, and when not a resident. The U.S. Census defines three broad categories of living arrangements: in a household, a group quarter, or an institution (U.S. Department of Commerce, 1970). Psychiatric hospitals, extended care facilities (such as homes for the aged), and prisons are sampled in the survey of treatment institutions. The residence for persons in treatment institutions is defined by their residence upon admission to the institution. Group quarters are transient residences like flophouses and YMCAs, but they also include halfway houses, college dormitories, military barracks, and general hospitals. Group quarters are sampled in the general population survey in two ways: either by listing the residential unit as dwelling unit and surveying it as usual (the procedure used, for example, for YMCAs and halfway houses), or by inquiring just before the household interview about other members of the household who are absent, and following them into the group quarters for an interview if necessary (the procedure used, for example, for college dormitories and general hospitals). In the second instance, the relevant group quarters are not included in the community survey, since residence is defined by the person's household address.

We expect the difference in the total true prevalence rate between the several ECA sites to be much smaller than differences between either institution rates or community rates between sites. Knowledge of the sizes of these differences will be very helpful in interpreting differences between various past studies, between various sociodemographic groups, and between ECA sites.

The sample size for the survey of treatment institutions has been tentatively set at 500. For most catchment areas, sampling at the same fraction as in the general population would yield an institutional sample of about 50. However, the prevalence in the institutions is much higher than in the general population. Sampling theory suggests that in this situation it is cost efficient to oversample this stratum; the result is a more precise estimate of the total true prevalence rate (Kish, 1965). As well as increasing the precision for the total rate, the sample size of 500 will yield rough estimates of the overall rate of mental disorders within each of the three major kinds of institutions (mental hospitals, homes for the aged, and prisons).

Incidence and Prevalence Data

Another aspect of the ECA Program is its emphasis on incidence. Incidence rates are superior to prevalence rates for the study of etiology. For diseases that are often fatal (for example, heart disease or cancer), the more important advantage of the incidence rate is that it is not contaminated by mortality; for chronic, nonfatal diseases (for example, diabetes and mental disorders), the more important advantage is that incidence rates are less contaminated by insidious onset and secondary complications. Mental disorders develop over extended periods, and a person's diagnosis and the severity of his or her disorder may shift from time to time in as yet unknown ways. Since the incidence rate gives the investigator the least contaminated look at the disorder, etiologic relationships should be more visible. If there is a precipitating event, the investigator should be able to discern it more easily than if it occurred in the distant past. Incidence rates and etiologic relationships are relevant to programs of primary prevention, but for planning of services and programs prevalence rates are superior because they are closer to an estimate of demand for treatment.

Incidence data require identification of new cases, and in effect this means monitoring a population for a period of time. In the past the closest approximation to incidence has come from statistics on admissions to treatment, in which new cases are those without prior treatment; in effect, the treatment system monitors the population continuously. However, monitoring the population for a period of time is much more costly when psychiatric treatment is not used as the criterion for casefinding, and in most community studies prevalence rates are estimated. The irony is that even though incidence data are much more relevant to etiology than prevalence data, as we have noted, community surveys are usually conducted by investigators interested in etiology.

The ECA Program requires two waves of interviews on the same persons in both the community and the institution surveys. Two waves are the minimum number required for identification of new cases. Furthermore, this two-wave design allows the study of relapse and remission.

Linkage with Service Utilization Data

Another fundamental innovation in the ECA Program is its provision for the systematic collection of survey data from people about their use of psychiatric, general health, and other human services. One goal of the Program is to determine why people use or do not use treatment facilities. Thus the objective is to ascertain how unmet need is generated and why some groups are underserved. The strategy is to analyze differences between the psychiatrically disordered persons who are in treatment and those with the same diagnoses who are not. Groups that include many people who meet the criteria for diagnosis but are not in treatment are "underserved"; areas where there are many such persons may need new treatment facilities. We suspect that two kinds of factors may be important here: *(a)* barriers to care, which include aspects of mental health services and programs that hinder treatment (such as long waiting times for appointments, long distances to treatment facilities, inadequate or understaffed facilities, and cost of care); and *(b)* illness behavior, which includes the individual's ability and willingness to identify psychiatric problems, attitudes toward help-seeking in general, and avoidance of psychiatric treatment due to stigma. In the first wave of interviews factors can be identified in the data analysis that are associated with barriers to care and/or illness behavior. These factors can then be used prospectively to predict utilization over the coming year.

A related goal of the ECA Program is to discover how people choose the specific locus of treatment and to assess the degree to which facilities are used appropriately. To enable us to understand better the pathways leading into the various kinds of services, utilization data will include the general health, specialty mental health, and human services sectors. By covering a broad range of facilities and having diagnostic data available, we can study issues related to duplication of services, inappropriate provision of services, and the use of multiple facilities for a single clinical episode—analyses that have major policy implications for the financing and operation of the mental health service system. This sort of data base is much stronger than the earlier case registers, which relied solely on treated cases (Bahn, 1965).

The Multisite Aspect

The ECA Program plan is to have five different sites of research and is designed to complement the psychiatric component of a large-scale national sample survey such as the National Center for Health Statistics Health Examination Surveys. Even though only a large-scale project such as the Health Examination Survey can provide nationwide estimates of prevalence, a multisite design such as the ECA program has many advantages that the large single-shot survey lacks. The major advantage is that it permits results from many sites of research to be compared. In the past there has been quite a disparity in results from different research sites, due, it is suspected, to the different orientations and methodologies of investigators (Dohrenwend and Dohrenwend, 1969). The disparity has led some researchers to become pessimistic about the possibility of ever obtaining the replicable results that are so necessary if we are to build a scientific foundation for the field of psychiatric epidemiology. Our hope in this project is to demonstrate which results are replicable and which depend on the specific research site. The results that occur repeatedly can contribute to the desired scientific foundation; the results that are observed at only one site or at only a few sites may provide etiological leads if methodological differences are examined and ruled out.

In the field of psychiatric epidemiology, a multisite design generates higher quality data than the large one-shot survey. To integrate the general population survey with an institutional survey on a national level is extremely difficult. Both the Census Bureau and the National Center for Health Statistics conduct their surveys of institutions separately from their general population surveys, because of this difficulty. To integrate the two surveys as carefully as is necessary requires intimate knowledge of the local institutions and the populations they treat. Coordinating the two surveys requires the explicit cooperation of every single institution in the area, which is difficult to obtain in a large-scale national effort. Furthermore, smaller, local sites of research allow considerably more involvement of high-level, professional researchers in the actual survey process than is usual for typical sample surveys. And participation of such researchers not only increases the probability of obtaining high-quality data, but should alert us quickly to shortcomings in the DIS or in the quality control process.

The five ECA sites are located in New Haven, Connecticut, at Yale University, with Jerome K. Myers, as principal investigator; Baltimore, Maryland, at Johns Hopkins University, with Morton Kramer as principal investigator; St. Louis, Missouri, at Washington University—St. Louis, with Lee N. Robins, as principal investigator; Raleigh-Durham, North Carolina, at Duke University with Dan Blazer as principal investigator; and Los Angeles, California, at the University of California, Los Angeles, with

Richard Hough as principal investigator. Multi-disciplinary teams of psychiatrists, social scientists, epidemiologists, and statisticians are involved at each site.

Although each site follows the standard research design outlined above, there has been the opportunity to take advantage of unique talents at one or the other universities, or to exploit local opportunities for innovative research. Johns Hopkins, Yale, and Duke, for example, have been able to heavily oversample the population over 65 years of age. Johns Hopkins, Duke, and Washington University are sampling large populations of blacks. UCLA has designed its sample to include about 1,500 Hispanics. There are special studies of the chronically mentally ill at Yale and Johns Hopkins, special studies of the mental health consequences of sexual assault at Duke and UCLA, plans to study the effects of stress from toxic environmental disaster that occurred in part of the St. Louis study area during the second wave of interviews, and many other small but important studies which are not common to all five sites but which add considerably to the value of the program as a whole. Early results from the first three sites of the Program are available in a recent series of five papers (Regier et al.; Eaton et al.; Myers et al.; Shapiro et al.; Robins et al., in press).

Summary

We hope that the ECA Program can make a unique contribution to the field of psychiatric epidemiology and mental health services research. The Program will provide total true prevalence data on mental disorders according to the latest diagnostic criteria, and that in itself will be a significant contribution. Such data should be of enormous benefit to those interested in etiology as well as those interested in health services research. For researchers interested in etiology, the data can be used to identify, by comparison, high-risk groups. For those interested in health services research, the results can serve as a health planning guide that does not depend on the presence or absence of treatment facilities in a given area.

Incidence data will be the second major contribution of the ECA Program. Its two-wave design enhances the study of incidence, etiology, and the natural history of disorders and also allows study of the social behavior of persons entering treatment for mental disorders—a subject important to health planners.

Finally, a significant result of the ECA Program may well be the development of a viable standardized methodology for the epidemiologic study of mental disorders, by means of which demonstrably replicable results can be produced. Once we demonstrate the equivalence of method and results, the stage is set for comparative studies of all sorts.

Acknowledgments

The Epidemiologic Catchment Area Program is a series of five epidemiologic research studies performed by independent research teams in collaboration with staff of the Division of Biometry and Epidemiology (DBE) of the National Institute of Mental Health (NIMH). The NIMH Principal Collaborators are Darrel A. Regier, Ben Z. Locke, and William W. Eaton; the NIMH Project Officer is Carl A. Taube. The Principal Investigators and Co-Investigators from the five sites are: Yale University, U01 MH 34224—Jerome K. Myers, Myrna M. Weissman, and Gary Tischler; Johns Hopkins University; U01 MH 33870—Morton Kramer, Ernest Gruenberg, and Sam Shapiro; Washington University, St. Louis, U01 MH 33883—Lee N. Robins, John Helzer, and Jack Croughan; Duke University, U01 MH 35386—Dan Blazer and Linda George; University of California, Los Angeles, U01 MH 35865—Richard Hough, Marvin Karno, Javier Escobar, and Audrey Burnam.

References

Bahn, A.K. (1965), Experience and philosophy with regard to case registers in health and welfare. *Com Ment Health J* 1:245-250.

Berger, P.A. (1978), Medical treatment of mental disorder. *Science* 200:974-981.

Dohrenwend, B.P. (1975), Sociocultural and social- psychological factors in the genesis of mental disorders. *J Health Soc Behav* 16:365-392.

Dohrenwend, B.P. & Dohrenwend, B.S. (1969), *Social Status and Psychological Disorder: A Causal Inquiry.* New York: Wiley.

Dunham, H.W. (1965), *Community and Schizophrenia: An Epidemiological Analysis.* Detroit: Wayne State University Press.

Eaton, J.W. & Weil, R.J. (1953), The mental health of the Hutterites. *Sci Am* 189:31-37.

Eaton, W.W., Holzer, C.E., Von Korff, M., Anthony, J.C., Helzer, J.E., George, L.K., Burnam, M.A., Boyd, J.H., Kessler, L.G., & Locke, R.Z. The design of the ECA surveys: The control and measurement of error. *Arch Gen Psychiatr,* in press.

Endicott, J. & Spitzer, R.L. (1978), A diagnostic interview. *Arch Gen Psychiatr* 35:837-844.

Hagnell, O. (1966), *A Prospective Study of the Incidence of Mental Disorder.* Stockholm: Strenska Bokforlaget.

Helzer, J., Robins, L., & Taibleson, M. (1977), Reliability of psychiatric diagnosis: a methodological review. *Arch Gen Psychiatr* 34:129-133.

Kadushin, C. (1969), *Why People Go To Psychiatrists.* New York: Atherton.

Kantor, M.E. (ed.) (1965), *Migration and the Major Mental Disorders.* Springfield, Ill.: Charles C. Thomas.

Kish, L. (1965), *Survey Sampling.* New York: Wiley.

Kitsuse, J. & Cicourel, A. (1963), A note on the use of official statistics. *Soc Prob* 11:131-159.

Locke, B.Z. & Gardner, E.A. (1969), Psychiatric disorders among the patients of general practitioners and internists. *Publ Health Rep* 3, 84:167-173.

Myers, J.K., Weissman, M.M., Tischler, G.L., Holzer, C.E., Leaf, P., Orvaschel, H., Anthony, J.C., Boyd, J.H., Burke, J.D., Kramer, M., & Stoltzman, R., Six month prevalence of psychiatric disorders in three communities: 1980-1982. *Arch Gen Psychiatr,* in press.

Regier, D., Goldberg, I., & Taube, C. (1978), The de facto mental health system. *Arch Gen Psychiatr* 35:685-693.

Regier, D.A., Myers, J.K., Kramer, M., Robins, L.N., Blazer, D.G., Hough, R.L., Eaton, W.W., & Locke, B.Z. The NIMH epidemiologic catchment area program: Historical context, major objectives, and study population characteristics. *Arch Gen Psychiatr*, in press.

Robins, L., Helzer, J., Croughan, J., Williams, J.B., & Spitzer, R.L. (1979), *The NIMH Diagnostic Interview Schedule*. Rockville, Md: National Institute of Mental Health.

Robins, L.N., Helzer, J.E., Weissman, M., Orvaschel, H., Regier, D.A. & Burke, J.D., Lifetime prevalence in three sites. *Arch Gen Psychiatr*, in press.

Scheff, T. (1966), *Being Mentally Ill: A Sociological Theory*. Chicago: Aldine.

Shapiro, S., Skinner, E.A., VonKorff, M., German, P.S., Tischler, G.L., Leaf, P., Benham, L., Cottler, L., Kessler, L.G. & Regier, G.A., Three epidemiologic catchment area sites. *Arch Gen Psychiatr*, in press.

U.S. Department of Commerce, (1970), *1970 Census Users' Guide*. Washington, D.C.: Government Printing Office.

Weissman, M.M. & Klerman, G.L. (1978), The epidemiology of mental disorder: Emerging trends. *Arch Gen Psychiatr* 35:705-712.

Weissman, M.M., Myers, J.K. & Harding, P.S. (1978), Psychiatric disorders in a U.S. urban community: 1975-1976. *Am J Psychiatr* 135:459-462.

Chapter 12

Expectancy and Outcome of Mental Disorders in Iceland

TÓMAS HELGASON

The purpose of the study reviewed here was to contribute to the descriptive and comparative epidemiology of mental disorders. The main questions considered were the magnitude of psychiatric morbidity in Iceland, its distribution according to diagnosis, its possible variation despite the homogeneity of the population among various demographic groups, and comparison with the morbidity in other countries. Subsidiary questions were related to mortality and outcome of mental disorders.

For a meaningful comparison with studies from other countries it was necessary to carry out a study according to the same method, and with the same intensity and diagnostic classification, as one of the available studies from other countries. Besides answering the special questions related to psychiatric morbidity in Iceland, such a study could also be of a more general and methodologic interest.

In selecting the method for the study, practical and theoretical aspects were taken into consideration. These also influenced the decision on selecting the measure to be used for expressing the morbidity rates. Obviously, the best method would have been a prospective study of a birth cohort followed over a sufficiently long period. This would have involved the professional lifetime of several psychiatrists succeeding each other seeing all the probands at frequent intervals. No such studies were available at the time when the Icelandic study was planned. Besides the financial difficulties involved in such studies, other practical problems would have been incurred, such as those relating to the orientation of psychiatrists of different generations. An intensive incidence study over a short period of time, but including a large sample of the population in all age groups, could also have been considered if sufficient psychiatric manpower had been available as well as other studies for comparison. An intensive prevalence study was not possible for the same reasons and an extensive prevalence study had already been attempted (Helgason, 1954).

The second best choice was a retrospective longitudinal study of a birth cohort. The advantage of this method is that health information is collected on every member of the cohort during his lifetime from all available resources and is evaluated by one psychiatrist. The limitations, on the other hand, are that the data collected are partly recorded and partly memorized by a number of individuals and thus need verification. Also it is very likely that minor disorders that the probands might have been suffering from long ago are forgotten. Two previous studies with this method were available, one from Munich by Klemperer (1933) and the other from Bornholm in Denmark by Fremming (1947, 1951). As the theoretical orientation of the author at the beginning of the study was similar to that prevailing in Denmark, the possibility for comparison with the latter study was thought to be fairly good.

Methods and Materials

The cohort was selected and investigated according to the principles of Klemperer's (1933) "biographical" method. This method is not applicable except under special external circumstances. Given these circumstances, as in Iceland, the method is effective and should give information for the determination of disease expectancy as reliable as possible in retrospective investigations. The essentials and main advantages of the method are:

1. The initial probands are an almost unbiased sample of children in the population to be investigated, i.e., persons who have not entered the usual manifestation period of the functional psychoses.
2. The health of each individual is investigated as thoroughly as possible during his lifespan or until he has passed the manifestation period of the disorders to be investigated.

The only bias in the sample itself is that all the probands belong necessarily to one age group, selected by the fact that those alive at the time of the investigation should have passed the manifestation period of the diseases in question. Therefore, it is not possible to draw the primary material by random sampling in many age groups, and a suitable number of probands born during one or as few years as possible has to be obtained, possibly by including every person born in these years. This selection is most helpful in collecting the necessary information about the probands. It makes possible the search of all official registers and hospital files, whereas this work would have been practically impossible if the initial study had been carried out for the same number of persons drawn completely at random.

Information is collected on each proband, living or dead, to find all those who may have been sick or abnormal during the observation period and to find out what they have suffered from, when their illness started, how long it has lasted, and how severely they were affected. Furthermore, information is collected on social status, family, and other aspects that might affect the health and development of the individual.

In longitudinal studies like this one, it is essential to compromise between two standpoints if the investigation is to achieve its purpose. On the one hand, the probands of the cohort have to be born so long ago that those still alive at the time of the investigation have passed the manifestation period of diseases to be investigated. As one of the main purposes of the present investigation was to find the disease expectancy for manic-depressive psychosis, the probands should preferably have been born 70-75 years before the time of investigation. This is also desirable for the investigation of the risk of senile dementia and other diseases that do not make their appearances until at an advanced age. On the other hand, it is important for the reliability of the information obtained that the number of probands who died long ago should not be too large.

In compliance with these considerations it seemed most appropriate to select probands who were born 60 years before the first study was carried out, although about onefourth of the probands who were in the age range of 13-15 years in 1910 would have been deceased by July 1, 1957, which was chosen as the cross-sectional date of the study. It could be expected that there would still be many persons alive who had known the dead probands well enough to give reliable information on their health. It was also considered more valuable to obtain information about major diseases appearing when the probands were in their fifties than to try to concentrate on minor disorders among those who died at any early age. Klemperer and Fremming selected their probands from birth registers, but only persons who had reached the age of 10 or more were included in the psychiatric survey. In the Icelandic study it was intended to proceed in the same way, but unfortunately some of the parish records that contained the necessary birth registers had been lost by fire. Therefore, the only way to obtain a complete sample of the population in the necessary age group was to draw the names of the probands from the population census registers. The census register from 1910 contained all the necessary identification data on each person. This register was therefore used to draw the sample: all Icelanders born in Iceland during the years 1895-1897 and living there on December 1st, 1910. The probands were thus 13-15 years of age at the beginning of the observation period. As the sample includes all Icelanders of a certain age group alive at a certain date, it is unquestionably representative of the nation.

The primary sources of information about the probands' health were the general practitioners who had been taking care of them. For the dead and emigrated probands, information was also collected from relatives and acquaintances as well as from various key informants in each community. Some probands were approached directly, either in writing or personally, and a number of probands, especially those with more serious psychiatric problems who were still alive, had been in psychiatric consultation. The information thus obtained was amplified and verified by searching the files of all hospitals in the country, both general and special, the files of the State Disability Insurance Board, the files of nursing and old age homes, the police records, the files of clinics for alcoholics, and the files of a psychiatrist who was in practice in Iceland during the latter two thirds of the observation period.

To further ensure that the diagnostic classification was comparable to the Danish diagnostic classification, the material was worked up at the Institute of Psychiatry in Århus during 1959-1962. The case histories and diagnoses were discussed intensively with three Danish psychiatrists. Although the author is responsible for the final diagnosis, it has to be stressed that the agreement between him and the Danish psychiatrists was extensive both on the diagnostic principles and on the diagnosis in individual cases. Diagnostic criteria follow European lines as given for example in Strömgren's (1956) textbook of psychiatry.

The study was initiated in 1956 by copying the names and birth dates of all Icelanders born during the years 1895-1897 from the original material of the population census taken in Iceland on December 1, 1910, and tracing the fate and whereabouts of the 5,395 probands born during these years according to the population register (table 1).

TABLE 1
Distribution of a Birth Cohort of Icelanders Alive in Iceland at the Age of 13-15 Years (in 1910) According to Sex and Survival Until the Age of 60-62 Years (in 1957).

Outcome	*Males(%) (n=2,729)*	*Females(%) (n=2,666)*	*Both Sexes(%) (n=5,395)*
Not traced	0.2	0.2	0.2
Disappeared alive, 1910-1957	0.8	0.8	0.8
Deceased, 1910-1957	30.7	24.8	27.8
Alive at the age of 60-62 years	68.3	74.2	71.2
TOTAL	100.0	100.0	100.0

During 1895-1897, 7,209 children were born alive in Iceland (Stjórnartiðindi, 1896-1898). Thus 74.8% of the birth cohort survived in Iceland until the age of 13-15 years.

Only 0.2% of the probands of the study could not be traced after 1910. With another 0.4% it was not possible to obtain sufficient information of psychiatric relevance, except that they had been functioning socially. During 1910-1957, 27.8% of the probands died, while 0.8% disappeared alive from observation. Emigration was minimal, only 4.5%, during this period. An attempt was made to collect as detailed information on those who had emigrated or disappeared during the observation period as on those still alive on July 1, 1957. However, it is obvious that symptoms and signs of minor disorders are more likely to be missed among those who have disappeared from observation at an early age than among those still alive.

In 1971 follow-up data were collected on those still alive in Iceland in 1957 until their death or until the age of 74-76 years. At the follow-up, 0.1% of those alive in 1957 could not be traced, and 27.4% died before July 1, 1971. The information in the follow-up study was collected very much in the same way as during the first stage, except that by this time a psychiatric register had been established. The register comprises those who have been seen by psychiatrists in Iceland from 1908 onwards, and those who have been admitted to departments of neurology and internal medicine and nursing homes after 1960 and assigned a psychiatric diagnosis. Probands who had emigrated were excluded from the follow-up study.

TABLE 2
Distribution of the Birth Cohort Whose Mental Health Had Been Studied Until the Age of 60-62 Years (in 1957) According to Sex and Survival 14 Years Later (in 1971).

Outcome	*Males(%) (n=1,864)*	*Females(%) (n=1,979)*	*Both Sexes(%) (n=3,843)*
Emigrated before 1957	2.5	4.6	3.6
Not traced after 1957	0.0	0.1	0.1
Deceased 1957-1971	32.7	22.3	27.4
Alive in 1971	64.8	72.9	69.0
TOTAL	100.0	99.9	100.1

Morbidity in the study is expressed as disease expectancy, defined as the probability that an individual of a given age will develop a specified disease at some time during life or prior to a certain later age, provided that he survives the manifestation period of the disease or lives to the specified age. Disease expectancy is thus an age-corrected expression of morbidity, independent of mortality in various groups at various times. Therefore, it is suitable for comparison of morbidity. The procedure used for estimating the disease expectancy in the present study is the summation expectancy measure (Goldhamer and Marshall, 1953), which is the principle underlying Strömgren's (1935) method for calculating the age-corrected population at risk (Bezugziffer). These methods are described in an earlier report on the study (Helgason, 1964).

Lifetime prevalence is the number of active and previously active cases in the population alive at a certain time. If there is no excess mortality among those contracting the disease, the lifetime prevalence should be the same as the disease expectancy. Otherwise the disease expectancy will be higher than the lifetime prevalence, provided the casefinding among the deceased is as efficient as among those alive. Should the casefinding among the deceased be less efficient, the lifetime prevalence in the rest of the cohort may be used as an approximation of the disease expectancy.

In the initial study, 1,543 probands were identified with mental disorders. In the follow-up study, an additional 539 cases were identified. In the analysis of the material, each proband appears only once, i.e., under his main diagnosis from either of the two phases of the study. The diagnoses are arranged in a hierarchical order with manic-depressive psychosis at the top, followed by schizophrenia, psychogenic psychoses, unclassified psychoses, "mild endogenous depressive syndromes," neuroses, alcoholism, organic mental disorders, intellectual subnormality, and personality disorders. The unspecified mental disorders were given the lowest priority.

Results

In the initial study (Helgason, 1964), which was purely retrospective, 1,543 probands were identified with mental disorder occurring before the age of 60-62 years or before the proband's disappearance from observation. The available information was sufficient to assign a diagnosis to the majority of these probands. Only 5.8% of them could not be given a specific diagnosis and were labelled unspecific mental disorder, which probably is most often some form of personality disorder. Besides this group there were 7.4% of the probands with mental disorders where there was some uncertainty as to which diagnostic category they belonged to. In the present paper they are included with the group that was thought to be the most likely. During the follow-up period, 56 new cases of psychosis were identified. The majority of these were manic-depressive psychosis. This called for a new estimate of the expectancy of psychoses. The new estimate is slightly higher than the previous one, although not to a statistically significant degree. This is caused mainly by a higher estimate of the expectancy of manic-depressive psychosis and of unclassified psychoses, both for men and women. Most of the new cases of manic-depressive psychosis were seen by a psychiatrist or admitted to a hospital during their illness. The new cases of unclassified psychoses include eight cases of paranoid psychoses, all but one among women. The expectancy of functional psychoses is considerably higher for women than for men (table 3).

Although the absolute numbers become small (Helgason, 1964) when divided between various demographic groups, expectancy rates were calculated for these and the following trends emerged. The expectancy of developing a psychosis is similar for adolescents residing in rural and urban communities. It is higher for nonmigrants, for persons staying on in rural communities, for those remaining in the lowest socioeconomic class, and for those remaining unmarried. The expectancy is lower for migrants and for those eventually settling in urban communities. It is also lower for persons who belong to the higher socioeconomic classes and for persons who have been married. This general description is rather more applicable to men than to women and is most typical for schizophrenia. The expectancy of manic-depressive psychosis is more evenly distributed, but with the same general trends except that it is slightly higher in the highest socioeconomic class, although the difference is not significant.

TABLE 3
Expectancy (% ± SE) of Developing Functional Psychoses Before the Age of 75 Years According to Sex and Diagnosis.

	Expectancy		
Disorder	*Males(n)*[a]	*Females(n)*	*Both sexes*
Manic depressive psychosis	2.77 ± 0.36 (58)	3.93 ± 0.42 (86)	3.36 ± 0.28 (144)
Schizophrenia	0.69 ± 0.17 (17)	1.10 ± 0.21 (27)	0.90 ± 0.13 (44)
Psychogenic psychoses	0.89 ± 0.20 (19)	1.51 ± 0.26 (34)	1.21 ± 0.16 (53)
Unclassified psychoses	0.39 ± 0.13 (9)	1.29 ± 0.25 (27)	0.85 ± 0.14 (36)
TOTAL	4.74 ± 0.46 (103)	7.83 ± 0.57 (174)	6.32 ± 0.37 (277)

[a]Number of cases in parentheses.

The expectancy for functional psychoses and other mental disorders is shown in table 4. During the follow-up study a total of 539 cases were identified, 298 of which were organic mental disorders of varying severity, while 241 were functional disorders. Thus 38.6% of the initial cohort aged 13-15 years developed a mental disorder before their death or before the average age of 75 years.

The 50 cases of mild endogenous depressions were identified through the general practitioners only. Although these are quite similar in symptomatology, course, and response to treatment to the depressive phase in manic-depressive psychosis, this group is kept separate as the severity of the illness was definitely less and did not call for treatment by a psychiatrist (Helgason, 1979).

According to table 4, every second member of the population who survives until the age of 74 years can be expected to experience some form of mental disorder during his lifetime. One-third of the expectancy is accounted for by the neuroses, one-fourth by the expectancy for organic mental disorders. Functional psychoses are the third large group and alcohol and drug abuse the fourth. Approximately one-half of the probands with neuroses have been treated only by general practitioners and the majority of the organic mental disorders have not been treated by psychiatrists. The concept of alcohol abuse is rather broad in accordance with what was defined by the World Health Organization (1951, 1952) as excessive drinking. About two-thirds would fall within WHO's narrow definition (1952) of alcoholism and accordingly need treatment. The number of probands with neuroses and unspecified mental disorder was proportionally lower among the deceased than among those alive at the age of 60-62 years. Therefore, the life-

TABLE 4
Expectancy (% ± SE) of Developing A Mental Disorder Before the Age of 75 Years According to Sex and Diagnosis.

Disorder	*Expectancy*					
	Males(n)[a]		***Females(n)***		***Both sexes(n)***	
Functional psychoses	4.74 ± 0.46	(103)	7.83 ± 0.57	(174)	6.32 ± 0.37	(277)
Mild endogenous depression (61-74 years)	1.05 ± 0.30	(22)	1.28 ± 0.30	(28)	1.17 ± 0.21	(50)
Neuroses[b]	12.77 ± 0.78	(247)	22.94 ± 0.96	(478)	18.01 ± 0.6	(725)
Alcohol and drug abuse	9.65 ± 0.61	(227)	1.05 ± 0.21	(25)	5.34 ± 0.3	(252)
Organic mental disorder	14.03 ± 0.85	(234)	12.28 ± 0.76	(227)	13.09 ± 0.5	(461)
Intellectual subnormality	2.90 ± 0.32	(79)	2.36 ± 0.29	(63)	2.63 ± 0.2	(142)
Personality disorder	1.76 ± 0.25	(48)	1.99 ± 0.27	(53)	1.87 ± 0.1	(101)
Unspecified mental disorder[b]	1.66 ± 0.30	(41)	1.59 ± 0.28	(33)	1.62 ± 0.2	(74)
TOTAL	48.56 ± 1.10	(1,001)	51.32 ± 1.09	(1,081)	50.05 ± 0.7	(2,082)

[a]Number of cases in parentheses.

[b]Based on lifetime prevalence at the average age of 61 years (187 men and 352 women with neuroses and 31 men and 28 women with unspecified mental disorder) plus incidence during the age period 61-74 years (46 men and 92 women with neuroses).

time prevalence at this age was considered as the best estimate of the expectancy of these disorders until the age of 60-62 years. The incidence rates in different age groups after that age were added to this rate to obtain the total estimate given in table 4.

The total expectancy of developing a mental disorder is similar among men and women, while the expectancy of developing different forms of illness is different between the sexes. This applies mainly to the functional disorders that are not considered congenital or as having developed during early childhood. The higher expectancy of women for developing psychoses has already been alluded to. The expectancy for women to develop neuroses is twice as high as that for men, while the expectancy for men of developing alcohol or drug abuse is ten times higher than that for women. The combined expectancy of neuroses and alcohol abuse is thus similar among men and women. Other epidemiologic findings for these disorders are similar except mortality, which is greater among the alcohol abusers, but could not be assessed for the neurotics in the initial study, and was similar to that of the general population during the follow-up study.

The overall expectancy of developing a mental disorder before the age of 61 years (Helgason, 1964) is higher in urban communities, especially in the largest town, in the lowest social class, and among the single, but lower in rural communities, in the higher social classes, and among those who have married. The difference between the expectancy of neuroses in social Class I and social Class III is small and insignificant, but tends to be higher among men in social Class I. This is also the case with regard to alcohol and drug abuse; however, the expectancy in social Class I is slightly higher than in social Class III although the difference is still not of a statistical significance. Other functional mental disorders, i.e., personality disorders, intellectual subnormality, and unspecified mental disorder, are most common in the lowest socioeconomic class, among the never-married and in the rural population. These, along with the psychoses, contribute mainly to the differential distribution of the expectancy according to demographic factors.

The expectancy of developing affective disorders before the age of 75 has been studied separately (Helgason, 1979), and found to be about 12% for men and women combined while it is 10% for men and approximately 15% for women. One-half of this expectancy is accounted for by expectancy of depressive neuroses. The total expectancy of affective disorders does not vary to a statistically significant degree according to social class. It is also similar among those who had never married and those who are married or have been married.

In the initial study, those who had been granted some form of social security assistance from the State Disability Insurance Board or were inpatients in institutions were considered disabled. When evaluating the outcome among the probands in 1971, disability was assessed in collaboration with the general practitioners as at this time the probands were receiving old age pension whether they were disabled or not. The patients were not classified as disabled unless their disability amounted to at least 50%, which would have entitled them to social security benefits at an earlier age. It was attempted to assess whether the main reason for disability were psychiatric symptoms or other symptoms.

In 1957, 1,552 of the probands or 28.8% of the cohort, had disappeared from observation, all but 54 by death. Of the 1,543 cases with mental disorder, 23.1% had died by 1957, while the corresponding figure for those without mental disorder is 31%. The lower percentage of deceased probands with diagnosis is caused by the low identification of cases of neuroses and of unspecified mental disorders and to a certain extent cases of personality disorder among the deceased. On the other hand, the percentage of dead probands in other groups was higher than that among those without mental disorders. Besides the 10.7% disabled on account of psychiatric symptoms,

7.4% of probands with psychiatric diagnosis were disabled on account of other symptoms, compared to 2.9% of the probands without psychiatric diagnosis.

The mortality of probands with psychiatric diagnosis can be inferred from Table 5 and Table 6. The latter shows that there is a higher percentage of probands who had been assigned a psychiatric diagnosis in the initial study who have died during the follow-up period of 14 years than in the group without psychiatric diagnosis. This applies to all diagnostic categories except unspecified mental disorders. However, the difference between those without mental disorders and those with neuroses and intellectual subnormality is small. Previously (Helgason, 1964) the decreased remaining mean life expectancy for probands with functional psychoses or alcohol abuse has been demonstrated. This was only 71-75% for men and women, respectively, of that of the general population for probands who had contracted functional psychoses and about 83% for probands with alcohol abuse.

During the 14-year follow-up period, the percentage of probands disabled on account of mental disorders has increased in all categories. Even among those who had not been diagnosed with a mental disorder at the age of 60-62 years, 3.5% are disabled on account of a mental disorder at the end of the follow-up period. These have developed their disorder during the follow-up period. Only 40.2% of the probands who were alive at the age of 60-62 years and who had had a mental disorder at that time were not disabled at the end of the follow-up period, while 60.5% of those without mental disorder were alive and not disabled.

Table 6 shows that only 25.5% of probands who had functional psychoses during their prime of life remain fit, and only 31.5% of those with alcohol or drug abuse do so until the advanced age of 74-76 years. The long-term prognosis for patients with mental disorders is thus gloomy, except for those with unspecified mental disorders and to some extent for those with neuroses.

Table 7 compares the outcome among probands with psychiatric diagnosis registered during the followup period with those who had no psychiatric diagnosis during this period. Only 38.2% of the probands with mental disorders are still alive and not disabled by the end of this period, compared to 63.5% of those who did not have any mental disorder. During this period, a group of patients were identified with mild endogenous depressions. A considerable number of these were identified during the latter part of the period. This partly explains the low percentage of dead probands in this group. But it is also possible that cases of this type have been missed, because it was not possible to have continuous registration of those who were seen by general practitioners on account of mental disorder during the whole period. Also, it is to be expected that the percentage of dead probands among those with organic mental disorder will increase steeply with longer observation periods. Disability other than psychiatric was rare in the group with functional psychoses, mild endogenous depression, and alcohol or drug abuse, while in the other diagnostic groups it was similar to that among those without mental disorder. Of course, the majority of the patients with organic mental disorder who were classified as disabled on account of their psychiatric symptoms could as well have been classified as physically dis-

TABLE 5
Distribution of Outcome in 1957 Among the Probands in a Birth Cohort Alive in 1910 at the Age of 13-15 Years According to Main Diagnosis.

	Outcome					
Main diagnosis	*Not disabled (%)*	*Psychiatric disability (%)*	*Other disability (%)*	*Dead (%)*[a]	*Total (%)*	*Number of probands*
Functional psychoses	35.7	27.6	4.1	32.6	100.0	221
Neuroses	76.2	8.0	7.2	8.6	100.0	584
Alcohol and drug abuse	57.8	4.3	3.0	34.9	100.0	232
Organic mental disorder	27.5	9.2	26.0	37.4	100.1	131
Intellectual subnormality	47.5	11.4	3.8	37.3	100.0	158
Personality disorder	52.8	13.4	7.9	26.0	100.1	127
Unspecified mental disorder	80.0	0.0	6.7	13.3	100.0	90
All mental disorders	58.8	10.7	7.4	23.1	100.0	1,543
Without mental disorder	66.1	0.0	2.9	31.0	100.0	3,852
TOTAL	64.1	3.1	4.2	28.8	100.1	5,395

[a]Includes 54 probands who disappeared alive.

TABLE 6
Distribution of Outcome in 1971 Among Probands Alive in 1957 in Iceland at the Age of 60-62 Years According to Main Diagnosis at That Time.

	Outcome					
Main diagnosis	*Not disabled* (%)	*Psychiatric disability* (%)	*Other disability* (%)	*Dead* (%)	*Total* (%)	*Number of probands*
Functional psychoses	25.5	31.0	6.2	37.2	99.9	145
Neuroses	49.4	12.2	10.1	28.3	100.0	526
Alcohol and drug abuse	31.5	12.1	4.0	52.3	99.9	149
Organic mental disorder	18.3	20.7	9.8	51.2	100.0	82
Intellectual subnormality	34.0	22.7	12.4	30.9	100.0	97
Personality disorder	34.9	20.5	6.0	38.6	100.0	83
Unspecified mental disorder	58.4	5.2	11.7	24.7	100.0	77
All mental disorders	40.2	16.1	8.8	34.9	100.0	1,159
Without mental disorders	60.5	3.5	10.5	25.5	100.0	2,543
TOTAL	54.2	7.4	10.0	28.4	100.0	3,702

TABLE 7
Distribution of Outcome in 1971 Among Probands Alive in 1957 in Iceland at the Age of 60-62 Years According to Main Diagnosis Registered During the Followup Period.

	Outcome					
Main diagnosis	*Not disabled* (%)	*Psychiatric disability* (%)	*Other disability* (%)	*Dead* (%)	*Total* (%)	*Number of probands*
Functional psychoses	30.7	32.8	2.2	34.3	100.0	137
Mild endogenous depression	63.5	21.2	3.8	11.5	100.0	52
Neuroses	49.5	13.8	13.3	23.3	99.9	390
Alcohol and drug abuse	31.5	10.4	1.6	56.5	100.0	124
Organic mental disorder	29.3	25.5	7.8	37.3	99.9	498
Intellectual subnormality	43.0	16.5	8.9	31.6	100.0	79
Personality disorder	32.8	18.0	13.1	36.1	100.0	61
Unspecified mental disorder	59.3	3.7	11.1	25.9	100.0	27
All mental disorders	38.2	20.1	8.5	33.1	99.9	1,368
Without mental disorder	63.5	0.0	10.9	25.6	100.0	2,334
Total	54.2	7.4	10.0	28.4	100.0	3,702

abled. However, their psychiatric symptoms were considered to contribute more to their disability and therefore were taken as the main cause of disability.

During the observation period from 1910 to 1971, 61 probands, 40 men and 21 women, committed suicide. Almost 90% of the probands who committed suicide had been mentally ill, 60% with some form of affective disorder.

From the available data, the expectancy of committing suicide before the average age of 75 years can be estimated to be approximately 2% for men and 1% for women.

TABLE 8
Number of Suicides According to Sex and Diagnosis.

Diagnosis	*Males (n=40)*	*Females (n=21)*	*Both sexes (n=61)*
Affective disorders	23	13	36
Other diagnoses	13	7	20
Without psychiatric diagnosis	4	1	5

Discussion

The method of the study has obvious limitations. The data were collected in two stages and in both instances retrospectively. Although they were collected from a number of sources, the general practitioners were of major importance for identifying possible cases. To a certain extent the G.P.s had the probands on their lists only for a short period. Although they knew the patients surprisingly well, it is obvious that some minor (psychiatric) illness periods that the probands might have experienced long ago, might easily not have come to the present G.P.s' notice. Also, it is likely that such episodes would be forgotten by relatives and key informants or ascribed as symptoms of the terminal illness of the proband. On the other hand, the fact that all the probands were born during a specified period of time made it possible to search manually the files of all institutions, including those of psychiatrists working outside of hospitals, where the probands might possibly have sought treatment or made other forms of contact on account of their disorder. The cross-checking of information from different sources was valuable in a number of instances and increased the efficiency of the case identification. In addition to the institutions mentioned earlier, where information was sought, an attempt was made to find the elementary school records of the probands and retrieve their grades at final examination. For a number of reasons these have not been used so far. As the probands finished their elementary school shortly after schooling became compulsory in Iceland, it was only possible to find the grades for about 70% of the cohort.

Because of the extensive sources of information it is unlikely that many probands with major disorders have escaped attention. On the other hand, it is likely that a number of minor illness episodes have not been registered, especially those occurring during the initial observation period. This is partly for the reasons mentioned and partly on account of the limited possibilities for special treatment, i.e., pharmacological treatment, that the G.P.s could offer. It is possible, for instance, that illnesses similar to the mild depressive episodes recorded during the follow-up period might also have occurred at an early age, but went unnoticed or unrecorded as no antidepressive drugs were available at that time. The estimate of disease expectancy given here should therefore be regarded as minimal rates.

In addition to the possible deficiencies in the case identification, some problems in the calculation of disease expectancy should be mentioned. The expectancy may be estimated for a certain age period, and a group of diseases such as functional psychoses may be treated as one disorder (Helgason, 1964, 1981). The expectancy may also be estimated for a lifetime, as in this paper, with regard to manic-depressive psychosis, schizophrenia, alcohol abuse, personality disorders, and subnormality (Helgason, 1964) and the total expectancy estimated as the aggregate of that of the specific disorders. This, of course, can give different results. The expectancy of developing a mental disorder before the average age of 61 years was estimated to be 34% (Helgason, 1964). The expectancy of developing a mental disorder identified from that age before the average age of 75 years is estimated to be 16.5% (Helgason, 1980). In the present paper the expectancy of developing a mental disorder before the age of 75 years is estimated for separate disorders and the aggregate expectancy for all mental disorders is estimated by adding the rates for the specific disorders and found to be 50%. The estimation of the expectancy would be more correct by excluding those who have already contracted a mental disorder from the population at risk. This is of minor importance when considering each disorder separately, but when considering all mental disorders together it has considerable influence on the estimate. The estimates of the risk of a previously mentally healthy person at the age of 61 years to develop a mental disorder before the age of 75 years would be 27%-28%, which is considerably higher than the estimate for the whole cohort mentioned above (Helgason, 1980). Due to the difficulties in identifying minor disorders and their age at onset in the initial study a similar calculation on the basis of the data collected in 1957 is of scant value.

Hagnell (1966), in his study of psychiatric morbidity in a small community in southern Sweden over a period of 10 years, estimated the disease expectancy from the inception rates among persons without known mental illness. Consequently, his estimates are higher than those based on the total population. But the majority of the difference between Hagnell's estimates and those reported here is accounted for by differences in research strategies. His approach will lead to identification of more mild cases because the observation period is much shorter and because he was able to interview all the probands alive personally.

The results of the present study and those of Fremming's study from the Danish island of Bornholm, which was carried out with the same methodology, proved to be very similar for comparable diagnostic categories. Although rigorously standardized techniques of history-taking and examination are the best methods of obtaining clinical data for comparative epidemiologic studies, the results of the present study and Fremming's study suggest that it is possible to obtain valid clinical data for such studies if the psychiatric-medical training of the clinicians collecting the data is similar.

"In psychiatry as in other branches of medicine, epidemiological inquiry is designed to measure the risk of attack by specific disorders within communities and to uncover clues about their origin and mode of spread. These clues are gleaned from the distribution of disease in relation to time and space or the distinguishing characteristics of the individuals or social groupings affected" (Reid, 1960). The results of the present study hardly go beyond the object of measuring the risk of attack by specific disorders in the community. This in itself is an important piece of information because it tells something about the magnitude of the problem, which in turn ought to alert those responsible for delivery of services and for education of doctors and other health workers to the necessity of increased service and better education about mental health and illness. It is also important to know the disease expectancy of the general population in order to be able to compare with the expectancy in high risk groups, e.g., relatives of patients with mental illness. Furthermore, a similar study of a younger cohort ought to give an idea of possible changes in frequency, patterns, and outcome of mental illness. Also, it will be possible to study the psychiatric morbidity among the descendants of selected groups within this cohort.

The comparison of expectancy rates between men and women shows that mental illness occurs with similar frequency among both sexes, but as different syndromes. This is reflected in the high expectancy of alcohol abuse and moderate expectancy of neuroses among men and high expectancy of neuroses and low expectancy of alcohol abuse among women. The obvious epidemiologic hypothesis is that these disorders have some common etiologic factors. This is not news to psychiatrists and it has been substantiated by clinical research long ago (Bleuler, 1955). This hypothesis could be tested by studying a new cohort that has been subject to different attitudes towards alcohol and increasing per capita consumption of alcohol. Thus studies of this type can be used to support or generate etiological hypothesis of psychiatric syndromes.

Summary

Psychiatric, medical, and demographic information has been collected for a cohort of 5,395 persons. The cohort consists of all Icelanders born 1895-1897, who survived until the age of 13-15 years. Information was initially collected until July 1, 1957, or until the probands' death. Information of psychiatric diagnostic relevance could be obtained for 99.8% of the cohort. Follow-up information has later been collected for those who remained alive in Iceland in 1957 until July 1, 1971, when those still alive were at the age of 74-76 years.

A total of 2,082 probands were identified as having had a mental disorder. From these data the disease expectancy for different diagnostic groups as well as for mental disorders in general was estimated. The latter is estimated to be about 50%, similar for men and women, while the expectancy for functional psychoses is estimated to be 4.8% for men and 7.8% for women. Mental disorders are a major cause of disability among those alive at the age of 60-62 years as well as among those alive at the age of 74-76 years. Most mental disorders except neuroses involve excess mortality.

Problems related to case identification in the study and to the estimation of disease expectancy are discussed briefly.

References

Bleuler, M. (1955), Familial and personal background of chronic alcoholics. In: *Etiology of Chronic Alcoholism*, ed. O. Diethelm. Springfield, Ill.: Charles C. Thomas.

Fremming, K.H. (1947), *Sygdomsrisikoen for Sindslidelser* (The expectancy of mental disorders). Copenhagen: Munksgaard.

Fremming, K.H. (1951), The expectation of mental infirmity in a sample of the Danish population. *Occasional Papers on Eugenics*, No. 7. London: Cassell.

Goldhamer, H. & A. Marshall (1953), *Psychosis And Civilization*. Glencoe, Ill.: Free Press.

Hagnell, O. (1966), *A Prospective Study of the Incidence of Mental Disorder*. Stockholm: Svenska Bokforlaget.

Helgason, T. (1954),Talning ge$\phi\phi$g taugasjuklinga 15. marz 1953 (Prevalence of nervous and mental disorder). Reykjavík, mimeographed, 1954.

Helgason, T. (1964), The epidemiology of mental disorder in Iceland. *Acta Psychiatr Scand*, Suppl 173.

Helgason, T. (1980), Epidemiological follow-up research within a geographically stable population. In: *Ziele, Methoden und Ergebnisse der Psychiatrischen Verlaufsforschung*, ed. G.W. Schimmelpenning. Bern: Hans Huber.

Helgason, T. (1979), Epidemiological investigation concerning affective disorders. In: *Origin, Prevention and Treatment of Affective Disorders*, eds. M. Shou & E. Stromgren. London: Academic Press.

Helgason, T. (1981), Psychiatric epidemiological studies in Iceland. In: *Longitudinal Research. Methods and Uses in Behavioural Science*, eds., F. Schulsinger, S. Mednick, and J. Knop. Boston: Martinus Nijhoff.

Klemperer, J. (1933), Zur Belastungsstatistik der Durchschnittsbevölkerung: Psychosenhaufigkeit unter 1000 stichprobenmässig ausgelesenen Probanden. *Z Ges Neurol Psychiat* 146:277-316.

Reid, D.D. (1960), Epidemiological methods in the study of mental disorders. World Health Organization, Public Health Paper No. 2.

Strömgren, E. (1935), Zum Ersatz des Weinbergschen "abgekürzten Verfahrens." *Z Ges Neurol Psychiat* 153:784-797.

Strömgren, E. (1956), Psykiatri, 5th Edition. Copenhagen: Munksgaard.

Stjórnartíðindi, C-deild (1896-1898), Mannfjöldi 1895-1897. (Population in Iceland). Reykjavık: Landshagskynslur.

World Health Organization (1951), Expert committee on mental health: Report on the first session of the alcholism subcommittee. World Health Organization Technical Report Series 42.

World Health Organization (1952), Expert committee on mental health: Alcoholism subcommittee, second report. World Health Organization Technical Report Series 48.

Chapter 13

Community Surveys of Emotional Disorders in Israel: An Updated Review

---

ITZHAK LEVAV
URI AVIRAM

Israel gained its independence only in 1948, but it is a state of people with an ancient history. This discontinuity is due to the destruction of the previous Jewish state by the Romans in 70 A.D., followed by dispersion of the population over almost the entire world. Although there has always been a remnant of the old community in the territory of what is today Israel, the majority have been in exile. Thus in 1882 it was estimated that only 0.3% of the world Jewry was living in the Holy Land. By the time of independence, that proportion had risen to 5.6%. Today it is over 20% (Central Bureau of Statistics, 1979). This increase in the population is due essentially to three immigratory waves: one, the return to the homeland promoted by Zionism, a movement aimed at the attainment of an independent Jewish State; second, to the large masses of former concentration camp survivors who left Europe for Israel at the end of World War II; and third, to the migration of nearly the entire population of Jews from Islamic countries shortly after independence.

By now, the Israeli Jewish population, which numbers slightly over 3 million, is equally divided between native and foreign born citizens. The paternal place of birth of the native born, which is an indication of origin, is as follows: 10.3%, Israel; 16.3% Europe and America; and 24.3% Asia and Africa. The origin of the foreign born is 22.1% from Asia and Africa and 27.0% from Europe and America.

Most of the Israeli Jewish population (90.6%) live in urban localities. The remainder 9.4% live in rural areas, mostly in cooperative settlements (4.4% live in moshavim and 3.3% in kibbutzim) (Central Bureau of Statistics, 1979; Weintraub, Lissak and Azmon, 1969).

This singular sociodemographic composition in a country of small dimensions (20,325 square kilometers, which is smaller than the state of New

Jersey), coupled with the availability of detailed population records, has turned Israel into a close-to-ideal laboratory for studies of psychiatric epidemiology. Of the long list of subjects bearing on substantive issues in this field, four suffice to illustrate the opportunities provided by such a research setting.

1. As the home of an unusually large number of ethnic groups of Jewish origin, which are culturally *(Encyclopaedia Judaica,* 1972) and genetically heterogeneous (Mourant, et al. 1978), Israel provides advantages to study issues regarding ethnicity and mental illness. The ethnic mosaic becomes even more varied among the Israeli minorities, who comprise close to 1/7th of the total population.
2. Opportunities for studying the effects of migration on mental health are enhanced by the fact that about 50% of the Israeli Jewish population is foreign born. Furthermore, factors of selection that contaminate most work on the effects of migration have not operated in some communities. In the case of the Yemenites, for example, the entire group left the country of origin, Yemen, to arrive at the same destination at one time.
3. Studies on the effects of the sociocultural environment on mental disorders (Dohrenwend and Dohrenwend, 1974) are greatly facilitated by the presence of contrasting social organizations. These range from the individualistic urban settings, to intermediate forms such as cooperative settlements (moshavim) in the rural areas, ending with the total collectivism of the kibbutzim (Weintraub, Lissak and Azmon, 1969).
4. Finally, the ongoing state of military-political hostility in the Middle East provides an opportunity to investigate the effects of a major stressor on an entire population (Breznitz, 1980).

Of the procedural and methodological factors that turn Israel into an advantageous site for epidemiologic research, the organization of medical services is noteworthy. This system, similar to the one in the United Kingdom, requires that the entire population be registered with a primary medical care clinic. Israeli researchers have capitalized on the resulting records and resources in order to conduct their studies.

Of further benefit to researchers is the Psychiatric Case Register, (Miller, 1964). This register, created in 1952, cumulatively records all admissions and discharges of inpatients in private and public psychiatric facilities nationwide. The statistics based on the register have supplied the raw material for a number of useful publications (e.g., Gampel, 1970, 1976; Mandel-Popper et al., 1971; Gershon and Liebowitz, 1975). With one exception, these papers are not reviewed here since they deal with treated prevalence rates only. It has been shown (Dohrenwend and Dohrenwend, 1969) that although treated rates of disorders may be derived from the clearest definition of what constitutes a case, they do not represent the total picture depicting the emotional burden on a community. That is because patient status depends on factors other than psychopathology, such as the attitudes of the public toward mental illness (Zohar, et al., 1974; Levav, et al., 1974); the knowledge, attitudes and practices of key referral agents such as general practitioners (Link, et al., 1982); the physical distance to a facility (Dunham, 1961); or simply the availability of services. As Cooper and Morgan (1973) very aptly put it, "treatment represents the assignment that a society makes of its gross national product to the care of its sick members."

Only studies based on community surveys are reviewed here, including six that have been reported in the literature (Maoz et al., 1966; Hoek et al., 1965; Abramson, 1966b; Polliack, 1971; Wamosher, 1972; Levav and Arnon, 1976) and one not yet in print (Menkes, unpublished). Despite the risk of inconsistency, one study based on first admissions of Jerusalem residents to the local inpatient psychiatric facilities will be included because of its special interest to epidemiologists. It provides data on demographic and sociocultural correlates of affective disorders (Gershon and Liebowitz, 1975), which are known to be higher among Jews than non-Jews (Malzberg, 1973).

The Studies

Table 1 summarizes the studies conducted so far: one in an immigrant town (Maoz, et al., 1966); three in the city of Jerusalem (Hoek et al., 1965; Abramson, 1966b; Gershon and Liebowitz, 1975); one in a neighborhood of a middle-size city (Polliack, 1971), and three in rural cooperative settlements (Wamosher, 1972; Levav and Arnon, 1976; and Menkes, unpublished).

Maoz and colleagues (1966) carried out the first community study in 1961. They surveyed the adult population of Kiryat Shmona, which was at the time a developing town mostly settled by newly arrived immigrants. Their casefinding method was based on data collected from medical and nonmedical agencies on recognized deviant behavior. The medical agencies constituted an excellent source since well over 90% of the population were insured in the Worker's Sick Fund of the General Federation of Labour. The majority of the cases were identified through the screening of the medical records. The case identification was completed by information obtained from other community agencies: public health nurses, police, welfare offices, and a probation agency. The disorders were classified according to the nomenclature of the American Psychiatric Association. Maoz et al. (1966) identified 247 cases, which yielded a prevalence rate of 4.5%.

Two years later Hoek et al. (1965) studied a subsection (a lower class immigrant housing development) of a neighborhood in Jerusalem. The community consisted of 963 adults aged 20 and over. The authors found 200 subjects who matched their operational definition of mental disorder, a prevalence of 20.8%.

The third survey was conducted in the same neighborhood and at about the same time as the Hoek study. It was the first door-to-door survey and it relied on the use of the full version of the Cornell Medical Index (CMI) as a method for case identification (Abramson, 1965). The prevalence, as defined by scores of 30 or above on this index for a random sample of 970

TABLE 1
Community Surveys of Emotional Disorders in Israel.

Author	Location	Population	Objectives	Method of Case Identification	Rates in %		
					Both	Men	Women
Maoz et al. 1965	Kiryat Shmona (immigrant town)	5,447 aged 20 and over	1. Prevalence of disorders 2. Association with ethnicity	Records search	4.5	4.2	4.9
Hoek et al. 1965	Kiryat Yovel (neighborhood in Jerusalem)	963 adults aged 20 and over	As above	G.P.'s appraisal	20.8	18.8	22.4
Abramson 1966	Kiryat Yovel (neighborhood in Jerusalem)	Random sample 970 respondents aged 20 and over	1. Prevalence of disorders 2. Association with status inconsistency	Full version of CMI[a]	45.5[b]	32.7	55.7
Polliak 1971	General practice in town of Herzlia	454 Married couples	1. Prevalence of disorders 2. Association with attendance at G.P. clinic	As above	43.0[b]	35.0	51.0

TABLE 1 (Continued)

Author	Location	Population	Objectives	Method of Case Identification	Rates in % Both	Men	Women
Wamosher 1972	General practice in three cooperative settlements (2 moshavim and 1 kibbutz)	778 Adults aged 20 and over	As above	1. G.P.'s recording of psychosis, neurosis, and personality disorders 2. Full version of CMI	37.8	25.2	49.8 (with CMI)
Menkes 1974	2 communal settlements (moshavim)	233 Adults aged 20 and over	Effect of community dis-organization on prevalence rates	1. Records search 2. 22 item Langner scale	Not reported		
Gershon & Liebowitz 1975	Jerusalem	Aged 15 and over	Association of affective disorders with sociocultural & demographic variables	First admissions (Psychiatric Case Register)	0.2[c] (all disorders) 0.04 (affective disorders)		
Levav & Arnon 1976	General practice in 6 cooperative settlements (moshavim)	896 Adults aged 20 and over	1. Prevalence of disorders 2. Association with attendance at G.P. clinic	1. Review of G.P.'s records 2. Shortened version of CMI	18.9	16.3	21.5 (both methods)

[a]CMI: Cornell Medical Index
[b]Calculated by us
[c]Figures are all for prevalence rates except for [c]which is an incidence rate.

respondents, was double the rate found in the study by Hoek et al. (1965)—45.5% (Abramson, 1966b).

The burden of the emotional disorders on a general practice was explored by Polliack (1971). His study was prompted by his impression that he was providing primary medical care to "consultation prone" families whose illness behaviors were, in all likelihood, reflecting an emotional disorder. Polliack also used the CMI as an instrument for case identification. The population he studied consisted 454 married couples who were insured members of the Worker's Sick Fund Clinic, for which Polliack was responsible. In this study, which was intended to relate prevalence rates to attendance at the clinic, he found the rate among men to be 35% and 51% among women; using the same cutoff as Abramson (1966).

Wamosher (1972) reported the first study conducted in rural settings—two moshavim and one kibbutz (the only one, to date, done in a kibbutz). The author was, at the time of the study, the general practitioner (GP) of those settlements and had been for the previous 10 years. He used a double method of case identification: (A) the complete CMI questionnaire and (B) notes he made in the medical records on the presence of neurosis, psychosis, and personality disorders. The population studied consisted of 769 adults. Wamosher, as all other authors, found that men scored lower than women (25.2% versus 49.8%).

Menkes studied a pair of rural villages settled by Jews of Kurdistan origin. She found that those two settlements were characterized by contrasting levels of social organization-disorganization, providing a suitable natural setting to investigate Leighton's theory on the relation between the social environment and mental illness (Leighton, 1966). Her study, which included 233 adults, used a double method of case identification: record searches in the medical clinics, psychiatric facilities, and welfare offices, as well as the administration of the 22-item Langner scale (Langner, 1962). She found a mean of 4.2 symptoms in the organized village, and 6.1 in the disorganized one. Twenty percent of the probands in the organized village had no symptoms on the Langner scale, compared with only 7.0% in the disorganized village.

Levav and Arnon (1976) studied the distribution of emotional disorders among 686 adults living in six villages (moshavim). They used both the medical records and a screening instrument consisting of two shortened versions of the CMI (Abramson, 1965; Eastwood, 1970; Levav, Arnon and Portnoy, 1977) to identify possible psychiatric cases. Combining both methods of case identification, they found a prevalence rate of 16.3% among the men and 21.5% among the women.

Finally, Gershon and Liebowitz (1975) reported their study based on the Psychiatric Case Register. It included all first admissions of Jerusalem residents suffering from primary affective illness during a period of 3 years. They found an average yearly treated incidence rate of 0.04% for the population 15 years of age and older.

Critical Analysis

The following discussion focuses on three aspects: the study objectives, the methods used and the results obtained.

Some general considerations first. Given the diversity of the country, it is noteworthy that no survey was conducted on a nationwide basis. It would seem that the community studies were almost all selected out of convenience rather than for their representativeness of the total Israeli population. This lack of representativeness, compounded by an unsatisfactory description of the populations in some studies, precludes generalizations of some of the findings. However, this limitation applies more to descriptive statistics such as prevalence of mental disorders rather than to theoretically relevant findings such as those of Abramson (1966b).

A second common feature of the studies is the lower age limit of the population under investigation—20 years. The only exception is the study by Gershon and Liebowitz (1975), which also included respondents 5 years younger. The cutoff age of 20 was chosen since that is approximately the age at which soldiers return home upon release from compulsory military service and records on them again become available. Therefore, the rates of the disorders that affect the younger population await investigation.

No survey has yet reported on the impairment of the social functioning caused by psychopathology (Dohrenwend and Dohrenwend, 1973); except, minimally, for Hoek et al.'s (1965) and Levav and Arnon's (1976) studies in which the association between the emotional status and the attendance rates to the social welfare office was, to some extent, investigated.

In some ways analogous to much of the work in the United States (cf., Weissman and Myers, 1978), community-wide prevalence of *specific* psychiatric disorders are unavailable in Israel. Maoz et al.'s study (1965) hardly constitutes an exception because it was based on recognized cases only. Furthermore, the diagnostic reliability never was spelled out.

Objectives of the Studies

Three of the surveys (Maoz et al., 1966; Wamosher, 1972; Levav and Arnon, 1976) specifically intended to establish overall prevalence rates of emotional disorders. These objectives were not always fully met however, except for Levav and Arnon's study (1976), because there was incomplete coverage of the full range of disorders (Maoz et al., 1966; Wamosher, 1972).

Review of the study aims shows that aside from descriptive purposes, several of them had built-in analytic objectives. Abramson's investigation (1966b) sought to establish the degree of association between emotional disorders and the status inconsistency created in the migratory process. Maoz et al. (1966), Hoek et al. (1965) and Gershon and Liebowitz (1975) sought to determine the role of ethnicity in the rate of disorders. The role of other universal variables such as age, sex, education, social class and length of stay in the country—a measure of acculturation—were also investigated. Menkes research (unpublished) attempted to test Leighton's theory of social disintegration.

Whether made explicit or only tangentially suggested, all the studies that were based on a general practice clinic (Hoek et al., 1965; Polliack, 1971; Wamosher, 1972; Levav and Arnon, 1976) had additional objectives such as the effect of the emotional status on the frequency of the contacts with the clinic.

Methods and Procedures

Israeli studies show marked differences in the prevalence rates of emotional disorder (see Results). It seems that such differences are largely accounted by the methods used for case identification. In this respect, Israeli community surveys have been affected by problems of measurement just as most studies conducted elsewhere. Indeed, Dohrenwend and Dohrenwend (1969), in their review of psychiatric epidemiological studies carried out in many countries over several decades, found that the prevalence of psychiatric disorders varied from 1% to 64%. It is clear from their analysis that those values were more a function of the methods used, particularly those to determine what constitutes a case and how to identify it, rather than a true expression of distribution of the disorders in the populations.

A review of the research design shows that except for two studies (Maoz et al., 1966; Gershon and Liebowitz, 1975) all obtained their data from surveys conducted in a community. Thus they are the only ones that meet the criteria for true prevalence studies. Although the authors in one of the studies (Maoz et al., 1966) claimed that they surveyed the total community, they actually relied on "known cases" and no method was used to uncover cases unknown to the agencies.

The methods of case identification used throughout the true prevalence studies can be grouped into two categories (see table 1). The first one relied on the judgment made by general practitioners as to the presence of an emotional disorder in the population they served. The other was based on the administration of the CMI. Two studies used a combination of both methods (Wamosher, 1972; Levav and Arnon, 1976), a strategy that reduced the number of "false positives" identified by either method. Thus it is no surprise that rates were lower when both methods were combined (men, 16.3%; women, 21.5%) as compared with results of one method only (men, 28.5%; women, 41.3%) (Levav and Arnon, 1976).

It is interesting that except for one community study (Levav and Arnon, 1976), where a psychiatrist made indirect assessments based on the GP's records, no psychiatrist was a member of the casefinding team, an issue which bears on validity (Cooper and Morgan, 1973) although in all the studies the general practitioners were well acquainted with their population. The neurotic label could easily be ascribed to a respondent (client) who is an "overuser" of the clinic, a behavior that might give rise to negative countertransference feelings on the part of the GP. On the other hand, an "underuser" could be spared such a label, though this behavior is far from being incompatible with emotional disorder (Shepherd et al., 1966). In short, studies have shown that cases can be missed since recognition depends in part on attitudinal factors as well as extensiveness of contact (Shepherd et al., 1966;

Link et al., 1982). Furthermore, the appraisal remains a private intellectual activity, and unless its process is made explicit, replication—a necessary condition in epidemiologic research—is prevented. The definition of how a case was appraised was fully made in Levav and Arnon's study (1976), only partially in Hoek et al.'s (1966), and was absent in Wamosher's (1972). Reliability tests were, however, somewhat deficient in all three.

The alternate method used for case identification in the Israeli surveys has been the CMI, either in its full (195 questions) or in two shortened versions (10 and 19 questions respectively). The CMI was widely used in the United States years ago (Brodman et al., 1952) and in England (Culpan, Davies and Oppenheim, 1960; Hamilton et al., 1962). Its merits range from the encouraging early reports to more sober ones such as Shepherd et al.'s (1966) in their study of general practices in London that reported unsatisfactory misclassification rates. It was introduced in Israel by Kark et al. (1963) in a study of the health of undergraduate students and has been used a number of times ever since (Abramson, 1966a).

Abramson et al. (1965) used general practitioners' appraisals as criteria for a validity test they conducted with the full version of the CMI. The sensitivity and specificity they obtained were considered adequate for use in epidemiologic studies. They also found that 13 of the 195 questions were at least 10 times more likely to be answered affirmatively by the group of "emotionally disturbed persons" as defined by GPs than by the group of "emotionally healthy" persons. After discarding three items that were noncontributory they found a moderate correlation (R = 0.63) between the number of positive replies to the ten questions and the total CMI score. The 10-item CMI questionnaire was subjected to a new validity test by Levav, Arnon and Portnoy (1977) and by Abramson and Levav (1978).

Levav et al. (1977) used two groups for a test of validity: treated patients and a psychiatrist's appraisal on the degree of "caseness" of the population (Leighton et al., 1963) as well as a grading of the emotional ill health (Abramson, 1965) made independently by the GP of the research team. The results show that the capacity of the shortened versions of the CMI was grossly affected by factors other than the respondent's emotional status. Females were more likely to give positive answers to CMI items than males at the same level of "caseness." Age also introduced an artifact, with older people giving a higher number of positive replies for the same psychiatric degree of "caseness." Ethnicity was the third factor that confounded the results, as African- and Asian-born respondents had higher scores in the CMI than the European- and the Israeli-born respondents, controlling for "caseness" rating. A later reexamination of the data by Abramson and Levav (1978) using analysis of variance essentially confirmed the above results. This reanalysis, however, unconfounded ethnicity and education by showing that the differences in ethnicity were largely a reflection of education. As for the contribution of the emotional ill health to the CMI scores, the further analyses showed that the variance explained by the CMI responses was only 3.6%, while the proportion reached 10.2% when no control was made of the other variables (age, ethnicity, sex, and education). All five factors accounted for 37.5% of the variance of the total scores. The authors conservatively concluded that it is "justifiable to use [the CMI] to measure emotional ill health in epidemiological studies, but they should be used only when better methods are not available."

Results

The Range in the Rates

Table 1 shows a considerable degree of variation in the prevalence of emotional disorders obtained in the studies under review. The highest one (Abramson, 1966b) was 10 times higher than the lowest rate (Maoz et al., 1966). As discussed earlier, chances are that the variation merely reflects the methods used for case identification. Indeed, the studies that used the CMI obtained higher rates than those that relied on other methods for case identification. In one study two sets of rates were obtained depending on the method used (Levav and Arnon, 1976).

Given those results, one should hope that a more accurate answer to the current puzzling picture as to the distribution of mental morbidity in the community will be rendered by the newly available screening and diagnostic instruments with higher validity and reliability (Dohrenwend et al., 1984).

Sex and Rate of Psychopathology

The overall prevalence of emotional disorders found in women was consistently higher than in men, similar to findings of other community studies conducted elsewhere (Dohrenwend and Dohrenwend, 1976). There are, however, methodologic issues to be solved before substantial conclusions can be reached: the higher rates among women could be the result of the use of an instrument more sensitive in eliciting responses from one sex than another (Dohrenwend and Dohrenwend, 1976). Indeed, the difference in the overall rates between the sexes was higher when the CMI was used for case identification.

As for specific disorders, both Hoek et al. (1965) and Maoz et al. (1966), found higher rates of neuroses among women and higher rates of personality disorders among men. Hoek et al. (1965) found 12.4% of neuroses among women compared with 3.7% among men, while personality disorders among men were almost three times higher than among women (8.5%; 2.8%). The prevalence of psychosis was negligibly higher among women (2.4%) than among men (2.0%). The sex difference in the rates of specific disorders was proportionally smaller in Maoz et al.'s study (1966) but nevertheless present. This finding is consistent with those reported in the literature (Dohrenwend and Dohrenwend, 1974).

Arnon and Levav (1979) recently reported findings on the rates of psychosomatic disorders made during the course of the epidemiologic study they conducted some years earlier (Levav and Arnon, 1976). Their operational definition of what constitutes a psychosomatic disorder was adopted from earlier British studies (Sainsbury, 1960; Kreitman et al., 1966). Though the conceptual domain of those disorders is ambiguous (Eastwood and Trevelyan, 1972), it is nevertheless interesting that Arnon and Levav found a differential distribution of the rates by sex, since the psychosomatic disorders are incorporated into the definition of "caseness" B and C according to Leighton et al. (1963). Such a definition was indeed followed by Levav and Arnon (1976) in their survey. It was precisely in degree of "caseness" B and C that they found higher rates for women, and that difference was largely due to the presence of psychosomatic disorders.

Finally, Gershon and Liebowitz (1975) found that the ratio of the incidence rates of affective disorders for women to men was 2:1 as in most other studies. The age of onset in women was earlier than in men.

Types of Psychopathology

Only three studies reported rates of specific disorder (Hoek et al., 1965; Maoz et al., 1966; Gershon and Liebowitz, 1975). All others applied methods with which diagnoses cannot be obtained.

Maoz et al. (1966) found a prevalence of 1.2% for psychosis, 1.5% for neuroses, and 1.1% for personality disorders. The authors indicated that their figures for psychoses and neuroses were lower than those found in other surveys. Here again the same methodologic issue raised earlier, namely, the problem of case identification, would serve as an initial explanation for the findings. However, other factors such as the cultural gap between physicians and patients could have affected the recognition and diagnosis of some disorders, as suggested by Shanan and Moses (1961).

Hoek et al. (1965) found a somewhat different distribution: 2.2% psychosis, 8.4% neurosis, 5.3% personality disorders, 0.4% organic disorders, and 4.4% psychophysiologic disorders. The proportion of the different types of psychopathology had a higher congruency with other findings than those above.

Gershon and Liebowitz (1975) reported an incidence of 0.2% for all disorders for the population aged 15 years and over. That figure is almost double that for Jews in New York State (Malzberg, 1973). However, the first admission rate for affective disorders in the Jerusalem study (0.04%) was similar to those reported in other countries such as the United States and Denmark.

Age and Rates of Disorders

In spite of its interest, the issue of age and rates of disorders remains inconclusive, largely because of methodologic problems. The studies that used the CMI were affected by an age-related bias of the instrument (Levav, Arnon and Portnoy, 1977). Also, those that used the GP's appraisal were not bias-free. It is quite reasonable to assume that when physical disorders were present—a common occurrence as age increases—along with emotional symptoms, the GP tended to concentrate on physical disorders in diagnosing, recording, and treating and to play down the importance of emotional symptoms. The only consistent findings for all the studies was that the youngest group ages 20 to 30 had the lowest rate of emotional disorders. The special disorders of the elderly (e.g., organic brain syndromes) have not been studied in community surveys in Israel, though the proportion of the aged in the general population has been rapidly increasing.

Rates by Place of Birth

Studies based on treated rates have reported higher figures for the native-born than for foreign-born (Murphy, 1961; Gershon and Liebowitz, 1975). Those results contrast with those obtained in community surveys. Thus Abramson (1966b) found a prevalence of 4% in the age group 20-29 among the Israeli-born while it was over 6 times higher for the foreign-born. The rates for Israeli- and foreign-born women in the same age group were 28% and 53% respectively. Abramson's results are of interest since place of birth was unconfounded with social class. Levav and Arnon (1976) controlled for education and sex when they compared rates between native and foreign-born. Their results were identical to those in the previous study, but the difference between both groups dropped when education was held constant.

On variations between ethnic groups, Abramson (1966b) found no consistent differences in the prevalence of high CMI scores when he compared respondents born in Europe, America, North Africa, and Asia. However, as noted earlier, there are serious reservations about the CMI as a screening device. Also, the appropriateness of grouping respondents whose ethnic-dependent status differ according to the specific country of origin must be considered (Peres, 1977).

Of major interest is the extent to which different types of psychopathology are distributed in various ethnic groups. Maoz et al. (1966) reported relevant data, though their grouping of the respondents into three large regions of origin—Europe, North Africa, and Asia—is questionable. They found a higher prevalence rate for all disorders among Asian immigrants than for those from Africa. But it was among the latter where rates of personality disorders were higher. Close to 60% of those diagnosed as having a personality disorder came from North Africa while the proportion of this group in the general population was 45%. Almost all the cases (80%) were men. The authors also mentioned that the high rate of neurosis among Asians found in their study was largely due to the high rates among immigrant women from Iran. These findings remain unexplained since they were not pursued beyond description.

Gershon and Liebowitz (1975) showed that affective disorders were significantly associated with European-American origin. The incidence found was 0.06% for this group, contrasting with the group of African-Asian origin for which it was one third lower. Rates are not available for the Israeli-born according to their ethnic ancestry, but the authors have argued that the findings for the native-born would in fact have replicated those for the foreign-born. Further analysis by the authors showed that ethnic origin, being part of two other sociocultural factors (socioeconomic and immigrant status), explained less of the variance than demographic variables such as age, sex, and marital status. But it was the single sociocultural variable that retained some effect after the others were controlled.

Rural-Urban Living and Rates of Emotional Disorders

There is a widely held belief that the social stress associated with urban living produces higher rates of psychopathology. Consistent with this, Dohrenwend and Dohrenwend (1974b) have carefully documented that the median rate for the studies conducted in urban settings was higher than for those in rural areas.

Three of the Israeli studies under review are susceptible to such comparison since all of them shared an identical casefinding method, the full version of the CMI. Two were carried out in a city (Abramson, 1966; Polliack, 1971) and one in a rural area (Wamosher, 1972). In the one in the rural area, the rate was somewhat lower (37.8%) than in the other two (45.5% and 43.0% respectively). However, before it is concluded that the rates are indeed a true reflection of reality, further tests are needed to eliminate the effect of spurious factors (e.g., educational level in the contrasting populations) that affect the interpretation of the data and to check on historical-genetic factors that bear on the explanation of the data. Fortunately, the recent constitution of the country and the availability of records and documents allow inquiry into factors that border on an explanatory hypothesis.

Social Class and Rate of Disorders

A most conspicuous result in psychiatric epidemiology studies has been the inverse relationship between social class and rates of disorders (Dohrenwend and Dohrenwend, 1969). The Israeli studies are no exception whether using the CMI in case finding (Abramson, 1966b; Polliack, 1971) or a "caseness" rating based on the examination of the medical records (Levav and Arnon, 1976). Polliack (1971), using occupation as an indicator of social class, found that the proportion of highest scores in the CMI ranged from a lowest 20% in the upper class to a highest 55%, in the lowest class. However, he did not unconfound ethnicity. Abramson (1966b), in addition to the overall result, found that the higher prevalence rates were associated with status inconsistency, a discrepancy between the educational level of the respondent and his/her occupational attainment. Levav and Arnon (1976), controlling for ethnicity as well as for age and sex, found marked differences in the rates especially when respondents with and without education were compared.

Conclusion

It was stated at the start that Israel constitutes a true social laboratory for psychiatric epidemiologic work. Has this natural setup been fully utilized by researchers? Let us summarize the partially affirmative answer this question deserves. Several studies have been conducted so far. They have shown higher rates of disorders for women, urban dwellers, lower classes, those with a discrepancy between education and occupation, those living in a disorganized community, and those in age groups older than 20-30 years.

They have also provided some evidence for differential distributions of psychopathology by ethnicity and by sex.

Regrettably, all the studies have been seriously affected by unsolved problems of reliability and validity in their methods. Previous reviewers (Aviram and Levav, 1975) have called for efforts to develop measures of untreated emotional disorders. Fortunately, there are now two screening instruments available for use in psychiatric epidemiology studies in Israel. One is the Psychiatric Epidemiology Research Interview (PERI), which has undergone stringent tests for internal consistency, reliability, and concurrent criterion of validity. The PERI has proved reliable in both sexes as well as in different ethnic and educational groups, a *sine qua non* for studies of communities of heterogeneous composition. The second instrument that has undergone a validity test is the Middlesex Hospital Questionnaire, which seems promising for use in general practice clinics (Dasbert and Shalif, 1978). However, more definitive results are still required from further methodologic work for this instrument. In addition to the screening devices, the Schedule for Affective Disorders and Schizophrenia (SADS) a diagnostic instrument for a large number of functional disorders (Spitzer and Endicott, 1978), can contribute to case identification and diagnosis in community surveys (Weissman and Myers, 1978). It is now available in a Hebrew version and has been tested in a methodologic study in Israel. SADS-L (a lifetime version of SADS) was found a reliable instrument, acceptable to community respondents as well as to patients (Dohrenwend et al., 1984).

Full advantage has not been taken of this readily available community laboratory. Original epidemiologic work is still wanting in all areas—psychosocial, cultural, demographic, familial-genetic—and research already done needs to be replicated. The recommendations made by Aviram and Levav (1975) saw a need for epidemiologic researchers to select theory-based issues in order to answer basic etiologic questions that continue to intrigue the mental health field. The challenge and the opportunities remain open in a most suitable place for research.

Acknowledgments

We thank Dr. B. P. Dohrenwend for his most useful comments on a first draft of this chapter.

References

Abramson, J. H., Terespolsky, L., Brook, J. G., & Kark, S. L. (1965), The Cornell Medical Index as a health measure in epidemiological studies. *Br J Prevent Soc Med* 19:105-110.

Abramson, J. H. (1966a), The Cornell Medical Index as an epidemiological tool. *Am J Publ Health* 56:287-289.

Abramson, J. H., (1966b), Emotional disorder, status inconsistency and migration: A health questionnaire in Israel, *Milbank Mem Fund Quart* 44:23-48.

Abramson, J. H. & Levav, I. (1978), Use of symptom inventories as measures of emotional ill-health in epidemiological studies, *Internat J Epidemiol* 7:381-383.

Arnon, A. & Levav, I. (1979), Psychosomatic disorders in a rural family practice, *Psychosomatics,* 20:483-491.

Aviram, U. & Levav, I. (1975), Psychiatric epidemiology in Israel: An analysis of community studies, *Acta Psychiatr Scand* 52:295-311.

Breznitz, S. (1980), Stress in Israel. In: *Selye's Guide to Stress Research,* Vol. 1, ed. H. Selye. New York: Van Nostrand-Reinhold.

Brodman, K., Erdmann, Jr., A. J., Lorge, F., Gershenson, C. P. & Wolff, H. G. (1952), The Cornell Medical Index Health Questionnaire III. The evaluation of emotional disturbances, *J Clin Psychol* 8:119-125.

Central Bureau of Statistics (1979), *Statistical Abstract of Israel, 1978,* Jerusalem: Central Bureau of Statistics.

Cooper, B. & Morgan, H. G. (1973), *Epidemiological Psychiatry.* Springfield, Illinois: Charles C. Thomas.

Culpan, R. H., Davies, B. M. & Oppenheim, A. N. (1960), Incidence of psychiatric illness among hospital outpatients: An application of the Cornell Medical Index. *Br Med J* 7:855-857.

Dasberg, H. & Shalif, I. (1978), On the validity of the Middlesex Hospital questionnaire: A comparison of diagnostic self-ratings in psychiatric outpatients, general practice patients, and 'normals' based on the Hebrew version, *Br J Med Psychol* 5:281-291.

Dohrenwend, B. P. & Dohrenwend, B. S. (1969), *Social Status and Psychological Disorder,* New York: John Wiley and Sons.

Dohrenwend, B. S. & Dohrenwend, B. P. (1973), Ability and disability in role functioning in psychiatric patients and nonpatient groups. In: *Roots of Evaluation: An Epidemiological Basis for Planning Psychiatric Services,* ed. J.K. Wing and H. Hafner. New York: Oxford University Press.

Dohrenwend, B. P. & Dohrenwend, B. S. (1974), Social and cultural influences on psychopathology, *Ann Rev Psychol* 25:417-425.

Dohrenwend, B. P. & Dohrenwend, B. S. (1974), Psychiatric disorders in urban settings. In: *American Handbook of Psychiatry,* 2nd Ed. Vol. 2, ed. S. Arieti and G. Kaplan. New York: Basic Books.

Dohrenwend, B. P., Levav, I. & Shrout, P. (1984), Screening scales from the Psychiatric Epidemiology Research Interview (PERI). In: *Community Surveys of Psychological Disorders,* eds. J.K. Myers and M.M. Weissman. New Brunswick, N.J.: Rutgers University Press.

Dohrenwend, B. P. & Dohrenwend, B. S. (1976), Sex differences and psychiatric disorders. *Am J Sociol* 81:1447-1454.

Dunham, H. W. (1961), Social structures and mental disorders: Competing hypotheses of explanation. In: *Causes of Mental Disorders: A Review of Epidemiological Knowledge.* New York: Milbank Memorial Fund.

Eastwood, M. R. (1970), Psychiatric morbidity and physical state in a general practice. In: *Psychiatric Epidemiology,* eds. E.H. Hare and J.K. Wing. London: Oxford University Press.

Eastwood, M. R. & Trevelyan, M. Y. (1972), Psychosomatic disorders in the community, *J Psychosomat Res* 16:381-386.

Encyclopaedia Judaica, (1972). Jersusalem: Keter Publishing House.

Gampel, J. (1970), *Official Bed Provision, Resident Patient and Total Patients in Care in Mental Hospital in Israel, 1948-1970.* Jerusalem: State of Israel, Ministry of Health, Mental Health Services.

Gampel, J. (1976), Epidemiological data on admissions for inpatient psychiatric care in Israel, In: *Toward Community Mental Health Services in Israel*, ed. I. Margulec. Jerusalem: Trust Fund for Development of Mental Health Services.

Gershon, E. S. & Liebowitz, J. H. (1975), Sociocultural and demographic correlates of affective disorders in Jerusalem, *J Psychiatr Res* 12:37-50.

Hamilton, N., Pond, D. A. & Ryle, A. (1962), Relation of CMI responses to some social and psychological factors. *J Psychosomat Res* 6:157-165.

Hoek, A., Moses, R. & Terespolsky, L. (1965), Emotional disorders in an *Israeli immigrant community, Israel Ann Psychiatr Rel Discip* 3:213-228.

Kark, E., Zaslany, A. & Ward, B. (1963), The health of undergraduate students on entry to the Hebrew University in Jerusalem. *Israel Med J* 22:5-8.

Kreitman, K., Pearce, K. I. & Ryle, Y. (1966), The relationship of psychiatric, psychosomatic and organic illness in a general practice. *Br J Psychiatr* 112:569-580.

Langner, T. (1962), A twenty-two item screening score of psychiatric symptoms indicating impairment. *J Health Hum Behav* 3:269-276.

Leighton, D. C., Harding, J. S., Macklin, D. B., MacMillan, A. M. & Leighton, A. H. (1963), *The Character of Danger.* New York: Basic Books.

Leighton, A. H. (1966), Psychiatric disorder and social environment: An outline for a frame of reference. In: *Issues and Problems in Social Psychiatry* eds. B.J. Bergen and C.S. Thomas. Springfield, Illinois: Charles C. Thomas.

Levav, I., Minami, H. & Adler, B. (1974), Mothers and daughters diagnose mental illness. *Israel Ann Psychiatr Rel Discip* 12:319-327.

Levav, I., & Arnon, A. (1976), Emotional disorders in six Israeli villages. *Acta Psychiatr Scand* 53:387-400.

Levav, I., Arnon, A., & Portnoy, A. (1977), Two shortened versions of the Cornell Medical Index: A new test of their validity. *Internat J Epidemiol* 6:135-141.

Link, B., Levav, I. & Cohen, A. (1982), The primary medical care practitioner's attitudes toward psychiatry: An Israeli study. *Soc Sci Med* 16:1413-1420.

Malzberg, B. (1973), Mental disease among Jews in New York State. *Acta Psychiatr Scand* 49:479-488.

Mandel-Popper, M., Gampel, J. & Miller, L. (1971), *Cases That Were Admitted to the Psychiatric Hospitals in Israel, 1966.* Jerusalem: State of Israel, Ministry of Health Services.

Maoz, B. S., Levy, S., Brand, N. & Halevi, H. S. (1966), An epidemiological survey of mental disorders in a community of newcomers to Israel. *J Coll Gen Pract* 77:267-284.

Menkes, A. (Mimeographed), Psychiatric Disorders in Two Comparable Kurdistan Communities in Israel.

Miller, L. (1964), A national programme in the epidemiology of mental disturbance in Israel. Preliminary Communications. *Israel Ann Psychiatr Rel Discip* 2:266-267.

Mourant, A. E., Kopec, A. C., Domaniewska-Sobczak, K. (1978), *The Genetics of the Jews.* Oxford: Clarendon Press.

Murphy, H. B. M. (1961), Social change and mental health. In: *Causes of Mental Disorders: A Review of Epidemiological Knowledge.* New York: Milbank Memorial Fund.

Peres, Y. (1977), *Ethnic Relations in Israel.* Tel Aviv: Sifriat Hapoalim (Hebrew).

Polliack, M. R. (1971), The relationship between Cornell Medical Index scores and attendance rates. *J Roy Coll Gen Pract* 21:453-459.

Sainsbury, P. (1960), Psychosomatic disorders and neurosis in outpatients attending a general hospital. *Psychosomat Res* 4:261-276.

Shanan, J. & Moses, R. (1961), The readiness to offer psychotherapy — its relationship to social background and formulation of complaints. *Arch Gen Psychiat* 4:202-212.

Shepherd, M., Cooper, B., Brown, A. C. & Kalton, G. W. (1966), *Psychiatric Illness in General Practice.* London: Oxford University Press.

Spitzer, R. L. & Endicott, J. (1978), A diagnostic interview: The Schedule for Affective Disorders and Schizophrenia. *Arch Gen Psychiatr* 35:837-844.

Wamosher, L. (1972), The relationship of emotional disorder to the consultation rate in family medicine. *Harefuah* 32:1-4. (Hebrew).

Weintraub, D., Lissak, M. & Azmon, Y. (1969), *Moshava, Kibbutz and Moshav,* Ithaca, N.Y.: Cornell University Press.

Weissman, M. M. & Myers, J. (1978), Affective disorders in a U.S. urban community: The use of Research Diagnostic Criteria in an epidemiological survey. *Arch Gen Psychiatr* 35:1304-1311.

Zohar, M., Floro, S. & Modan, B. (1974), The image of mental illness and the mentally ill in the Israeli society. *Harefuah* 86:8-10 (Hebrew).

Chapter 14

Epidemiologic Surveys of Mental Health of Geographically Defined Populations in Europe

A. JABLENSKY

The term *survey* in this review refers to investigations of mental health and mental morbidity that produce prevalence, incidence, and other data describing geographically defined populations. A population so studied can be large or small, representative or nonrepresentative of a larger universe, but in every case it forms a natural demographic unit based on a delimited territory, rather than a social, ethnic, or occupational category. Studies of mental disorders in particular occupational groups such as students and migrants, will not be reviewed, although the term *survey* can also be applied to them. This restriction is necessary to highlight better a particular type of research that has a longstanding tradition in European psychiatry, parallelled by a similar tradition of enquiry focused on the concept of "community" in European sociology.

Probably more than 100 studies that have taken place in Europe since the end of the 19th century meet the above criterion. A comprehensive review of this material is hardly possible, because not all studies have been published in easily accessible sources. Some selection was therefore unavoidable in this review, but an attempt was made to include both landmark studies in the epidemiologic field and less well-known but original studies. Table 1 lists the main descriptive features of 58 surveys that, in the opinion of the author, are examples of characteristic approaches or have produced results of special interest.

Since the scope of this review is defined by the criterion of a geographically defined population as the object of study, a simple typology of the investigations reviewed can be based on the characteristics of the epidemiologic denominator and the sampling strategy chosen by the investigators. Such a typology is not very different from classifications used in other reviews of the applications of the epidemiologic method in psychiatry (e.g., Reid,

TABLE 1

Descriptive Data on 57 Surveys of Geographically Defined Populations in Europe.

Type of study, author & year of publication	*Country*	*Type and size of population studied*	*Target group or sample investigated*	*Conditions investigated*	*Case-finding approach*	*Method of assessment and diagnosis*	*Remarks*
Birth cohort studies							
Klemperer (1933)	Germany	Urban (city of Munich)	Randomly selected birth cohort 1881-1890 (N=1,000)	Psychoses, mental retardation, epilepsy	Tracing of all probands attempted (44% traced)	Personal examination or key informant interview (271 examined)	
Fremming (1947)	Denmark	Rural, island of Bornholm* (N=40,000)	Full birth cohort 1883-1887 (N=5,500)	All mental disorders	Tracing of all probands (92% traced)	Personal examination	*Same population surveyed by Strömgren (1938)
Helgason, T. (1964)	Iceland	Mixed total (N=85,183 in 1910)	All members of the birth cohort 1895-1897 who were alive in 1910	All mental disorders	Tracing of all probands 99.4% traced)	Hospital records and personal examination	

TABLE 1 (Continued)

Type of study, author & year of publication	*Country*	*Type and size of population studied*	*Target group or sample investigated*	*Conditions investigated*	*Case-finding approach*	*Method of assessment and diagnosis*	*Remarks*
Census & longitudinal studies of whole populations							
Lewis, E.O. (1929)	England and Wales	3 Urban and 3 rural areas (N=600,000)	All persons "suspect" for "mental defect"	Mental retardation, all grades	Screening of schools and institutions; key informants	Group testing of children, personal examination of adults	
Brugger (1931)	Germany (Thuringia)	Mixed (N=37,561)	All persons "suspect" for mental disorder	All mental and certain neurological disorders	Records and key informants consulted to detect "suspects"	Personal examination of all "suspects" and of a sample of "healthy" persons	
Brugger (1933, 1938)	Germany (Bavaria)	2 Rural areas (N=5,425 and 3,203)	All inhabitants	Psychoses, "hysteria," mental retardation, psychopathy, alcoholism	Door-to-door interviewing	Personal examination (semistructured interview)	

TABLE 1 (Continued)

Type of study, author & year of publication	*Country*	*Type and size of population studied*	*Target group or sample investigated*	*Conditions investigated*	*Case-finding approach*	*Method of assessment and diagnosis*	*Remarks*
Strömgren (1938)	Denmark	Rural, island of Bornholm* (N=40,000)	All inhabitants	Psychoses, mental retardation, psychopathy	Key informants; door-to-door interviews in a sample area	Personal examination	*Same population studied by Fremming (1947)
Sjögren (1948) Larsson and Sjögren (1954)	Sweden	Rural, 2 islands off the west coast (N=8,736)	All persons born or resident on the islands	Psychoses, mental retardation, severe psychopathy, suicide	Door-to-door interviewing, parish records*	Personal examination	*Longitudinal data covering 45 years collected
Mayer-Gross (1948)	Scotland	Rural (N=56,000)	"Nucleus of cases" for past 100 years	All mental disorders	Records and key informants	Study of records	
Bremer (1951)	Norway	Rural (N=1,325)	All inhabitants	All mental disorders	Door-to-door interviewing	Personal examination	

TABLE 1 (Continued)

Type of study, author & year of publication	*Country*	*Type and size of population studied*	*Target group or sample investigated*	*Conditions investigated*	*Case-finding approach*	*Method of assessment and diagnosis*	*Remarks*
Böök (1953) Böök et al. (1978)	Sweden	Rural* (N=8,891 in 1949; N=5,748 in 1974)	All inhabitants; focus on pedigrees	Psychoses, mainly schizophrenia	Door-to-door interviewing	Personal examination; biochemical tests on subsample in 1974-77	*Genetic isolate
Essen-Möller et al. (1956)	Sweden	Rural* (N=2,550)	All inhabitants	All mental and physical disorders; personality traits	Door-to-door interviewing	Personal examination	*Same population later surveyed by Hagnell (1966)
Hagnell (1966, 1970, 1975)	Sweden	Rural (N=2,550 + 1,013 new residents)	All inhabitants	All mental disorders	Door-to-door; out-migrants also interviewed; 10 and 25 year followup	Personal examination	*Same population as above

TABLE 1 (Continued)

Type of study, author & year of publication	*Country*	*Type and size of population studied*	*Target group or sample investigated*	*Conditions investigated*	*Case-finding approach*	*Method of assessment and diagnosis*	*Remarks*
Brevik (1975)	Norway	Rural (N=600)	All inhabitants	Consultation behaviour; social variables	"Participant-observer" method (author was general practitioner in the area)	Personal examination	
Fugelli (1975)	Norway	Rural, 2 islands (N=1,700)	All inhabitants	Consultation behaviour; psychotropic drug consumption	Monitoring of GP contacts; additional screening of 81% of population	Personal examination	
Bjarnar et al. (1975)	Norway	Rural* (N=1,800)	All inhabitants	All mental disorders	Combined (door-to-door, Leighton's questionnaire, key informants)	Personal examination; psychol. tests in subsample	*Same population studied by Bremer (1951)

TABLE 1 (Continued)

Type of study, author & year of publication	*Country*	*Type and size of population studied*	*Target group or sample investigated*	*Conditions investigated*	*Case-finding approach*	*Method of assessment and diagnosis*	*Remarks*
Andersen (1975)	Norway	2 Rural communities: Norwegian (N=1,043) and Lapp (N=1,074)	All inhabitants	Psychoses and neuroses	Leighton's questionnaire	Analysis of questionnaire responses; some personal examinations	
Bernsen (1976)	Denmark	Mixed (N=233,162)	Children under 15	Severe mental retardation	Screening of all relevant agencies' records	Personal examination, psychological tests	
Rotstein (1977)	USSR	4 Urban and 1 rural area (N=35,590)	All inhabitants	All mental disorders	Door-to-door interviewing	Personal examination by group of psychiatrists	
Guntern (1978)	Switzerland	Rural (N=895)	All inhabitants	"Indicators of stress" (symptoms, syndromes, alcohol consumption)	"Participant-observer" method combined with sample in-depth interviewing	Personal examination	

TABLE 1 (Continued)

Type of study, author & year of publication	*Country*	*Type and size of population studied*	*Target group or sample investigated*	*Conditions investigated*	*Case-finding approach*	*Method of assessment and diagnosis*	*Remarks*
Takala et al. (1979)	Finland	Urban (N=2,431)	All inhabitants aged 40-64	"Psychological symptoms"	Self-administered general health questionnaire	Self-rating	
Sample surveys							
Kay et al. (1964)	England	Urban, 5 electoral wards (N=9,031)	Random sample (N=309) of persons aged 65+ and census of institutions	Old age disorders	Interviewing by social worker	Psychiatric examination of "cases" by psychiatrists	
Brunetti (1964, 1978)	France	Rural (N=714)	Random sample (N=102); later a comparison urban sample (N=75)	Psychological symptoms and impairments	Personal examination, Leighton's questionnaire		
Hare (1965)	England	Urban, 2 contrasting areas	2 Random samples (N=1,900 and 1,250)	Psychological symptoms, "neuroticism"	Interviewing, personality inventory		

TABLE 1 (Continued)

Type of study, author & year of publication	*Country*	*Type and size of population studied*	*Target group or sample investigated*	*Conditions investigated*	*Case-finding approach*	*Method of assessment and diagnosis*	*Remarks*
Piotrowski et al. (1967)	Poland	Mixed, 2 contrasting areas	2 Random samples (N=1,251 and 1,643)	All mental disorders	Interviewing by research assistants	Psychiatric diagnosis based on questionnaire	
Fülöp (1968)	Hungary	Rural (N=15,952)	Random sample (N=1,903)	All physical and mental disorders	Screening by a medical team	Personal examination by psychiatrist	
Crocetti et al. (1971)	Yugoslavia	Mixed* (N=400,000)	Household cluster sample (N=9,201)	Psychoses	Screening interviews by research assistants	Personal examination of "cases" by psychiatrists	*Area known for high prevalence of psychoses
Predescu et al. (1974)	Romania	Urban (N=202,224)	Random sample (N=11,729)	All mental disorders	Screening questionnaire, self-administered	"Caseness" judged by psychiatrists on basis of questionnaire	

TABLE 1 (Continued)

Type of study, author & year of publication	*Country*	*Type and size of population studied*	*Target group or sample investigated*	*Conditions investigated*	*Case-finding approach*	*Method of assessment and diagnosis*	*Remarks*
Jablensky and Oshavkov (1975)	Bulgaria	Mixed (N=8.5 mln)	Random sample (N=18,994) from total population aged 16+	All physical and mental impairments	Personal examination by general practitioner, laboratory tests	Impairments scored by psychiatrist	
Rutter et al. (1975)	England	A rural (Isle of Wight) and an urban (London) area	Random samples of high scorers on a screen (N=104 and 159) and controls (N=107 and 106), children aged 10	Childhood mental disorder, learning disability, school performance	Screening questionnaire to teachers	Interviewing of parents, school records	
Brown et al. (1975)	England and Scotland	An urban (London) and a rural (North Uist island) area	Random samples (N=458 and 154) of women	Neurotic disorders in women	Interviewing, short PSE	Personal examination	

TABLE 1 (Continued)

Type of study, author & year of publication	*Country*	*Type and size of population studied*	*Target group or sample investigated*	*Conditions investigated*	*Case-finding approach*	*Method of assessment and diagnosis*	*Remarks*
Giel et al. (1978)	Netherlands	Rural (N=2,527)	Random sample (N=255)	Neurotic and personality disorders, impairments	Interviewing, self-rated questionnaire	Judgement on "caseness" by psychiatrists	Followup
Lehtinen et al. (1978)	Finland	Mixed, 2 contrasting communities (N=9,590 and (6,825)	Stratified random samples (N=2×500), age 15-64	Major categories of psychiatric conditions, impairments	Interview, psychological tests, records	95% Examined by psychiatrist	
Gavrilova (1979)	USSR	Urban	2 Random samples (N=1,020 and 468 aged 60+)	Old age mental disorders	Door-to-door interviewing	All examined by psychiatrist	
Binder and Angst (1981)	Switzerland	Mostly urban (Canton of Zurich)	Stratified random samples of males born in 1959 (N=300) and females born in 1953 (N=300)	Minor psychiatric disorders, alcohol and drug abuse	Screening by self-related questionnaire (SCL-90R) followed by structured interview	Personal examination at the second stage	Several followup examinations envisaged

TABLE 1 (Continued)

Type of study, author & year of publication	*Country*	*Type and size of population studied*	*Target group or sample investigated*	*Conditions investigated*	*Case-finding approach*	*Method of assessment and diagnosis*	*Remarks*
Surveys based on service contacts							
Dahlberg and Stenberg (1931)	Sweden	City of Stockholm	All first admissions (N=2,458) during 1903-1929	Psychoses		Hospital diagnosis	
Ödegaard (1946)	Norway	Whole country	All first admissions (N=14,231) during 1926-1935	All mental disorders		Hospital diagnosis	
Hare (1955)	England	City of Bristol	All first admissions (N=1,264) over 5-year period, males only	Psychoses		Hospital diagnosis	
Shepherd (1957)	England	County of Buckingham-shire (N=400,000)	All first and readmissions for 1931-1933 and 1945-1947	Psychoses		Hospital diagnosis, grouped by author	

TABLE 1 (Continued)

Type of study, author & year of publication	*Country*	*Type and size of population studied*	*Target group or sample investigated*	*Conditions investigated*	*Case-finding approach*	*Method of assessment and diagnosis*	*Remarks*
Carstairs and Brown (1958)	South Wales (UK)	2 Contrasting communities (N=19,722 and 4,621)	All psychiatric contacts, age 15+, over 5-1/2 years	All mental disorders suicide, offenses	Hospital outpatient and police records		
Norris (1959)	England	Catchment area (N=1,661,000) in London	All persons admitted in 1947-1949	All mental disorders	Tracing of records, 2-year followup		
Wing, L. et al. (1967)	England, Scotland and USA	3 Catchment areas (London, Aberdeen, Baltimore)	All persons in episodes of contact on census day	All mental disorders	Case registers	Diagnosis made at facility	
Adelstein et al. (1968)	England	City of Salford (N=150,000)	All persons in "inception episodes" of contact	All mental disorders	Case register		

TABLE 1 (Continued)

Type of study, author & year of publication	*Country*	*Type and size of population studied*	*Target group or sample investigated*	*Conditions investigated*	*Case-finding approach*	*Method of assessment and diagnosis*	*Remarks*
Strotzka (1969)	Austria	Town of Krems (N=23,000)	Random sample (N=515 adults, 319 children)	Mental disorders offenses, school problems	Screening of records of agencies		
Walsh (1969)	Ireland	City of Dublin (N=720,000)	All first admissions (N=1,427)	All mental disorders		Hospital diagnosis	
Hafner and Reimann (1970)	Fed. Rep. of Germany	City of Mannheim (N=330,000)	All first contacts with specified services	All mental disorders, topographic distribution of cases		Diagnosis made at facility	
Liebermann (1974)	USSR	District of Moscow (N=248,000)	All onsets for period 1910-1964	Schizophrenia	Dispensary register	Records and personal examination of uncertain cases	

TABLE 1 (Continued)

Type of study, author & year of publication	*Country*	*Type and size of population studied*	*Target group or sample investigated*	*Conditions investigated*	*Case-finding approach*	*Method of assessment and diagnosis*	*Remarks*
de Alarcon et al. (1975)	England	Towns of Chichester (N=94,500) and Salisbury (N=88,000)	All "new" cases not seen by psychiatrist in previous 6 months	All mental disorders	Case register	Special form filled on each referral	
Chanoît et al. (1975)	France	Sector of Paris	Cohort of first admissions (N=1,200)	All mental disorders	Records	Hospital diagnosis	
Weeke et al. (1975)	Denmark	County of Aarhus (N=175,000)	All service contacts, age 15+	Depressive disorders	Case register	Hospital diagnosis	
Strömgren (1968) Nielsen (1976)	Denmark	Island of Samsö (N=6,823)	All service contacts over 18 years	All mental disorders	General practitioners, case register, census in 1964	Records; personal examination at census	
Helgason, L. (1977)	Iceland	Whole population (N=212,100) in 1973	All first admissions (N=2,388) over 10 years	All mental disorders	Case register	Hospital diagnosis	

TABLE 1 (Continued)

Type of study, author & year of publication	*Country*	*Type and size of population studied*	*Target group or sample investigated*	*Conditions investigated*	*Case-finding approach*	*Method of assessment and diagnosis*	*Remarks*
Dilling and Weyerer (1978)	Fed. Rep. of Germany	Mixed (a community in Bavaria*)		All mental disorders	Through inpatient and outpatient services		*Same area studied by Brugger in 1933
Ouspenskaya (1978)	USSR	Comparison of a Moscow district with 3 other urban areas in different parts of USSR	All registered cases	Schizophrenia	Dispensary registers	Records reclassified according to standard diagnostic scheme	
General practice surveys							
Shepherd et al. (1966)	England	Urban (12 "practices" in London)	Subjects registered with general practitioners (N=14,697)	a) "Formal" psychiatric illness b) "Psychiatric associated" conditions	General practice records and special forms	Independent assessments by GPs and by study teams	

TABLE 1 (Continued)

Type of study, author & year of publication	*Country*	*Type and size of population studied*	*Target group or sample investigated*	*Conditions investigated*	*Case-finding approach*	*Method of assessment and diagnosis*	*Remarks*
Eastwood (1970)	England	Urban (London borough)	Random sample N=1,500), age 40-64	Neurotic, psychosomatic and physical disorders	General practice records, CMI*	Subjects classified into "cases" and "controls" (CMI score)	*Cornell Medical Index
Ballinger (1975)	Scotland	Urban	Random sample (N=760) of women, age 40-55	Mental disorder in menopause	Postal survey, GHQ*	Subjects classified into "cases" and "non-cases"	*Goldberg's General Health Questionnaire

1960; Lin and Standley, 1962; Cooper and Morgan, 1973), but it has the advantage of ordering the material along a single axis, regardless of other characteristics of the study design. The main types of surveys are: birth cohort studies; census and longitudinal studies of whole populations; sample surveys; surveys based on service contacts; and general practice surveys.

Historical Note

The origins of the psychiatric epidemiologic survey can be traced back to the last decades of the 19th century. At that time the disease concept in psychiatry already played a prominent role, influenced by the advances of the experimental method in medicine and by a philosophy of mechanistic materialism, which came as a reaction to the earlier doctrine of "moral treatment" of mental illness. Mental disease was regarded as a "thing" residing within the affected individual; cases could therefore be counted in the same way as in the epidemiology of physical disease. At the same time, reforms in the administration of psychiatric services (e.g., the assumption by the state of the reponsibility for mental hospitals) increased the need for statistics and paved the way for epidemiologic studies.

Reviews of the early psychiatric population studies have been published by Lemkau et al. (1943) and by Strömgren (1950). Both papers stress the influence of the theory of hereditary pathology on the emerging research style of psychiatric epidemiology: "When. . . Mendelian ideas became generally recognized, numerous attempts were made to demonstrate simple Mendelian factors as the hereditary basis for mental disorders. . . . These attempts, with few exceptions, were unsuccessful." (Strömgren, 1950). The primary aim of the early surveys was to determine the "empirical genetic prognosis" of the mental disorders, and researchers were mainly interested in conditions for which a hereditary basis was postulated, like severe mental retardation and dementia praecox. A second source of influence was the social hygiene movement which was in ascendancy in pre-World War I Germany. The social hygienists fought for progressive public health reforms and emphasized the importance of social factors in the epidemiology of diseases. In the sphere of mental health, however, their ideas were greatly influenced by eugenics. Even a figure of the stature of Grotjahn (1923) regarded "the majority of the mentally ill" as a "deadweight of considerable size which has to be dragged along by public welfare." According to Grotjahn, "insanity will hardly be prevented to any extend worth mentioning through improvements of social conditions. Only eugenics can act in a preventive manner, but its applications are entirely in the realm of the future." A third source of influence was the development of empirical sociology in Europe (Durkheim published his *Rules of the Sociological Method* in 1895), which applied techniques essentially akin to epidemiological procedures.

Finally, a fourth source was the development of statistical correlation and sampling methods first applied to the measurement of psychological characteristics by Galton (1879, 1888).

Examples of early epidemiologic inquiries are the studies of Jost (1896) who, at the instigation of Kraepelin, investigated the psychiatric morbidity in the pedigrees of a sample of 200 presumably healthy people (and found the frequency to be about 2%) and Koller (1895) who compared the occurrence of mental diseases in relatives of samples of "sane" and of "mentally ill" subjects (370 in each group) in the canton of Zurich.

After World War I, epidemiologic research was under the strong influence of the Munich school of population genetics (Rüdin, 1916), which added considerable methodologic sophistication to epidemiology by introducing the "genealogical random test" and applying statistical methods to estimate individual morbid risks. Klemperer (1933) introduced the birth cohort method and a number of researchers carried out prevalence and genealogic studies based on defined populations (Panse, 1929; Graemiger, 1931; Brugger, 1931, 1933 and 1938; Boeters, 1936). In the late 1930s however, the ideas of the hereditary school and eugenics found ominous applications in the Nazi practices of forced sterilization and, later on, physical extermination of some 50,000-60,000 mentally ill patients (Schipkowenski, 1977).

In contrast to this tragic postscript to the German hereditary pathology school, socially useful applications of the survey method in that period can be illustrated on the examples of the survey of mental deficiency in England and Wales (Lewis, 1929), which provided the basis for a reform of the education facilities for mentally retarded children. The results of various studies in the USSR (e.g., Khotzyanov, Singerman, 1927) and in Scandinavia (e.g., Dahlberg and Stenberg, 1931; Strömgren, 1938) helped the planning of comprehensive mental health care.

The population surveys in Europe in the period after World War II were characterized by several new developments. First, the spectrum of mental morbidity that was investigated expanded considerably, due to an increased interest in the "minor psychiatric disorders," i.e., the neuroses, psychosomatic conditions, and milder varieties of personality disorders, which had been largely ignored in earlier surveys. Second, the assessment of social and other environmental correlates of mental illness assumed a greater importance than in the past. Third, there was an increased emphasis on the standardization of research methods and the reproducibility of results. The development of national health services and community mental health facilities, especially in Eastern Europe and in several West European countries, made it possible to use the service infrastructure for epidemiologic research, and also stimulated such research in a more general way, because of the need for planning and rational allocation of resources.

European psychiatric epidemiologic research in the post-World War II period retained a certain continuity with the nosological orientation of the earlier period. However, the disease concept became a less central preoccupation of the investigators, while measurement of social functioning and adjustment and evaluation of the needs for different types of care gained in importance. Technically, some of the more recent studies rely on such innovations as computerized population and morbidity registers. These technical aids, however, do not remove the new obstacles that have appeared, such as the increasing mobility of populations and transnational migration. The task of carrying out a community mental health survey today demands as much dedication and persistence on the part of the investigator as it did half a century ago.

Methodologic Aspects of Mental Health Surveys

The methodologic problems that have to be tackled in psychiatric epidemiologic research have been reviewed by an Expert Committee of the World Health Organization (WHO, 1960) which pointed to: *(a)* the existence of "individual factors in the causes and manifestations of many psychiatric diseases which, for instances, because they belong to the sphere of values cannot be fully quantified"; *(b)* the "essentially multifactorial" nature of the etiology of mental disorders, complicated by the fact that "in few branches of medicine are genetic, physiological and psychological factors as evenly distributed in the origin and evolution of disease as in psychiatry"; *(c)* the "incongruities in the diagnostic appraisal in different countries and schools" and a "tendency to use technical terms in different senses according to the theory favored"; *(d)* the presence of "considerable social and cultural differences in what is considered psychically abnormal in different surroundings, and in the way such abnormality is treated"; and (e) the problems of "infinite variations" in human character and behavior deviations, "ranging from severe psychosis to mild personality disorders which many would not consider to be the concern of psychiatry." The Committee concluded that "these problems may make it difficult to advance the study of epidemiology of mental disorders as quickly and consistently as might be hoped." It is important to examine how these problems have been tackled in psychiatric surveys of geographically delimited populations.

Selection of a Population for Study

The populations which have been the subject of epidemiological surveys in Europe fall into several categories.

1. *Rural Communities.*—Single villages or larger rural areas have been a favored object of study, although the proportion of rural population in Europe has been steadily declining since the beginning of the century. By 1973, it exceeded 50% in only a few countries, being of the order of 9%-33% in most parts of the continent (Cole, 1979). The earlier German studies, most of the Scandinavian studies, and a number of other surveys listed in table 1, focused on rural populations of varying size, ranging from 714 inhabitants of a commune in France (Brunetti, 1964) to over 40,000 on the island of Bornholm (Strömgren, 1938; Fremming, 1947). The advantage of studying rural populations is in their compactness, low geographic mobility, simple social organization, and stable way of life and little change from one generation to another. Although these features of rural life are gradually disap-

pearing, the advantages they still offer have been used in two kinds of study: those aiming to establish genetic risks of mental disorders through investigations of pedigrees (e.g., Larsson and Sjörgren 1954; Böök, 1953, 1978), and those aiming to examine the impact of social change on a traditional microecology (e.g., Brown et al. 1977; Guntern, 1978). A particularly effective approach is the *repeat survey*, in which the same population is reexamined after an interval during which social change has occurred (e.g., the complete followup by Hagnell in 1957 and 1972, of the population originally studied by Essen-Möller in 1947; or the followup by Böök et al., 1978, of the population studied by the same investigator 25 years earlier).

A disadvantage of the rural survey is the limited generalizability of its results. Precisely those factors which are minimally interfering in a rural survey (population mobility, social change and social organization) may be implicated in the causation and pathoplastic modification of many mental disorders. From this point of view, the sedentary, agricultural populations which have been spared the effects of "modernization," are atypical. Of course, in some instances, precisely the "atypism" of a population can be a reason for its selection for study, as in Böök's (1953) survey of a genetic isolate in Northern Sweden, or Guntern's (1978) survey of a small village in the Swiss Alps whose traditional way of life had been abruptly changed by the construction of a road.

2. *Island Populations.*—As most islands are rural, the study of island populations offers the same advantages and disadvantages as the study of rural areas. An additional attraction stems from the "captivity" of island population and the greater likelihood that they maintain a traditional way of life. Island populations, however, may be exposed to particular stresses, and this observation has led some authors to postulate a specific "insular pathology" (Jeanneau and Jeanneau, 1969). Examples of island studies include Strömgren (1938), Fremming (1947), Sjögren (1948) and Larsson and Sjögren (1954), T. Helgason (1964), Rutter et al. (1975), Brown et al. (1977), and L. Helgason (1977).
3. *Urban Populations.*—Urban areas are demographically and socially heterogeneous and the problem of delimitation of "natural" communities (in the sociological sense of "Gemeinschaft"—Tönnies, 1887) within them is difficult to resolve. The differences in life style between small towns (e.g., Mayer-Gross, 1948; Strotzka, 1969) and large cities (e.g., Norris, 1959; Walsh, 1969; Häfner and Reimann, 1970; Predescu et al., 1974; Lieberman, 1974; Chanoît et al., 1975) may be as important as those between rural and urban areas. Such differences may require the use of different sampling and assessment methods in studies of small towns and large cities.

However, with all the difficulties that urban studies present, their results are nevertheless more generalizable to other urban areas because of a certain uniformity of urban lifestyles. In addition, the presence of considerable ecologic and social contrasts between subsections of the urban populations allows environmental factors that may play a role in mental morbidity to be brought into sharper focus.

4. *Mixed Urban/Rural Areas and Comparisons Between Rural and Urban Areas.*—In many surveys the area selected for study includes an urban agglomeration and a surrounding rural area. This type of study should be distinguished from surveys in which populations or samples from two contrasting areas, one urban and one rural, are studied in a comparative manner (e.g., Rutter et al., 1975; Brown et al., 1977; Lehtinen et al., 1978; Brunetti et al., 1978). The methodologic merits of the latter approach are considerable in view of the ecological variation and contrasts that can be explored.
5. *Large Populations.*—Surveys of large demographic units, for example, the entire population of a country, are only feasible (excluding very small countries) through sampling, e.g., in general health surveys, or use of health service statistics. However, neither general health surveys, which may include mental health items, nor routine statistical reports from the mental health authorities qualify for inclusion in this review, the former because of lack of valid diagnostic information and the latter because of the usual incompleteness of service coverage. On the other hand, studies like those by Ödegaard (1946) and L. Helgason (1977), although based primarily or exclusively on treated morbidity, are in fact epidemiologic surveys. Ödegaard used case register data for the whole of Norway over the period 1926-1935, and Helgason included an additional search for undetected cases to produce incidence rates for the entire population of Iceland. Such estimates of morbidity appear to be close to those that can be obtained with more intensive case finding methods. An example of the sampling approach is a large scale sociomedical study in Bulgaria in which a multistage probability sample of 18,994 individuals drawn from the entire population of the country (8.5 million) was assessed for presence and degree of physical and mental disability (Jablensky and Oshavkov, 1975). Provided that an adequate sampling strategy can be designed, studies of large populations give the most accurate estimates of morbidity rates. However, important local variations of disease rates may be missed in this approach.

Goals of Surveys and the Definition of a Case

The goals of population surveys and the definitions of what is considered a "case" are interrelated. The early surveys aimed to estimate how many chronically ill or disabled individuals were in need of institutional care, financial support from public funds, or legal protection; to determine the "hereditary prognosis" of the psychiatric disorders; and to further the understanding of the causes of "insanity" through establishing its patterns of inheritance. Definitions of "caseness" in the early studies were sketchy or altogether absent, but it is now clear that the investigators were interested only in the severe cases of psychoses, mental retardation, epilepsy, alcoholism, and personality disorder ("psychopathy"), i.e., in conditions that were regarded as constitutional and largely "incurable." The neurotic illnesses were almost entirely outside the focus of interest, and diagnostic categories for the various situational reactions, adjustment problems, and "borderline" mental or behavioral pathology did not yet exist.

The studies of Koller (1895) and Jost (1896), in which the authors collected data on the occurrence of mental disorders in the relatives of "sane" individuals and hospitalized psychiatric patients, are examples of such early surveys. The Munich school of psychiatric genetics, which developed a more rigorous diagnostic assessment of dementia praecox (schizophrenia) and manic-depressive psychosis, remained limited in its concept of "caseness" to the severe and chronic conditions.

Authors rarely reported their diagnostic criteria and case definitions, but it seems that there was a close similarity between German and Scandinavian studies in the post-World War I period regarding the diagnostic criteria of the major psychotic disorders. In this group of disorders, at least, European diagnostic concepts have not apparently changed much until today. Diagnosis was made primarily on the basis of manifest clinical symptoms. Degree of functional impairment and disability were not explicit criteria in defining a "case," nor was subjective distress. Although psychiatrists were clearly aware of "all the possible transitions between mental health and severe mental illness. . ." (Ödegaard, 1946), they drew a rather sharp line of demarcation between "cases" and "noncases," leaving practically no "grey zone" between the two categories.

Several kinds of change occurred in the post-World War II period regarding the goals of population surveys and the concept of "caseness." As a wider range of treatments and services became available to populations, there was an increased interest in identifying not only the severe, but also the "minor" psychiatric conditions (neuroses, personality disorders, psychosomatic disturbances, drug-related problems). The demographic aging of populations and the growing awareness of the social problems of the aged stimulated the study of the psychiatric morbidity of the elderly. Advances in child psychiatry brought under the scrutiny of psychiatric epidemiology the conduct and neurotic disorders of childhood, specific learning disabilities, and related problems. Generally, there was an increased interest in the role of social factors in the etiology, pathogenesis, and prognosis of psychiatric disorders, and more systematic attempts were made to assess the social environment. The post-World War II epidemiologic work also showed a greater awareness of methodologic issues, for example the problems of reliability of psychiatric diagnosis. Case definition in population surveys could no longer be taken for granted.

The following three main approaches to case definitions have been applied in population surveys:

1. *Referral Behavior as a Criterion of "Caseness."* —Ödegaard's view that all patients with severe mental disorders are likely to make a contact with a service, provided that services are easily available (Ödegaard, 1946), has found some support in several experiments with "unlimited access to psychiatric consultation," given to defined populations. Referral was a criterion of "caseness" in the Samsö project (Strömgren, 1968; Nielsen, 1976), where the population of that Danish island was provided free and easily accessible psychiatric consultation over a

number of years. The incidence of psychiatric contacts increased initially, then stabilized at the level of 17.9 per 1,000 per year for all contacts, and 12.2 per 1,000 per year for first contacts (age groups 15 and over). A census study of the same population validated the expectation that very few, if any, psychiatric cases would fail to consult a doctor. A similar approach has been used by Bjarnar et al. (1975) in the repeat survey of a Norwegian fishing village, which had originally been studied by Bremer (1951).

Referral behavior, however, can be a valid criterion of "caseness" only under special circumstances. The factors that influence the probability that individuals suffering from mental disorder will consult a medical service have been classified by Svendsen (1952) into three groups: *(a)* population-related (e.g., population size, rate of growth, age structure); *(b)* nosocomial (related to the service itself, e.g., the number of available beds or the number of health personnel); and *(c)* threshold-related (e.g., severity of the condition and the tolerance of the social environment). These factors vary considerably even in areas with a high density of services, as is the case in many parts of Europe. A survey of a random sample of the population aged over 60 in a Moscow district, where an outpatient (dispensary) service had been in existence over several decades, revealed that 1.5% of the sample had had a diagnosable mental disorder (mostly mild forms of functional psychoses) but had never consulted a psychiatrist (Gavrilova, 1979). Similar findings with regard to severe mental retardation were reported by Bernsen (1976) for the county of Aarhus in Denmark, where almost 20% of the severely retarded children of school age had not been registered with the specialized services despite the availability of such services.

2. *Clinical Judgment as a Criterion of "Caseness."* —This approach has been advocated by a WHO Expert Committee, which proposed that a "case" be defined as a "manifest disturbance of mental functioning, specific enough in clinical character to be consistently recognizable as conforming to a clearly defined standard pattern and severe enough to cause loss of working or social capacity, or both, of a degree that can be specified in terms of absence from work or of the taking of legal or other social action" (WHO, 1960).

   By and large, this clinical approach to case definition has been inherent in most of the epidemiologic work in Europe. Since in many European studies case identification involved a personal examination of subjects by an experienced psychiatrist, clinical judgment, even without formal standardization, could be expected to have considerable validity. Problems arise, however, with conditions on the borderline between recognizable clinical syndromes and normal variation, with subjective complaints that do not present as clear-cut symptoms, and with behavior that deviates from the social norm but cannot be classified as symptomatic of a specific disorder. Such states form a large periphery around the core of clear-cut cases, and their identification and classification on clinical grounds is uncertain.

A rule-of-thumb criterion based on clinical common sense may be the best guide in such circumstances, provided the procedure is clearly described.

In a survey of women living in a London borough and on the island of North Uist, Brown et al. (1977) applied the criterion that "a psychiatrist would be surprised to see a woman defined as a *case* in an outpatient clinic and...would be likely to regard the woman as benefiting from some form of psychiatric treatment." A similar approach had been applied by Hagnell (1966) in the survey of a Swedish community where the investigator personally examined every inhabitant and made a clinical judgment about "caseness," supplemented by a separate rating of the degree of his own certainty. The reliability of the clinical approach to case definition can be enhanced by standardization, for example, by provision of vignette descriptions of symptoms and behaviors characteristic of "cases" and "noncases," by consensus judgment by two or more experienced investigators, and by operationalization of the judgment process. An example of the latter approach is the development of an index of definition (Wing, 1976) for use in conjunction with a standardized clinical interview (Present State Examination—Wing et al., 1974). The index of definition is a procedure for classifying mental state data into several levels according to the presence or absence of diagnostically important symptoms and the total number of symptoms present. Above a certain cutoff point of intensity and specificity, the symptoms form clinically meaningful syndromes and nosological categories. Since the whole sequence of steps can be written as a computer program, the technique is of considerable value in uniformly classifying survey data. It bypasses the conceptual difficulty of demarcating caseness from noncaseness by providing the investigator with several options of cutoff points. The choice of a particular cutoff point can be determined by the purpose of the study.

Another approach to the operationalization of judgment about caseness is the RIDIT method used in epidemiologic surveys in the United States, a technique that has been applied in a secondary analysis of a subsample of Hagnell's Lundby data (Leighton et al., 1971).

3. *Self-Reports as a Criterion of "Caseness."*—Self-reporting questionnaires are practical, low-cost tools for case finding, but their construction and application rest on assumptions about caseness that have to be validated against referral behavior and clinical judgment. Among the many self-reporting instruments, the Cornell Medical Index and Goldberg's General Health Questionnaire (GHQ) have been used in more than one survey in Europe. Most of the self-reporting questionnaires identify likely cases on the basis of a score derived by a simple summation of the positive answers given by the respondent. The case definition underlying the construction of the General Health Questionnaire (Goldberg, 1972) presupposes a "single axis ranging from a normality to severe disturbance" on which an individual's position determined by his score would be a "quantitative estimate of that individual's

degree of psychiatric disturbance." It should be noted that the GHQ was designed for detecting nonpsychotic illnesses and that the dimensional model on which it rests is not applicable to psychoses or organic mental disorders. The cutoff points for defining caseness have been derived by calibrating the instrument against three groups of subjects: a "severely ill" group (inpatients on a disturbed admission ward of a mental hospital), a "mildly ill" group (psychiatric and outpatients) and a "normal" group (selected from a community survey).

The dimensional approach to case definition, such as the one adopted by Goldberg, does not necessarily clash with the nosologic approach that has always been prominent in European research. The view that mental disorders are heterogeneous and not a single continuum has always prevailed in Europe and, as a rule, frequency data on mental disorders are reported in terms of diagnostic categories. At the same time, dimensional approaches are used increasingly to characterize the severity of conditions and the degree of functional impairment.

Survey Design and Case Finding

The various case finding strategies employed in European studies fall into six categories.

1. *Birth Cohort Surveys.*—This method was first used by Klemperer (1933), who selected from the birth register of the city of Munich a random sample of 1,000 individuals born between 1800 and 1890 but succeeded in tracing and examining only about 30% of them. Later, the same approach was used with greater success by Fremming (1947) who collected life history data on 92% of the 5,500 persons born on the island of Bornholm in the period 1883-1887. A more recent application of this method is T. Helgason's study in Iceland (Helgason, 1964) in which all births in the country for the period 1895-1897 were identified through screening of the parish records, then a list was compiled of those individuals still alive on December 1, 1910. This cohort, consisting of 5,395 individuals who had survived into adulthood, was traced until 1957, and life history and psychiatric data were obtained for 99.4% of them from admission records and interviews.
2. *Surveys of Whole Communities.*—This type of study is one of the characteristic contributions of European psychiatric epidemiology. Essentially, the method involves: *(a)* selection of a study population (usually geographically compact, of a small to moderate size); *(b)* collection of background information on the demography, geography, history, and current social and economic characteristics of the area; *(c)* collation of a comprehensive list of all residents living and, in some cases, those born in the area during a specified period; *(d)* search for medical and psychiatric records, key informant data, and other sources that might facilitate the detection of both current and past cases; (e) personal interviewing of every person alive on a census day; and (f) search of the persons born in the area who had migrated. The advantages of this type of study lie in the completeness of coverage, and

they can be exploited best if a repeat survey of the area is envisaged. The disadvantages, besides the cost and amount of effort required, include the risk that a population, even if thoroughly surveyed, may not be sufficiently representative and general conclusions based on such findings may be misleading.

The comprehensive survey method presupposes the existence of certain conditions which cannot be easily met. For example, the reliable estimation of lifetime prevalence and morbid risk depends on the availability and quality of demographic statistics. No less important are the skills, time available, patience, and general attitudes of the investigator who has to spend long periods as a "participant observer" in the community whose confidence he should be able to win. The administrative conditions that would allow such a research style to be practiced include relative freedom of the investigator from administrative chores and from pressure to publish circumstances that are not at present widely prevalent. It is not surprising that, after the pioneering work of Brugger (1931, 1933) in Thuringia and Bavaria, a major share of such studies have taken place in the Scandinavian countries (table 1), which have had excellent population statistics at least since the beginning of this century (Strömgren, 1938; Sjögren, 1948; Essen-Möller, 1956; Bremer, 1951; Hagnell, 1966, 1970, 1975).

A special variety of the comprehensive survey is the *period* survey which, in addition to a census investigation, includes either a retrospective data collection covering a specified period, or a followup. Examples of the former are the studies by Strömgren (1938) and Larsson and Sjögren (1954). The best known example of a prospective followup design is the Lundby survey (Essen-Möller, 1953; Hagnell, 1966, 1970, 1975). All the surviving inhabitants of the rural community originally surveyed by Essen-Möller in 1947, as well as all the newcomers to the area, were personally examined 20 years later by Hagnell and again, after another 15 years, by the same investigator. A similar design was employed by Böök (1953) and by Böök et al. (1978) who reexamined a North Swedish genetic isolate after an interval of 20 years, and by Bjarnar et al. (1975) who studied the population of a Norwegian village 30 years after the survey carried out by Bremer (1951). The studies by Dilling and Weyerer (1978, 1980), who surveyed treated psychiatric morbidity in the Bavarian communities of Traunstein and Rosenheim, once the site of Brugger's investigations, should also be mentioned in this context.

3. *Sample Surveys.*—Sampling techniques were developed as early as the 1880s but only around and after World War I were sampling strategies systematically employed. A special variety of the sampling approach, the *genealogical random test,* was used by Rüdin (1916) in epidemiologic-genetic studies. The technique involved the selection of a random sample of "normal" individuals *(propositi)* and the collection of data on the mental morbidity of all their first-degree relatives. Such data allowed the estimation of prevalence, incidence, and morbid risk. The "standard" figures on the risk and incidence of the major psychoses reported in the post-World War I German literature were

derived in this way. This method, however, has been criticized by Strömgren (1950) on grounds of small sample sizes and biased selection (e.g., in some instances the "propositi" were chosen among patients in somatic wards, or among hospital personnel). Nevertheless, the incidence figures for schizophrenia obtained through the genealogical random test were in surprisingly good agreement with data collected later with more accurate methods.

Another method, designed specifically for population genetic studies, was the *pedigree sample* technique, which aims to reconstruct the morbidity history of several generations of individuals related by blood or marriage and to trace the origin of a hereditary trait or disorder to one or several common ancestors. This method was applied successfully by Sjögren (1948) in a Swedish island population, and by Böök (1953) who related the unusually high current incidence of catatonic schizophrenia in a genetic isolate in Northern Sweden to three families who had moved into the area two centuries earlier.

Probability sampling, in its different varieties (stratified or unstratified, multifocal, etc.) is at present the most widely used sampling method. Since each person in a population has an equal chance of being selected, the technique makes it possible to study representative collections of individuals and to generalize the results to the population at large. An effective strategy is the simultaneous or consecutive study of probability samples drawn from socioeconomically contrasting geographic areas as, for example, in the study by Lehtinen et al. (1978) who compared mental morbidity to one northern and one southern community in Finland by investigating random samples from the two areas, each including 300 urban and 200 rural inhabitants. A prospective psychiatric study of a representative sample of 300 males and 300 females aged 20-21, drawn from the total population in that age group in the Canton of Zurich (Switzerland) has been reported by Binder and Angst (1981). Random sampling from large population aggregates helps to avoid the "ecological fallacy," which manifests itself in spuriously high levels of intercorrelation of variables measured in a population sharing a common ecology.

4. *Screening Techniques and Multistage Surveys.*—One of the post-World War II innovations in epidemiologic research technology has been the development of screening procedures for the rapid identification, in the general population, of a subset of individuals in whom mental disorder can be suspected. The suspects can then be given a more detailed clinical examination resulting in a diagnosis. An illustration of the application of the two-stage method can be found in the epidemiologic study of psychoses in Croatia, Yugoslavia (Lemkau et al., 1971; Kulcar et al., 1971; Crocetti et al., 1971). In this survey, a group of medical students who had received brief training as research assistants, performed a first-stage screening by personally interviewing the members of sampled clusters of households and identified potential cases which were then examined and diagnosed by experienced psychiatrists.

5. *General Practice Surveys.*—The first epidemiologic survey of mental morbidity in a community by a general practitioner was carried out by Bremer (1951), but the development of the general practice survey as a specific epidemiologic method started with the pioneering study by Shepherd et al. (1966). That study demonstrated that during a one-year period 14% of the individuals on the lists of general practitioners developed at least one episode of mental disorder, but only 1 of 20 persons with mental disorder was receiving specialist care. With the growing role of primary health care, epidemiologic investigations of samples of general practice populations have become an increasingly useful approach to the estimation of mental morbidity and the needs for treatment and care. An approach combining case finding by a general practitioner and direct service provision in the form of "unlimited" access to psychiatric consultation, has been maintained over a number of years on the Danish island of Samsö (Strömgren, 1957; Nielsen, 1976).
6. *Surveys of "Declared" Psychiatric Morbidity.*—Although the existence of unrecognized psychiatric morbidity in the community has been well documented, the importance of epidemiologic investigations of "declared" cases, i.e., those admitted as inpatients or outpatients to a treatment facility, has not diminished. Surveys based on service contacts can answer questions about the pathways leading to treatment, about the efficacy of treatment and management, about the social and personal consequences of being diagnosed as mentally ill, and also, in areas of sufficient density of treatment facilities, about incidence and prevalence. A carefully designed survey of service contacts, in which not only psychiatric but also any other facilities that may be used by patients are covered, can be a reasonable approximation to a door-to-door survey or even a substitute for it. A technical innovation, introduced in the Scandinavian countries after World War I, and later in other European countries is the centralized *cumulative psychiatric case register,* which keeps an ongoing record of persons resident in a given area and of their contacts with various services. A very similar approach to cumulative recording of mental morbidity, introduced in the Soviet Union in the 1920s and the East European countries after World War II, is the *dispensary registration list (dispansernyj uchet).*

Assessment and Diagnosis of Cases

Methods of case assessment used in epidemiological surveys of mental morbidity fall into three groups.

1. The *personal examination* of every inhabitant or of every potential case has been a feature of a number of European studies. In the absence of any biologic or other independent validating criteria for the majority of the disorders seen in the community, clinical judgment remains the most valid approach to the assessment of psychopathology. However,

the clinical interviews and diagnosis give rise to problems of reliability, and assessment techniques can be ranked according to the degree of their standardization. At one end of the scale are the unstructured techniques used by earlier investigators. At the other extreme are the more recent, standardized interviewing techniques which have been extensively tested for interrater reliability and repeatability. Among them, the Present State Examination (PSE-Wing, et al., 1974) represents a semistructured interview guide in which ratings of presence and intensity of symptoms are made on the basis of the interviewer's clinical judgment. This instrument has been translated into more than 25 languages and used in major cross-cultural studies (WHO, 1973; 1979). A short version of the PSE for interviewing in the community is also available. An intermediate position on this dimension is occupied by the semistandardized interviewing methods used mainly by Scandinavian investigators. The assessment methods used in the Lundby study (Essen-Möller, 1956; Hagnell, 1966) deserve special mention. In addition to a psychiatric interview which had an initial, free-flowing part and a second, semistructured part, the investigators made ratings on personality traits using the dimensional model of Sjobring (1974). Generally, the Scandinavian surveys are characterized by extraordinary thoroughness of clinical assessment. On the other hand, they have been criticized for rarely reporting reliability data and for the difficult to translate terminology in which clinical findings are often formulated.

2. Interviewing by *research assistants* in psychiatric surveys has been a less frequent procedure in Europe than in the United States. A rare example of the use of research assistants (medical students) is the study of psychoses in Croatia, Yugoslavia (Crocetti et al., 1971).
3. The uses of *self-administered questionnaires* in community surveys have been reviewed by Goldberg (1972). The data reported in the literature on the use of instruments such as the Cornell Medical Inventory (CMI), Saslow's New Psychiatric Screening Test, Zung's Self-Rating Depression Scale, Fould's Personal Distress Scale, and a number of others, led to the conclusion that "no scale at present in use is really satisfactory for the purpose of case identification and that most of them do not distinguish between personality traits and symptoms." Among the reasons for this were the low reliability of the informants, the reluctance of subjects to reveal their inner experiences (or, the opposite tendency to overreporting in "polysymptomatic hypochondriacs"), and the effects of the "social desirability" response set. These shortcomings, however, do not disqualify self-reporting techniques, and some of the difficulties can be overcome, as the development and subsequent use of Goldberg's General Health Questionnaire (GHQ) have demonstrated.

Since findings in most epidemiologic surveys are reported in terms of some kind of diagnostic categories, a comparison of results obtained in different studies can only be as meaningful as a comparison between the diagnostic and classification criteria employed by different investigators. The degree to which diagnostic concepts may vary between different countries and schools of psychiatry has been extensively documented (Cooper et al., 1972; WHO, 1973). The sources of diagnostic variation in epidemiologic surveys of mental disorders include: *(a)* differences in the accuracy and reliability of primary data, due to the variety of information sources used in surveys (records, self-rating questionnaires, key informant data, personal examination); *(b)* varying degrees of standardization of the data collection process and lack of uniform methods of data recording; and *(c)* variation of the disease theories and diagnostic concepts over time and among different schools of psychiatry. Work undertaken jointly by the World Health Organization (WHO) and the Alcohol, Drug Abuse, and Mental Health Administration (ADAMHA) of the United States (WHO, 1981, 1982) has helped considerably in elucidating current differences between major schools and traditions in psychiatry with regard to diagnosis. There is no single solution for all these difficulties, but recent methodological advances related to the standardization of assessment methods, the development of uniform recording techniques, and the compilation of glossaries and operational definitions of syndromes, suggest that many of the obstacles can be overcome.

Epidemiologic Indexes

The results of community surveys are usually reported in terms of prevalence (point-period and lifetime), incidence, and morbid risk (expectancy).

1. *Point prevalence,* i.e., the number of "active" cases identified per 1,000 population on a given census day, can be expressed as a ratio of cases to: *(a)* the total population or *(b)* the population at risk. The point prevalence rate may underestimate conditions that are either of short duration or have an episodic course and may not be "active" on the census day. Since many of the frequent psychiatric disorders fall into this category, the attempts to correct this bias of the point prevalence rate have led to various modifications of the definition of an "active" case. Unless the precise definition of the active case is known, the interpretation of the rates will not be reliable. In studies where an indirect method of case assessment is employed, a case may be considered active on a given census day if the subject has been in treatment on that day or if he had made two or more contacts with a psychiatric service during a 6-month interval with the census day as a midpoint (Wing et al., 1967; Temkov et al., 1975).
2. *The period prevalence rate* represents the number of cases (per 1,000) that have been active at any time during a specified period, usually one year. It does more justice to the episodic or periodic patterns of illness than the point prevalence rate.
3. *Lifetime prevalence* is the count of all persons in a population, alive on a given census day who had experienced at least one episode of mental disorder at any time in their lives. In surveys that combine the cross-sectional census with a "period" retrospective investigation, both

lifetime prevalence and point prevalence are determined on the basis of data obtained through interviewing or search of records.

4. *Incidence,* i.e., the number of new cases (inceptions) per 1,000 population at risk during a defined period, is a particularly valuable index because it can provide clues to etiologic and pathogenetic factors. Incidence, however, is more difficult to determine because of uncertainties about the definition and detection of the point of onset, particularly in conditions of insidious beginning such as schizophrenia. This problem has resulted in a distinction between true onset (inception) and "social onset" (Ödegaard, 1946), the latter being the point at which a contact with a treating agency is made for the first time in life. The question about the extend to which the incidence of social onsets in a population can be used as an estimate of the true inception rate of psychotic disorders is perhaps impossible to answer in a general way, since the probability that an incipient case would contact a service without much delay is likely to vary considerably from one setting to another, and in the same setting over time. Incidence is usually determined by: (a) a prospective monitoring of social onsets in a given area (e.g., by means of a psychiatric case register); *(b)* a retrospective reconstruction of the past history and identification of the point of onset of disorders identified in a period-type study; or *(c)* a repeated census of all members of a defined population some time after a baseline census has been carried out. All three methods have been used in European surveys, but the followup census approach, as used by Hagnell, 1966, 1975 at 10-year and 25-year points after the initial survey, is perhaps the most accurate among them.
5. The *morbid risk,* or *expectancy,* is an index that expresses the probability that an individual belonging to a given population will develop a specified psychiatric condition, assuming that he reaches a defined age. Morbid risk can be computed for any age period, and for the entire lifespan of a population ("total" risk). The most frequently calculated index is the *aggregate morbid risk,* which is obtained by summing up the risks determined for successive age periods. The mathematical method employed since the 1920s, is represented in the formula:

$$q = \frac{d_x}{W_x n_x}$$

where q is the aggregate morbid risk expressed as a probability, d is the number of individuals in a population who have developed the condition at a given age x, n is the difference between the number of individuals who have "entered" observation at age x and the number of those who, for any reason, have disappeared from observation by that age, and w is a weight expressing the probability of developing the condition *before* age x as a proportion of the probability of developing the condition at all.

The same formula can be written simply as

$$q = \frac{D}{N},$$

where D would equal the number of all cases found in a given population (i.e. the prevalence count), and N is what in German epidemiology has been called *Bezugsziffer*—reference figure—that is, population at risk. The problem of obtaining reliable weight coefficients (w_x) for the latter has been extensively debated in the epidemiologic literature, and several modifications have been proposed. The simplified approach first proposed by Weinberg (1925) and known as *Weinberg's abridged method* is based on the assumption that a "risk zone" can be defined for every condition. The age-specific probability of developing the condition is then assumed to be 0 for persons who have passed the period of risk, 1 for persons who have not yet entered the period of risk, and 0.5 for persons within the period at risk. Weinberg's method has been criticized for some of its assumptions, but in sufficiently large populations the results of the abridged method are only negligibly different from those obtained with exact lifetable methods.

Overview of Results

A comprehensive presentation of the results obtained in epidemiologic studies of geographically defined populations in Europe is not possible within the limits of this review. A brief summary, however, is given of the most important findings, especially those that illustrate trends or raise questions that can only be answered by further research.

Schizophrenia

The most striking finding concerning schizophrenia (table 2) is the relatively good agreement between the rates of prevalence, incidence, and morbid risk obtained in different surveys, regardless of the arguments about the definition of the concept of schizophrenia and the repeated revisions of its boundaries. In most population studies the point prevalence of schizophrenic disorders has been found to be within the range 2.5-3.3 per 1,000. Lower rates have been reported by Brugger (1931) in his Thuringia survey and more recently by Dilling and Weyerer (1980) in Bavaria. In both surveys, however, failure to identify some schizophrenic patients in institutions outside the study area could not be excluded. Higher-than-average prevalence rates have been found by Essen-Möller (1956) in South Sweden and particularly by Böök (1953, 1978) in a genetic isolate in Northern Sweden. High prevalence rates of schizophrenia (and of other psychoses) have also been found in a coastal area in Croatia, Yugoslavia (Crocetti et al., 1971). The population of the latter area was much larger than the one studied by Böök, and consanquinity did not appear to be plausible explanation. No clear-cut support has been

TABLE 2

Occurrence of Schizophrenic Disorders in Geographically Defined Populations (Data from 26 Surveys in Europe).

Author, year	*Country*	*Point prevalence (per 1,000)*	*Incidence (per 1,000)*	*Morbid risk (per 100)*	*Remarks*
Birth cohort studies					
Klemperer (1933)	Germany	10.0*	—	1.40	* Estimated with correction for cohort attrition
Fremming (1947)	Denmark	—	—	0.90	
Helgason (1964)	Iceland	—	—	0.57-0.69 (M)*	
		—	—	0.90-1.02 (F)*	* Up to age 61
Census studies					
Brugger (1931)	Germany	2.4* (1.9**)	—	0.38	* Per 1,000 aged 10+ ** Per 1,000 all ages
Brugger (1933)	Germany	2.2*	—	0.41	* Per 1,000 all ages
Brugger (1938)	Germany	2.3* (1.8**)	—	0.36	* Per 1,000 aged 10+ ** Per 1,000 all ages
Strömgren (1938)	Denmark		—	0.58	
Sjögren (1948) and Larsson & Sjögren (1954)	Sweden	4.6	—	1.60*	* Equal for M and F
Böök (1953)	Sweden	9.5	—	2.66*	* Age 15-50
Böök (1978)	Same population	17.0	—	2.68 (M) 2.27 (F)	* Genetic isolate

TABLE 2 (Continued)

Author, year	*Country*	*Point prevalence (per 1,000)*	*Incidence (per 1,000)*	*Morbid risk (per 100)*	*Remarks*
Essen-Möller et al. (1956)	Sweden	6.7 (3.9*)	—	—	* Psychotic on census date
Hagnell (1966)	Same population	4.5			
Crocetti et al. (1971)	Yugoslavia*	5.9	—	—	* Area known for high rate of psychosis
Lehtinen et al. (1978)	Finland	15.0	—	—	
Rotstein (1977)	USSR	3.8	—	—	
Service contact studies					
Ödegaard (1946)	Norway	—	0.24*	1.87	* Age 10+
Norris (1959)	United Kingdom	—	0.17		
Adelstein et al. (1968)	United Kingdom	—	0.35* (M) 0.26* (F)		* Age 15+
Walsh (1969)	Ireland	—	0.57* (M) 0.46* (F)		* Age 10+
Hafner & Reimann (1970)	Fed. Rep. of Germany	—	0.54		

TABLE 2 (Continued)

Author, year	*Country*	*Point prevalence (per 1,000)*	*Incidence (per 1,000)*	*Morbid risk (per 100)*	*Remarks*
Lieberman (1974)	USSR	—	0.20 (M) 0.19 (F)		* Patients with onset in 1950-1964 personally investigated by author
Temkov et al. (1975)	Bulgaria	2.8			
Nielsen (1976)	Denmark	2.7*	0.20	—	* Census on 1 Jan 1964
Ouspenskaya (1978)	USSR	5.3*			* Lifetime prevalence, per 1,000 age 14+
Helgason L. (1977)	Iceland	—	0.27	0.43 (M) 0.54 (F)	

found for a hypothesis of negative selection through outmigration of the healthier individuals.

Information on the incidence of schizophrenia (i.e., the annual rate of new onsets) has been obtained mainly in studies utilizing first-admission or first-contact data. The rates vary within the range 0.17-0.57 per 1,000 per year. The extent to which incidence rates determined on the basis of service contacts are biased because of nosocomial and threshold factors can be estimated from the results of intensive sample surveys (Gavrilova, 1979). A number of schizophrenic patients never consult a psychiatrist and therefore are missed in surveys where case finding is limited to service contacts. There is also a time lag averaging 2.1 years between the onset of schizophrenia and the first contact with a psychiatric service. In settings where the services experience administrative changes, the time lag may fluctuate considerably from year to year and the incidence rates obtained in any single year may be unreliable. In stabilized situations the annual first contact or referral rate is likely to be a very close estimate of the "true" incidence rate.

Morbid risk for schizoprenia is perhaps the most informative index if genetic isolates are excluded. The estimates of risk (mostly using Weinberg's abridged method) vary between 0.36% and 1.87% for the general population. Even if allowance is made for registration bias, distorting effects of the study design, or differences in the methods of computing risk, the variation between the different estimates obtained in European studies deserves attention. The birth cohort method tends to produce higher risk figures than the census/period. However, there was a fourfold difference between morbid risks estimated for the not too dissimilar populations of Norway and Iceland in two thorough investigations using very similar designs (Ödegaard, 1946; Helgason, 1977). This raises the possibility that a real decrease in the morbid risk for schizophrenia may have occurred during the 30 or more years that separate the two cohorts.

The data on the frequency of schizophrenia in different communities are probably among the best documented evidence in psychiatric epidemiology, yet they leave many questions about the nature of this disorder unanswered. The extent of variation of the morbid risk in different populations is not sufficiently well known. The similarity of the prevalence, incidence, and expectancy rates of schizophrenia found in different populations is sometimes seen as evidence strongly favoring a predominantly genetic cause of the disorder. There is, however, no a priori reason to assume that a genetic predisposition to schizophrenia should be evenly distributed across different populations. Environmental causation (which does not have to rule out a significant genetic contribution) is no less compatible with similar rates of manifestation of the disorder in geographically different locations. The epidemiologic indexes of the frequency of schizophrenia, taken in isolation from other evidence, are therefore irrelevant to the "nature/nurture" argument about the etiology of schizophrenia, unless epidemiologic data are collected to test specific hypotheses. One such hypothesis (Böök, 1953) proposes that the operation of an environmental etiological factor would be manifested, *inter alia*, in disproportionately elevated morbid risks for the first-degree relatives of schizophrenics in settings characterized by higher than average incidence rates. Such increases of the morbid risks for relatives have not yet been demonstrated. Böök's own data indicate that the exceptionally high incidence of schizophrenia in the genetic isolate studied by him was not accompanied by an increase of the relative risks for siblings, parents and children of schizophrenics. Nevertheless, the further testing of this, and of related hypotheses, may be a promising line of research.

Affective Psychoses

The main findings are summarized in table 3. There is a general trend for higher rates to be reported in more recent studies, but it is difficult to disentangle the effects of changes in the diagnostic approaches to affective disorders (widening of the scope of the diagnostic category) from real increases in their incidence, prevalence, and morbid risk. The lack of clearcut phenomenological discontinuities between the "endogenous" depressions and the various neurotic and reactive depressive illnesses complicates the problem of comparing results of individual studies.

Neurotic Conditions

The epidemiologic picture presented by survey results (table 4) is difficult to interpret, and the discrepancies between individual studies in regard of the prevalence of neuroses are striking.

Several reasons can be advanced to account for this phenomenon. First, the concept of neurosis was not widely used in clinical psychiatry before World War II, despite the ground it had gained in psychotherapy. Epidemiologically oriented psychiatrists either excluded neurotic disorders altogether from consideration (Strömgren, 1938; Larsson and Sjögren, 1954) or counted only the severe cases. In Brugger's surveys (Brugger, 1931, 1933, 1938) cases of "neurasthenia" were identified at the unlikely low rate of 0.4-0.8 per 1,000 (point prevalence). A possible reason for finding such low rates could be in the high threshold of severity at which a neurotic symptom would be considered worthy of reporting or recording in an epidemiologic investigation. It is quite likely that an occasional hallucinatory "voice" speaking to the patient would have been recorded even if it occurred very rarely, while reports of mild anxiety, fatigue, and difficulty in concentration might have been regarded as "normal" physiologic responses. However, even if possible threshold effects on reporting and recording are discounted, the differences between earlier and recent studies are striking. Some recent investigations have established a point prevalence of neuroses of the order 100-400 per 1,000. It seems unlikely that several decades ago experienced clinicians would have simply missed a large proportion of psychologic morbidity in the community. Considering the meticulous interviewing methods used in some of the earlier surveys, failure to recognize neurotic disorders in the community is difficult to accept as an explanation. This leaves the possibility that the incidence and prevalence of neurotic disorders were really lower in earlier periods (at least in the populations studied). Such a possibility would be in agreement with certain recent findings (Brown et al., 1977; Brunetti, 1974) which suggest a low rate of

TABLE 3
Selected Survey Data on Affective Psychoses.

Author, year	*Country*	*Point prevalence per 1,000*	*Incidence per 1,000/year*	*Morbid risk %*	*Remarks*
Dahlberg & Stenberg (1931)	Sweden			0.16(M), 0.30(F)	Manic-depressive psychosis
Brugger (1933)	Germany	2.0		0.31-0.42	Manic-depressive psychosis
Brugger (1938)	Germany	0.3 - 0.4		0.6	Manic-depressive psychosis
Strömgren (1938)	Denmark	1.3(+1.4 "suspect")		0.23-0.26	Manic-depressive psychosis
Ödegaard (1946)	Norway			0.70	Manic-depressive psychosis (first admissions)
Larsson & Sjögren (1954)	Sweden			0.90(M), 1.20(F)	Manic-depressive psychosis
Helgason T. (1964)	Iceland			2.18(M), 3.23(F)	Affective psychoses
Crocetti et al. (1971)	Yugoslavia	4.2			Manic-depressive psychosis
Nielsen (1976)	Denmark	13.1	1.1-2.7		Affective psychoses
Rotstein (1977)	USSR	1.91			Manic Depressive psychosis
Helgason L. (1977)	Iceland		0.42(M), 1.23(F)	1.20(M), 3.17(F)	Affective psychoses
Jablensky, Milenkov & Temkov (1981)	Bulgaria		0.27		Affective psychoses

TABLE 4
Selected Survey Data on Neurotic Disorders.

Author, year	*Country*	*Point prevalence per 1,000*	*Other prevalence per 1,000*	*Incidence per 1,000/year*	*Morbid risk %*	*Remarks*
Brugger (1933)	Germany				0.13 (hysteria) 0.16 (neurasthenia)	
Helgason T. (1964)	Iceland				9.50(M), 18.04(F)	
Hagnell (1966)	Sweden		131.0 (lifetime prevalence)			
Piotrowski et al. (1967)	Poland	72.1				
Väisänen (1975)	Finland	182.0 (neuroses) 383.0 (milder neurotic disorders)				
Nielsen (1976)	Denmark	65.9(M), 162.6(F)		2.9-5.5		
Rotstein (1977)	USSR	16.9*				*Includes neuroses and personality disorders
Helgason L. (1977)	Iceland		2.25(M), 4.06 (F)	3.92(M), 6.90(F)		

depressive neuroses among women living in socially cohesive, traditional rural areas. Brown proposed that an increased frequency of depression may be a response to the stresses and strains of urban life, to which women may be particularly vulnerable. Anxiety states may be a response of traditional communities experiencing incoming modernization and social change as threat to their values.

The main epidemiologic findings about neurotic disorders, obtained in the recent studies, can be summarized as follows. The annual incidence is about 7.5 per 1,000 according to followup census data (Hagnell, 1970). The point prevalence data, however, can be confusing. On the one hand, there are reports of extremely high rates (113 per 1,000, Nielsen, 1976; 182 per 1,000 Lehtinen et al., 1978; 210 per 1,000, Takala et al., 1979). On the other hand, a number of studies indicate a point prevalence of the order of 7 to 43 per 1,000. Despite the variation and lack of standardization of diagnostic criteria in this field, it is likely that these findings actually refer to two different categories of conditions. One category probably includes clear-cut syndromes that can be diagnosed in field studies by the same criteria as in a clinical setting. The second category is a collection of ill-defined syndromes, symptoms, and complaints that may be subjectively distressing and mildly disabling but lack the symptom specificity required for making a diagnosis. This uncertain, or ill-defined group may be excluded in some surveys but reported in others.

Another problem encountered in field surveys is the association between neurotic and physical morbidity. Surprisingly, the number of studies in which data or combined physical and psychiatric morbidity have been collected is very small. All the evidence available indicates that the frequency of physical disease in persons with psychiatric disorders (and vice versa) is increased (Shepherd et al., 1966). Essen-Möller (1953) collected such data systematically in the process of personally examining every inhabitant of Lundby and found that the age-specific point prevalence of combined physical and psychiatric morbidity was 159 per 1,000 for age groups 15-39, 312 per 1,000 for age groups 40-59 and 413 per 1,000 for age groups 60 and above. The prevalence of physical illnesses only in the same groups was 130, 170 and 212 per 1,000 respectively. Similarly, in an investigation of a random sample (n=1,500) from a general practice population, Eastwood (1970) found that 35.1% of the men and 33.3% of the women with neurotic disorders had at least one associated physical condition; most of the physical conditions were cardiovascular disorders. In contrast, physical disease only was present in 13.5% of the men and 12.5% of the women. Data of this kind raise important questions about the nature of "psychosomatic" morbidity and the pathogenesis of certain physical and psychiatric disorders. Such data can also be highly relevant to the planning of primary health care. It seems, however, that the lack of a suitable classification and diagnostic tests, confounded by the traditional split between the medical disciplines and psychiatry, have impeded the epidemiologic study of the relationship between soma and psyche.

Mental Retardation

Mental retardation presents fewer difficulties with regard to case definition and case identification, and the results of different epidemiologic surveys are not discrepant. The variation of reported rates is considerable for mild mental retardation but less pronounced for the moderate and severe grades. For severe mental retardation, Brugger found a prevalence rate of 5.4 per 1,000 in his first survey (1931) and 15.9 per 1,000 in the second survey (1933). The prevalence rates of severe retardation (per 1,000 of the population up to age 15) found by different authors are not very dissimilar: 4.2 (Strömgren, 1938), 5.7 (Sjögren, 1948), 9.8 (Essen-Möller, 1953), and 2.5 (Rotstein, 1977). A particularly thorough search for cases of severe mental retardation in the community of Aarhus, Denmark, revealed a prevalence of 3.38 per 1,000 (Bernsen, 1976). About 23% of the cases in the latter survey were identified as Down's syndrome, which gives 0.77 per 1,000 prevalence of this condition in the population. The genetic factors involved in severe mental retardation have been explored by Sjögren (using the pedigree method) who established a significantly higher degree of consanguinity in such pedigrees (5.6%) than in the total population of the islands surveyed by him (3.0%).

Total Psychiatric Morbidity of Populations

Considering the limited comparability of data collected by different investigators using different methods in different populations, the rates of total mental morbidity (table 5) should be viewed with caution. Since the neurotic conditions make up a large proportion of the total morbidity, but are also the least reliably identified group of conditions, they are likely to be the most important source of bias in total estimates. Nevertheless, the epidemiologic study of total mental morbidity suggests new and useful ways of looking at psychiatric morbidity in the community, which are different from a simple addition of the rates for individual disorders.

One way of analyzing total incidence and prevalence data would be to aim to identify "natural" groupings. Such groups may cut across nosologic boundaries and not be apparent if only rated for individual categories of conditions are examined. A "periodic" survey, or a repeated census like Essen-Möller's (1953) and Hagnell's (1966, 1970, 1975) investigations of the Lundby population, offer particularly favorable possibilities for this. Hagnell has indeed identified two major groups of illnesses in the general population: *(a)* a "middle-years-maximum" group (MYM) that included mainly neuroses, and *(b)* a "rising-with-age" group (RWA) consisting predominantly of organic conditions. These two groups are sufficiently important because of their size. However, they also raise the question whether the clustering of illnesses at particular stages of the life cycle may also reflect the existence of a common pathogenetic mechanism.

Another approach to the study of total psychiatric morbidity involves assessment of psychologic impairment and social disability associated with various conditions. This approach presupposes the construction of scales of psychologic and social functioning and the development of operational definitions and concepts that should be complementary to those describing

TABLE 5
Selected Survey Data on Total Psychiatric Morbidity in Defined Populations.

Author, year	*Country*	*Point prevalence per 1,000*	*Other prevalence per 1,000*	*Incidence per 1,000*	*Morbid risk %*	*Remarks*
Mayer-Gross (1948)	Scotland, UK	90.0*				*Persons considered "abnormal"
Essen-Möller et al. (1956)	Sweden	123.0(M), 149.0(F)				
Helgason, T. (1964)	Iceland		293.5(M)*,323.4(F)*		32.5(M)**, 35.3(F)**	*Lifetime prevalence **Until age 61
Hagnell (1966, 1970)	Sweden			113.0(M)*, 204.0(F)*	43.4(M)** 73.0(F)**	*10-year incidence **Until age 60
Shepherd et al. (1966)	UK		97.9(M)*,175.0(F)*	52.0**		*Annual consulting rate **Inception rate (1st consultation in the year)
Bjarnar et al. (1975)	Norway		205.0*			*Lifetime prevalence
Nielsen (1976)	Denmark	254.0(M),303.0(F)		12.2*		*Mean annual rate of first referrals for age groups 15+

TABLE 5 (Continued)

Author, year	*Country*	*Point prevalence per 1,000*	*Other prevalence per 1,000*	*Incidence per 1,000*	*Morbid risk %*	*Remarks*
Jablensky & Ochavkov (1976)	Bulgaria	51.2*				*Psychological impairment
Brown et al. (1977)	UK		a) 170.0*(F) b) 360.0**(F)			*Annual prevalence of "cases" **includ. "borderline" case
Helgason, L. (1977)	Iceland			5.06(M)*, 7.07(F)*		*Annual incidence
Rotstein (1977)	USSR	51.4(M) 53.4(F)				
Lehtinen et al. (1978)	Finland	a) 597.0(M)*, 696.0(F)* b) 140.0**				*Including cases of "mild psychological disorder" and "borderline states" **Psychological impairment

psychopathology. Examples of the application of an approach of this kind are the surveys by Lehtinen, et al. (1978) and Jablensky and Oshavkov (1976). In the Finnish survey, the prevalence of all grades of impairment was 140 per 1,000, that of severe impairment, 27 per 1,000. In the Bulgarian survey, in which a random sample of 18,994 persons was examined, the prevalence of all grades of impairment was 51 per 1,000. Differences in scale definition probably account for a proportion of the differences in rates.

Conclusions: Contributions of Survey Investigations in Europe to Epidemiologic Knowledge

In a book that has become a classic in its field, Morris (1975) distinguished seven major uses of the epidemiological method: *(a)* historical study of health and disease; *(b)* community diagnosis; *(c)* study of the working of health services; *(d)* determination of individual chances and risks; *(e)* identification of syndromes; *(f)* completing the clinical picture of diseases; and *(g)* search of causes of conditions. It seems appropriate to examine and sum up the European contribution to epidemiological knowledge under these seven headings.

Study of Historical Trends

The question: "Are mental disorders on the increase?" has been asked by generation after generation in Europe. More than 100 years ago, Henry Maudsley (1872) wrote: "There is always a large number of persons who are prompt enough to grumble at the age in which they live. . . . We need not wonder, therefore, if the alleged increase of insanity is accepted without sufficient proof. . . . The fast pace of living, and the strain of eager competition at the present day, are sure to find out the weak members of the community, and to try them severely. . . . Still it seems to me that there is a tendency to overlook the countervailing advantages of modern life. By the exercise of a little ingenuity, it would be possible to adduce as many theoretical arguments to prove that insanity need not, as can be brought forward to prove that it must increase."

The community survey should be one of the methods best suited to provide answers to questions like this, yet the answers that can actually be derived are not clear and simple. The history of community mental health research in Europe spans almost a century. However, methodologic problems preclude meaningful comparison between studies done at different times with the exception of the instances where the same community has been examined more than once by the same investigators, or where a psychiatric case register has been run with unchanged rules for a sufficiently long period of time. Comparisons between other kinds of studies can only be indirect and inferential. Nevertheless, the balance of the evidence points to the following conclusions:

1. The incidence and morbid risk for the *major psychoses* have not increased over time. On the contrary, there is some evidence (Weeke and Strömgren, 1978) that the incidence of schizophrenia as measured by the first admission rate, may be decreasing in some age groups. The prevalence of chronic psychotic conditions in the population has increased slightly, as a result of the demographic aging of populations and the diminishing mortality of the mentally ill.
2. No valid conclusion can be made about trends or changes in the incidence of neurotic disorders because of the lack of comparability of case definitions and diagnostic criteria. However, the possibility that the incidence of *neurotic disorders* may have increased over the last several decades cannot be ruled out.
3. Certain categories of mental morbidity (e.g., those associated with syphilis and other infections of the nervous system), which made up a significant proportion of the total burden of disease found in earlier surveys, have practically disappeared. Also, the frequency of the most severe and dramatic forms of psychosis, e.g., catatonic states in schizophrenia, delirium tremens, and severe depression ("melancholia"), has apparently decreased.
4. *Drug and alcohol abuse* appear to be increasing with "modernization." The picture, however, is far from uniform, especially regarding alcohol, and there are regions and communities where the frequency of alcohol abuse has been decreasing over time, while in other parts of the continent it has been on the increase.
5. The prevalence of *mental disorders of old age* is increasing, perhaps at a faster rate than any other category of mental morbidity. This is due to the combined effect of the growing proportion of elderly people in the population and the decrease in the formerly excessive mortality of old people suffering from mental disorder.

Community Diagnosis

Community surveys in Europe have demonstrated that:

1. Mental disorders constitute a major proportion of the total morbidity of populations. Depending on the case definition adopted, 5%-30% of the members of a community are suffering from mental disorder at any time, and the risk for an individual surviving until the age of 60 to develop at least one episode of mental disorder at any time may be as high as 43% for men and 73% for women.
2. The most important mental health problem in the community with regard to its frequency is neurosis (lifetime prevalence about 13%-14% and morbid risk, according to conservative estimates, 9%-10% for men and 17%-19% for women). The major psychoses have a lifetime prevalence of 1%-2% and morbid risk 3.5%-4.7% for men and 3.6%-6.9% for women.
3. The association between physical and mental disease is common and its frequency is higher than the product of the rates for physical and

mental disorders. The association between neurotic and cardiovascular disorders is particularly conspicuous.

4. Between 4% and 14% of the population is at any time functionally and socially impaired because of mental illness.

At the same time, the community diagnosis provided by the epidemiologic survey method remains incomplete. Most of the available data have been obtained in studies of relatively stable populations that have not been exposed to severe strains and crises. Such data cannot be extrapolated to other communities, especially those most affected by social change, urbanization, industrialization, and migration.

Working of the Health Services

There are considerable variations within Europe of the provision of psychiatric beds and other facilities per 1,000 population, the ratio of psychiatrists and other mental health workers to population, and the patterns of organization and administration of mental health care. Regardless of such variation, the results of epidemiological surveys indicate the following:

1. The proportion of mental morbidity requiring treatment in specialized facilities is very small in comparison with the total prevalence of mental health problems. The risk of ever being admitted to a mental hospital up to the age of 60 is 3%-4% for men and 5%-6% for women, in settings with easy availability of psychiatric beds.
2. The need for a psychiatric consultation on an outpatient basis, is much higher than the need for institutional treatment. Where enough psychiatrists are available to the population, about 30% of the men and about 42% of the women reaching the age of 60 will have seen a psychiatrist at least once. In some populations, the need for psychiatric treatment has been estimated as "evident" in as much as 8% of the total population at any given point in time.
3. The majority of people with mental health problems consult a general practitioner. Up to 15%-20% of the general practice clientele in some countries present with psychiatric problems but only 1 out of 20 cases is ever referred to a psychiatrist for specialist treatment and management. Even in countries with extensive coverage of the population by specialized psychiatric services, between 17% and 50% of the cases identified in community epidemiologic surveys are unknown to the psychiatric service.
4. There is no support for the assumption that the introduction of easily available and accessible mental health services in the community reinforces the "illness behavior" of its members and leads to unlimited and costly growth of the demand for care. Where unlimited access to psychiatric services has been offered, the demand has reached a plateau at the level of about 10 consultations per 1,000 children up to the age 14 per year and 17-18 consultations per 1,000 adults per year. It has

been estimated that about 28 psychiatrist's work days per year could meet the total needs of 1,000 of the general population. This amount of psychiatric work days can be shared between psychiatrists and general practitioners in various ways, depending on the system of organization of health care.

Determination of Individual Chances and Risks

The study of morbid risks for various psychiatric conditions has been one of the main objectives of the survey method. Actuarial risks (i.e., expectancy of developing a specified disorder on the assumption that an individual will reach a certain age) have been calculated for "average" individuals selected at random from the general population; men and women; and siblings, parents, and offspring of persons suffering from mental disorders. The figures concerning the general risk of developing mental illness have been quoted above, and the risk data for schizophrenia are presented in table 2. Most of these investigations have been undertaken under the influence of eugenic ideas that today attract less scientific and public health interest than in the first decades of this century. Regardless of some dated theoretical assumptions underlying the studies of morbid risk, two general conclusions can be made.

1. There is a gradient of increasing risk of developing a psychosis with the increasing genetic relatedness of an individual to an index case of psychosis. The size of this gradient however, is relatively small. In the instance of schizophrenia, the risk increases from about 1% in the case of an individual having no relative suffering from the disorder, to about 10%-11% in the case of a person who has a schizophrenic parent.
2. Women have higher morbid risks than men for total psychiatric morbidity, particularly the risk for neuroses and affective disorders. The sex differences in morbidity are consistent in all communities studied, including communities that are historically, socially, and culturally different or even contrasting. This fact suggests that the origin of such differences cannot be explained only in terms of social conditioning.

Identification of Syndromes

The investigation of psychiatric conditions in the community, being free of the effects of selection factors that influence hospital-based studies, has resulted in the description of new syndromes, as well as in the identification of "nonsyndromes" (Mörris, 1975). The following examples illustrate this point:

1. One of the most significant findings of epidemiologic surveys has been the discovery of a higher-than-chance frequency of syndromes of associated mental and physical morbidity.
2. A number of conditions for which no appropriate classification and diagnostic provisions exist at present have been found to be highly

prevalent in the general population. These conditions range from ill-defined neurotic complaints (e.g., "irritability," "nervousness," "fatigue"), to clear-cut syndromes (e.g., a "neurocardiovascular," syndrome which may be present in up to 24% of some populations).

3. Some clinical hypotheses about syndromes or diagnostic entities have been corroborated, and some refuted by survey data. Thus the existence of a disease entity that combines the features of schizophrenia and mental retardation ("Pfropff-Schizophrenie") and is more frequent than a chance combination of the two disorders has been supported by Sjögren's (1948) data. On the other hand, the notion of age-specific *involutional* mental morbidity has not found strong epidemiologic support.
4. Certain patterns of symptoms and behaviors have been described that appear to be closely connected with lifestyles and environmental factors prevalent among specific population groups. For example, an endemic peak of psychotropic drug consumption has been observed in fishing communities in Northern Norway (Fugelli, 1975). This behavior was found to coincide with a cyclic increase of the community's "normal" anxiety about the outcome of the fishing season, and not with the advent of the polar night, as formerly believed.

Completing the Clinical Picture of Mental Disorders

Community surveys have been particularly productive in this respect, enabling investigators to collect unbiased data on both symptomatology and "natural history" of psychiatric disorders. A few examples include the following:

1. Neurotic disorders, the most frequent category of mental morbidity in the community, have their peak of onsets in early middle age. In contrast to impressions formed in clinical and psychotherapeutic settings, more than one-third of the neuroses are self-limited illnesses (up to 4 months) regardless of treatment, and less than one-fifth of them progress for 3 or more years.
2. Schizophrenic disorders have extremely varied patterns of courses ranging from complete recovery through episodic symptoms to chronic disability; as many as 0.5%-1.5% of the population aged 60 and above, i.e., those who have passed the entire morbid risk period for schizophrenia, have had one or more episodes of schizophrenia or "schizophrenic spectrum" conditions and a considerable proportion of those have never been diagnosed or treated.
3. Neurotic and affective disorders can have their first onset much later in life than formerly accepted; up to 5% of the elderly people (aged 65 and over) in the community develop neurotic or affective illnesses late in life. The clinical manifestations of such disorders often present diagnostic difficulties and can mimic organic deterioration. They are, however, reversible and respond to appropriate treatment.

Search for Causes of Mental Disorders

So far, the application of the survey method to the study of the etiology of mental disorders has been less successful than the other uses of the method. After the discovery of the etiology of pellagra and the associated psychosis, no major causal factor involved in the etiology of the common or severe psychiatric conditions has been identified to date in surveys of the mental morbidity of geographically defined populations. This negative conclusion is underscored by the fact that the search for genetic etiological factors has been one of the principal objectives of the survey method since its inception. With regard to the "nature-nurture" paradigm in psychiatry, the results of epidemiologic surveys suggest the following:

1. Genetic factors play a role in the etiology and pathogenesis of schizophrenic psychoses and affective disorders, but the nature of this role is not fully understood. The occurrence of schizophrenia in populations does not follow the Mendelian rules of inheritance. The presence of a genetic predisposition is certainly not a sufficient cause for the development of a schizophrenic illness; it is not known whether it is a necessary cause. The majority of people who develop schizophrenia have no relatives suffering from schizophrenia, and the majority of the individuals who have a genetic loading for the disease (including the offspring of *two* schizophrenic parents) never develop schizophrenia. On the other hand, no single environmental factor of a psychosocial, physicochemical, or biological nature has been found to be specifically associated with the occurrence of schizophrenia. Repeated studies of the same population have failed to demonstrate any influence of social change on the incidence of schizophrenia. Of course, the possibility that the hypothetical environmental causal factors are too subtle to be captured by the present-day methods of investigation cannot be ruled out.
2. The existence of nosologically nonspecific risk factors for a variety of mental disorders has been demonstrated repeatedly in community surveys. Sex and age are consistently associated with particular patterns of morbidity. In addition, higher than average risks have been identified for the following groups: *(a)* widowed, divorced, and single individuals (aged widowers seem to be especially vulnerable); *(b)* those exposed to chronic stressful situations; *(c)* individuals with recently "changed status," including migrants, unemployed, sedentarized nomads (e.g., the Lapps in Norway). Where comparisons between rural and urban areas have been made, the morbidity rates in the former have usually been found to be higher (mainly due to negative selection through out-migration). The inverse relation between socioeconomic status and mental morbidity has been confirmed in Finnish studies but the opposite pattern has been found in Sweden, a fact that suggests that social class may be associated with different predisposing factors in different types of communities.

Despite its long history and successes, the method of the epidemiologic mental health survey of geographically defined populations has not yet exhausted its potential to contribute to knowledge. The lack of major achievements in psychiatric epidemiology in recent years is partly due to: *(a)* the absence of a common language in matters of case definition, diagnostic criteria, and classification of data; *(b)* the lack of agreed, standardized, widely acceptable, and reliable assessment tools; and *(c)* the lack of common analytical techniques and uniform ways of data presentation that would allow secondary analysis by other researchers. Many of these obstacles can be overcome, and if adequate administrative and financial support for community mental health research in European countries is ensured, the future may see the emergence of new, fresh approaches and advances in knowledge.

References

Adelstein, A. M., Downham, D. Y., Stein, Z. & Susser, M. W. (1968), The epidemiology of mental illness in an English city. *Soc Psychiatr* 3:47-59.

Andersen, T. (1975), Physical and mental illness in a Lapp and a Norwegian population. In: *Social, Somatic and Psychiatric Studies of Geographically Defined Populations,* eds. Anderson, T., Astrup, C., & Forsdahl, A. *Acta Psychiatr Scand* Suppl 263.

Ballinger, C. B. (1975), Psychiatric morbidity and the menopause; screening of a general population sample. *Br Med J* 3:344-346.

Berger, M., Yule, W. & Rutter, M. (1975), Attainment and adjustment in two geographical areas: II. The prevalence of specific reading retardation. *Br J Psychiatr* 125:510-519.

Bernsen, A. H. (1976), Severe mental retardation among children in the county of Aahus, Denmark: a community study on prevalence and provision of service. *Acta Psychiatr Scand* 54:43-66.

Binder, J. & Angst, J. (1981), A prospective epidemiological study of depressive, psychosomatic and neurotic disturbances (Switzerland). In: *Prospective Longitudinal Research,* eds. Mednick, S.A. & Baert, A.E. Published on behalf of the World Health Organization Regional Office for Europe. London: Oxford University Press.

Bjarnar, E., Reppesgaard, H. & Astrup, C. (1975), Psychiatric morbidity in Berlevåg. In: *Social, Somatic and Psychiatric Studies of Geographically Defined Populations,* eds. Andersen, T., Astrup, C. & Forsdahl, A. *Acta Psychiatr Scand* Suppl. 263.

Boeters, D. (1936), Belastungsstatistik einer schelesischen Durchschnittsbevölkerung. *Neurol Psychiatr* 155:675-701.

Böök, J. A. (1953), A genetic and neuropsychiatric investigation of a North Swedish population (with special regard to schizophrenia and mental deficiency). *Acta genet* 4:1-100.

Böök, J. A., Wetterberg, L. & Modrzewska, K. (1978), Schizophrenia in a North Swedish geographical isolate, 1900-1977. Epidemiology, genetics and biochemistry. *Clin Genet* 14:373-394.

Bremer, J. (1951), A social-psychiatric investigation of a small community in Northern Norway. *Acta Psychiatr Neurol Scand* Suppl. 62.

Brevik, J. I. (1975), The "Tromvika" project In: *Social, Somatic and Psychiatric Studies of Geographically Defined Populations*, eds, Andersen, T., Astrup, C. & Forsdahl, A. *Acta Psychiatr Scand* Suppl. 263.

Brown, G. W., Davidson, S., Harris, T., Maclean, V., Pollock, S. and Prudo, R. (1977), Psychiatric disorder in London and North Uist. *Soc Sci Med* 11:367-377.

Brugger, C. (1931), Versuch einer Geisteskrankenzählung in Thüringen. *Neurologie Psychiatr* 133:352-390.

Brugger, C. (1933), Psychiatrische Ergebnisse einer medizinischen, anthropologischen und soziologischen Benölkerungsuntersuchuing. *Z Neurol Psychiatr* 146:489-524.

Brugger, C. (1938), Psychiatrische Bestandesanfnahme im Gebiet eines medizinisch—anthropoligischen Zensus in der Naue von Rosenheim. *Z Neurol Psychiatr* 160:189-207.

Brunetti, P. M. (1964), A prevalence survey of mental disorders in a rural commune in Vaucluse: methodological considerations. *Acta Psychiatr Scand* 40:323-358.

Brunetti, P. M, Dacher, M. & Sequeira, S. (1978), Prevalence of psychological impairment in city and in country samples. *Acta Psychiatr Scand* 58:369-378.

Carstairs, G. M. & Brown, G. W. (1958), A census of psychiatric cases in two contrasting communities. *J Ment Sci* 104:72-81.

Cassou, B., Schiff, M. & Stewart, J. (1979), Génétique et schizophrénie: ré-évaluation d'un consensus. *L'évolution Psychiatrique* 44:733-748.

Chanoït, P., de Barsey, D., de Traversa, B. C., Perseil, A. & Douarin, J. (1975), Approche épidémiologique de la pathologie mental d'un secteur géographique (bilan d'une année). *Ann Méd Psychol* 133:712-724.

Cole, J. P. (1979), *Geography of World Affairs*, 5th Edition. Penguin Books.

Cooper, B. & Morgan, H. G. (1973), *Epidemiological Psychiatry*. Springfield, Illinois: Thomas.

Cooper, B., Fry, J. & Kalton, G. (1969), A longitudinal study of psychiatric morbidity in a general practice population. *Br J Prev Soc Med* 23:210-217.

Cooper, B., Eastwood, M. R. & Sylph, J. (1970), Psychiatric morbidity and social adjustment in a general practice population. In: *Psychiatric Epidemiology*, eds. Hare, E.H. & Wing, J.K. London: Oxford University Press.

Cooper, J. E., Kendall, R. E., Gurland, B. J., Sharpe, L., Copeland, J. R. M. & Simon, R. (1972), *Psychiatric Diagnosis in New York and London*. Maudsley Monographs No. 20. London: Oxford University Press.

Crocetti, G. J., Lemkau, P. V., Kulcar, A. & Kesic, B. (1971), Selected aspects of the epidemiology of psychoses in Croatia, Yugoslavia. III. The cluster sample and the results of the pilot survey. *Am J Epidemiol* 94:126-134.

Dahlberg, G. & Stenberg, S. (1931), Eine statisticsche Untersuchung über die Wahrscheinlichkeit der Erkrankung an verschiedenen Psychosen *Z Neur* 133:477-482.

De Alarcon, J. G., Sainsburg, P. & Constain, W. R. (1975), Incidence of referred mental illness in Chichester and Salisbury. *Psychol Med* 5:32-54.

Dilling, H. & Weyerer, S. (1978), *Epidemiologie psychischer Störungen und psychiatrische Versorgung.* München u. Wien: Urban & Schwarzenberg.

Dilling H. & Weyerer, S. (1980), Incidence and prevalence of treated mental disorders. Health care planning in a small-town rural region of Upper Bavaria. *Acta Psychiatr Scand* 61:209-222.

Durkheim, E. (1964), *The Rules of Sociological Method.* London: Macmillan.

Eastwood, M. R., (1970), Psychiatric morbidity and physical state in a general practice population. In: *Psychiatric Epidemiology,* eds. Hare, E.H. & Wing, J.K. London: Oxford University Press, pp. 291-298.

Essen-Möller, E., Larsson, H., Uddenberg, C. E. & White, G. (1956), Individual traits and morbidity in a Swedish rural population. *Acta Psychiatr Neurol Scand,* Suppl 100.

Fremming, K.H. (1947), *Sygdomsrisikoen for sindslidelser og andre sjaelelige abnormtilstande i den Danske Gennemshitbefolkning. Paa grundlag af en katamnestisk underøgelsse af 5500 personer født i 1883-87.* Copenhagen: Munksgaard.

Fugelli, P. (1975), Mental health and living conditions in a fishing community in Northern Norway. In: *Social, Somatic and Psychiatric Studies of Geographically Defined Populations,* eds. Andersen, T., Astrup, C. & Forsdahl, A. *Acta Psychiatr Scand,* Suppl 263.

Fülöp, T. (1968), Komplex epidemiologiai vizsgalatok falusi lakossag Köreben (complex epidemiological studies in a rural population). Nepegeszegugy 49:20-34.

Galton, F. (1888), Correlations and their measurement, chiefly from anthropometric data. *Proc Roy Soc* 15:135-145.

Galton, F. (1879), Psychometric experiments. *Brain* 2:149-162.

Gavrilova, S. I. (1979), Schizophrenic disorders not registered by the dispensary and identified in a clinical-epidemiological study of elderly age-groups in a general population. *Zh Nevropatol Psihiat* 79:1366-1372.

Giel, R., Ten Horn, G. H. M. M., Ormel, J., Schudel, W. J. & Wiersma, D. (1978), Mental illness, neuroticism and life events in a Dutch village sample: A followup study. *Psychol Med* 8:235-243.

Goldberg, D. P. & Blackwell, B. (1970), Psychiatric illness in a general practice. A detailed study using a new method of case identification. *Br Med J* 2:439-443.

Goldberg, D. P. (1972), *The Detection of Psychiatric Illness by Questionnaire,* Maudsley Monographs No. 21. London: Oxford University Press.

Graemiger, O. (1931), Beitrag zur Frage der Haufigkeit der Psychosen und der erblichen Belastung. *Schweig Med Wschr* 1:561-569.

Grotjahn, A. (1923), *Soziale Pathologie. Dritte Auflage.* Berlin: Julius Springer.

Guntern, G. (1978), *Alpendorf: Transactional Processes in a Human System. A Followup Study About Social Change, Tourism, Stress and Mental Health in a Tourist Resort of the Swiss Alps.* Reports from the Laboratory for Clinical Stress Research, Karolinska Institute, Stockholm, No. 76.

Häfner, H. and Reimann, H. (1970), Spatial distribution of mental disorders in Mannheim, 1965. In: *Psychiatric Epidemiology,* eds. Hare, E.H. & Wing, J.D. London: Oxford University Press, pp 342-354.

Hagnell, O. (1966), *A Prospective Study of the Incidence of Mental Disorder*. Lund, Sweden: Svenska Bokförlaget.

Hagnell, O. (1970), The incidence and duration of episodes of mental illness in a total population. In: *Psychiatric Epidemiology*, eds. Hare, E.H. & Wing, J.K. London: Oxford University Press, pp 213-232.

Hagnell, O. & Öjesjö, L. (1975), A prospective study concerning mental disorders of a total population investigated in 1947, 1957 and 1972. In: *Social, Somatic and Psychiatric Studies of Geographically Defined Populations*, eds. Andersen, T., Astrup, C. & Forsdahl, *A. Acta Psychiatr Scand*, Suppl 263.

Hare, E. H. (1955), Mental illness and social class in Bristol. *Br J Prevent Soc Med* 9:191-195.

Hare, E. G. & Shaw, G. K. (1965), *Mental Health on a New Housing Estate*, Maudsley Monographs No. 12. London: Oxford University Press.

Helgason, T. (1964), Epidemiology of mental disorders in Iceland, *Acta Psychiatr Scand* Suppl 173.

Helgason, L. (1977), Psychiatric services and mental illness in Iceland. *Acta Psychiatr Scand* Suppl 268.

Jablensky, A. & Ochavkov, J. (1975), Health and disability in a total population. In: *Health, Medicine and Society*, eds. Sokolowska, M., Holowka, J. & Ostrowska, A. Dordrecht: Reidel.

Jablensky, A., Milenkov, K. & Temkov I. (1981), Depressive disorders and depressive symptoms among patients making their first contact with a mental health service. In: *Prevention and Treatment of Depression*, eds. Ban, T.A., Gonzalez, R., Jablensky, A., Sartorius, N. & Vartanian, F.E. Baltimore: University Park Press.

Jeanneau, A. & Jeanneau, S. (1969), Existe-t-il une pathologie insulaire? Essai de géographie psychiatrique. *Ann Med Psychol* 127:804-810.

Jost, H. (1896), Quoted from Strömgren (1950).

Kastrup, M., Nakane, Y., Dupont, A. & Bille, M. (1976), Psychiatric treatment in a delimited population—with particular reference to outpatients: a demographic study. *Acta Psychiatr Scand* 53:35-50.

Kay, D. W. K., Beamish, P. & Roth, M. (1964), Old age mental disorders in Newcastle upon Tyne. *Br J Psychiatr* 110:146-158.

Khotzyanov, L. K. (1927), Quoted from Model (1957).

Klemperer, J. (1933), Zur Belastungsstatistik der Durchschnittsbevölkerung. Psychosenhäufigkeit unter 1,000 stichprobenmässig ausgelesenen Probanden. *Neurol Psychiatr* 146:277-316.

Koller, J. (1895), Beitrag zur Erblichkeitsstatistik der Geisteskranken im Kanton Zurich. *Arch Psychiatr* 27:268-294.

Krasik, E. D. (1965), Study on prevalence based on registration of patients by psychiatric dispensary (district of Ryazan). *Zh Nevropatol Psihiat* 65:608-616.

Kulcar, Z., Crochetti, G. M., Lemkau, P. V. & Kesic, B. (1971), Selected aspects of the epidemiology of psychoses in Croatia, Yugoslavia. II. Pilot studies of communities. *Am J Epidemiol* 94:118-125.

Larsson, T., & Sjögren, T. (1954), A methodological, psychiatric and statistical study of a large Swedish rural population. *Acta Psychiatr Neurol Scand*, Suppl 89.

Lehtinen, V., Väisänen, E., Alanen, Y. O. & Tienari, P. (1978), Preventive implication of a social-psychiatric survey of the Finnish population. *Psychiatr* Fennica 1978, 143-151.

Leighton, D. C. Hagnell, O., Leighton, A. H., Harding, J. S., Kellert, S. R. & Dauley, R. A. (1971), Psychiatric disorder in a Swedish and Canadian community: An exploratory study. *Soc Sci Med* 5:189-209.

Lemkau, P., Tietze, C. & Cooper, M. (1943), A survey of statistical studies on the prevalence and incidence of mental disorder in sample populations. *Pub Health Rep* 58:1909-1927.

Lemkau, P. V., Kulcar, Z., Crocetti, M. & Kesic, B. (1971), Selected aspects of the epidemiology of psychoses in Croatia, Yugoslavia. I. Background and use of psychiatric hospital statistics. *Am J Epidemiol* 94:112-117.

Lewis, E. O. (1929), Report on an investigation into the incidence of mental deficiency in six areas, 1925-1927. *Report of the Mental Deficiency Committee of the Board of Education and Board of Control, Part IV.* London: HMSO.

Lieberman, Y. I. (1947), On the problem of incidence of schizophrenia (material from a clinical-epidemiological investigation). *Zh Nevropatol Psihiatr* 74:1224-1232.

Lin, T. Y. & Standley, C. C. (1962), *The Scope of Epidemiology in Psychiatry,* Public Health Papers No. 16, Geneva: World Health Organization.

Maudsley, H. (1872), Is insanity on the increase? *Br Med J* i:36-39.

Mayer-Gross, W. (1948), Mental health survey in a rural,area a preliminary report. *Eugenics Rev* 40:140-155.

Model, A. A. (1957), Disorders of the nervous system in Kolkhoz farmers. *Zh Nevropatol Psihiatr* 57:57.

Morris, J. N. (1975), *Uses of Epidemiology,* 3rd Edition Edinburgh: Churchill Livingstone.

Nielsen, J. (1976), The Samsϕ project from 1957 to 1974. *Acta Psychiatr Scand* 54:198-222.

Norris, V. (1959), *Mental Illness in London,* Maudsley Monographs No. 6 London: Chapman and Hall.

Ödegaard, Ö. (1946), A statistical investigation of the incidence of mental disorder in Norway. *Psychiatr Quart* 20:381-401.

Ouspenskaya, L. Y. (1978), Some aspects of the method of comparative epidemiological study and the characteristics of the spread of schizophrenia in different areas of the country. *Zh Nevropatol Psihiatr* 78:742-748.

Panse, F. (1929), Beitrag zur Belastungsstatistik einer Durchschnittsbevölkerung. *Z Neurol Psychiatr* 194-222.

Piotrowski, A., Henisz, J. & Gnat, T. (1967), Individual Interview and clinical examination to determine prevalence of mental disorders. Methodology and results of mental health survey in Poland. In: *Proceedings, Fourth World Congress of Psychiatry, Madrid, 5-11 Sept. 1966, Part 4.* Amsterdam: Excerpta Medical 2477-2478.

Predescu, V., et al. (1974), Metodologia depistarii active a bolilor psihice in populatia urbana. *Igiena* 23:361-368.

Reid, D. D. (1960), *Epidemiological Methods in the Study of Mental Disorders,* Public Health Papers No. 2. Geneva: World Health Organization.

Rotstein, V. G. (1977), Results of a psychiatric examination of samples of adult population in a number of areas in the USSR. *Zh Nevropatol Psihiatr* 77:569-574.

Rüdin, E. (1916), *Zur Vererbung und Neuentstehung der Dementia praecox.* Berlin: Juluis Springer.

Rutter, M., Cox, A., Tupling, C., Berger, M. & Yule, W. (1975), Attainment and adjustment in two geographical areas: I. The Prevalence of psychiatric disorder. *Bri J Psychiatr* 126:493-509.

Rutter, M., Yule, B., Quinton, D., Berger, M. & Yule, W. (1975), Attainment and adjustment in two geographical areas: III. Some factors accounting for area differences. *Br J Psychiatr* 125:520-533.

Schipkowenski, N. (1977), *Iatrogenie oder befreiende Psychotherapie?* Basel and Stuttgart: Schwabe & Co.

Shepherd, M. (1957), *A Study of the Major Psychoses in an English County*, Maudsley Monograph No. 3. London: Chapman & Hall.

Shepherd, M., Cooper, B., Brown, A. C. & Kalton, G. (1966), *Psychiatric Illness in General Practice.* London: Oxford University Press.

Singerman, N. I. (1927), Quoted from Model (1957).

Sjobring, H. (1974), Mental constitution and mental illness. In: *Themes and Variations in European Psychiatry*, eds. Hirsch, S. R. & Shepherd, M. Bristol: John Wright & Sons.

Sjögren, T. (1948), Genetic-statistical and psychiatric investigations of a West Swedish population. *Acta Psychiatr Neurol* Suppl. 52.

Slater, E. (1935), The incidence of mental disorder. *Ann Eugen* 6.

Strömgren, E. (1938), Beiträge zur psychiatrischen Erblehre, auf Grund von Untersuchungen an einer Inselbevölkerung. *Acta Psychiatr Neurol*, Suppl. 19.

Strömgren, E. (1950), Statistical and genetical population studies within psychiatry: methods and principal results. *Proc. First Internat. Congress of Psychiatry*, Vol. VI, Paris: Herman & Cie, pp. 155-192.

Strömgren, E. (1968), Contributions to psychiatric epidemiology and genetics. *Acta Jutlandica* 40:41-86.

Strotzka, H. (1969), *Kleinburg: eine sozialpsychiatrische Feldstudie*, Österreichischer Bundesverlag für Unterricht, Wissenschaft und Kunst, Wein-München.

Svendsen, B. B. (1952), Psychiatric morbidity among civilians in wartime. On trends studies in general and a trends study of Danish psychiatric hospital admissions 1939-1948. *Acta Jutlandica* 24, Suppl. A.

Takala, J., Sievers, K. & Takala, A. (1978), A multiphasic screening programme at the health centre level; Säkylä-Köyliö project. The variables, methods and participation. *Scand J Soc Med* 7:87-91.

Takala, J., Räkkölainen, V., Salminen, J. & Sievers, K. (1979), Mental health in the middle-aged population. *Acta Psychiatr Scand* 59:294-305.

Temkov, I., Jablensky, A. & Boyadjieva, M. (1975), Use of reported prevalence data in cross-national comparisons of psychiatric morbidity. *Soc Psihijat* 3:111-117.

Tönnies, F. (1887), *Gemeinschaft und Gesellschaft.* Berlin.

Väisänen, E. (1975), Psychiatric Disorders in Finland. *Acta Psychiatr Scand* Suppl. 263, pp. 22-33.

Videbech, T., Bille, M., Dupont, A. & Juel-Nielsen, N. (1970), A survey of mental illness in a Danish County. The Aarhus County investigation *Acta Psychiatr Scand,* Suppl 217.

Walsh, D. (1969), Mental illness in Dublin—first admissions. *Br J Psychiatr* 115:449-456.

Weeke, A., Bille, M., Videbech, Th., Dupont, A. & Juel-Nielsen, N. (1975), Incidence of depressive syndromes in a Danish County. *Acta Psychiatr Scand* 51:28-41.

Weeke, A. & Strömgren, E. (1978), Fifteen years later. A comparison of patients in Danish psychiatric institutions in 1957, 1962, 1967 and 1972. *Acta Psychiatr Scand* 57:129-144.

Weinberg, W. (1925), Methoden und Technik der Statistik mit besonderer Berücksichtigung der Sozialbiologi. In: *Handbuch d. sozial. Hygiene und Gesundheitsfürsorge, Bd.I.* 71-148, Berlin: Springer.

Wing, J. K. (1976), A technique for studying psychiatric morbidity in inpatient and outpatient series and in general population samples. *Psychol Med* 6:665-671.

Wing, J. K., Cooper, J. E. & Sartorius, N. (1974), *The Measurement and Classification of Psychiatric Symptoms.* Cambridge University Press.

Wing, L., Wing, J. K., Hailey, A., Bahn, A. K., Smith, H. E. & Baldwin, J. A. (1967), The use of psychiatric services in three urban areas: An international case register study. *Social Psychiatr* 2:158-167.

World Health Organization (1960), *Epidemiology of Mental Disorders.* Eighth Report of the Expert Committee on Mental Health. Technical Report Series No. 185. Geneva: WHO.

World Health Organization (1973), *Report of the International Pilot Study of Schizophrenia, Vol. I.* Geneva: WHO.

World Health Organization (1979), *Schizophrenia. An International Follow-up Study.* Chichester: John Wiley & Sons.

World Health Organization (1981), *Current State of Diagnosis and Classification in the Mental Health Field.* A report from the WHO/ADAMHA joint project on diagnosis and classification of mental disorders and alcohol-and drug-related problems, Geneva: World Health Organization.

World Health Organization (1982), *International Conference on Diagnosis and Classification of Mental Disorders and Alcohol-and Drug-Related Problems.* Workshop reports and panel discussions, MNH/82/52 Rev. 1. Geneva: World Health Organization.

Zharikov, N. M. (1965), Epidemiological study of mental morbidity. *Zh Nevropatol Psihiatr* 65:617-623.

Zharikov, N. M. (1968), Epidemiological study of mental illness in the USSR. *Social Psychiatr* 3:135-138.

Zharikov, N. M., Kalachev, V. F. & Sokolova, E. D. (1979), Comparative clinical-epidemiological study of schizophrenic patients in central districts and in the extreme North-East of the USSR. *Zh Nevropatol Psihiatr* 79:453-460.

Part Two

Defining a Case

Chapter 15

What Do Instruments Like the 22-Item Screening Score Measure? A Look at Correlates and a Review of Construct Validity

THOMAS S. LANGNER

In 1962 a paper called "A Twenty-Two Item Screening Score of Psychiatric Symptoms Indicating Impairment" was published in the Journal of Health and Human Behavior (Langner, 1962). Some similar instruments, such as the Health Opinion Survey (HOS) (MacMillan, 1957) had been used in several studies. In fact, such screening checklists go back as far as Woodworth (1917) or perhaps earlier. Hundreds of similar tests are listed in the Mental Measurements Yearbook (Buros, 1959). For some unknown reason, a few of these instruments became more widely used than others. The distinction should be made between such global or overall measures as the HOS, the 22-Item Screening Score, the General Well-Being Schedule (Dupuy 1973), and construct-specific scales purporting to measure anxiety, depression, satisfaction, self-control, etc. What is becoming clear, however, is that global measures of impairment, symptom level or mental health often have a strong bias toward particular types of items. They generally emphasize anxiety, depression, somatization, and tension. They typically avoid questions having to do with antisocial behavior. They seldom have large numbers of questions concerning delusions, hallucinations, depersonalization, or relatively rare symptoms such as formication or trichotillomania. In the 1962 paper, I said "We suspect that it (the 22-item score) does not screen persons with organic brain damage, the mentally retarded, and the sociopaths. It does, however, provide a rough indication of where people lie on a continuum of impairment in life functioning due to very common types of psychiatric symptoms."

The global screening instruments, then, seem to account pretty well for the middle range of emotional disorders, but certainly not for the extremes such as the psychoses. They were never meant to be used for the positive identification of individuals for treatment or intervention. They were usually constructed with the purpose of comparing large subgroups of people and for identifying a potential high risk group whose individuals could then be classified on the basis of further examination.

In trying to define what the 22-Item Screening Score and some similar scales measure we can use several approaches. These are usually called content validity, construct validity, criterion (known groups) validity, discriminant validity, and predictive validity. These types of validity translate into rather specific operations.

1. The content of scale items is examined, and the face validity of the scale determined.
2. The correlations of the particular scale with other scores are examined. There should be a theoretical framework, and the correlation of the criterion with other behaviors or conditions should support the hypotheses in magnitude and direction.
3. Criterion validity compares the scale with a previously validated measure of the same construct. Very often global measures have used a group of known ill, such as inpatients or outpatients in psychiatric treatment, and compared them with a screened well group. That was one of the procedures used in validating the 22-Item Screening Score (see text). Unfortunately, mental hospital patients are a heterogeneous group, and we are left with a scale that discriminates between patients and nonpatients, but still don't know what particular construct it measures, except a global illness or impairment. A criterion group of diagnosed depressed patients, or a group observed to be highly anxious, often helps to define what the scale in question is really measuring. Unfortunately, visits for psychiatric or similar treatment do not constitute a very good criterion. A large proportion of the population with serious symptomatology remains untreated. For example, in the Family Research Project, a longitudinal study of over 2000 families on which I shall draw for correlates of the 22-Item Screening Score, only half of the children and adolescents aged 6-18 who were rated 4 or 5 (severely impaired or incapacitated) on a five-point scale of psychiatric impairment by psychiatrists working from a detailed mother's report of the child's behavior, were *ever referred* for treatment, much less actually treated. Many field studies of adults support the idea that treatment itself is only a moderately good criterion against which to test measures for use in community studies.
4. Discriminant validity is often used as a term describing the ability of a scale or measure to discriminate between a treated and untreated group, or between a diagnosed group (or groups) and known "wells" (or community controls, who tend to have a fair amount of serious psychopathology).
5. Divergent validity is seldom found for global instruments and is fairly rare even in the case of construct-specific scales. This describes the ability of a scale to relate positively to the measure, which it should by reason of the hypothesized underlying construct, and by the same token, the ability to not relate or relate inversely to a measure that

opposes that construct. For example, a dependency scale should show high scores in a group of younger children judged to be dependent, but low scores in a group of adolescents judged to be antisocial or delinquent. What is striking about so many measures is that they discriminate between "wells" and patients, but not between types of patients. For example, when the CES-Depression scale was administered to alcoholics, depressives, ex-depressives, and other types of patients, all of the diagnosed groups scored quite high, while controls did not (Weissman et al., 1977). It is plausible that people in mental hospitals and even outpatient services are generally depressed. What is disappointing is that there are not some diagnostic groups which can be shown to be pathologically elated, or even within the normal range of depression-elation.

6. Predictive validity adds some assurance over concurrent validity since the time span allows us a better approach to teasing out causal relationships. A theoretical framework usually involves assumptions about causal direction. Cross-lagged analysis and path analysis offer some grip on directionality. Without longitudinal studies, we are caught in a web of concurrent associations. If we can say with some confidence, for example, that *prior* undesirable life events are associated with later depression, or that *prior* physical punishment by parents is associated with later delinquency, we have made a little step forward in understanding our depression and delinquency measures. A review of the types of information that help in construct validation is given in Ware et al. (1979), along with a helpful discussion of the problems of construct-specific validity. They also review construct validity findings for a large series of studies involving the types of measures we are discussing here, and more specific measures such as anxiety and depression. I will refer again to their review, especially as it pertains to the Screening Score.

Studies Using the 22-Item Screening Score

I have not made a thorough search of the literature on the 22-Item Score, since the purpose of this paper is to look for the meaning behind a scale that is typical of so many others, and so highly intercorrelated with them. In the Family Research Project, my colleagues and I have steered away from monolithic measures and have used multivariate dependent variables (at least 18 factored dimensions). (Langner, McCarthy, Gersten, Simcha-Fagan & Eisenberg, 1979; Langner, Gersten & Eisenberg, 1977). In a screening instrument for children and adolescents, we used seven orthogonal dimensions, so that there would be adequate coverage of key behavior domains (Langner, Gersten, McCarthy & Eisenberg, et al., 1976). I am clearly not arguing for the use of global measures, but given the wide use of the 22-Item Screening Score and similar measures, it seems necessary to pursue the will-o-the-wisp of its "true meaning."

Here, not necessarily in any order, are a few of the studies using the 22-Item Score: Langner (1962, 1965), Haberman (1964), Phillips (1966), Fabřega & McBee (1970), Summers, Seiler & Hough (1971), Dohrenwend (1973), Radloff (1977), Mueller (1980), Edwards et al. (unpublished), Haese & Meile (1967), Edgerton, Bentz & Hollistter (1970), Phillips & Segal (1965), Yancy et al. (1972), Meile & Haese (1969), Manis et al. (1964), Gaitz & Scott (1972). Quite a few studies have been done in foreign countries such as Canada and France. Ware (1979), Dohrenwend et al., (1980), and Radloff (1977) give descriptions of some of these studies, which I will not repeat here. They also give correlations of the 22-Item Score with other measures, which will be helpful in unraveling its content.

Face Validity

On their face, the items (see reprinted text) fall into several domains. "Nervous," "restlessness,"and "worrying type" seem to be anxiety items. "Trouble getting to sleep," "in low or very low spirits," "wonder if anything is worthwhile," "nothing turns out the way I want it," and "can't get going" are more like depression items. While sleep problems are usually associated with depression, they are also psychophysiological and could be included in that rubric. The psychophysiological items are "appetite poor," "cold sweats," "heart beats hard," "sour stomach," "hands tremble," "shortness of breath," "fainting a few times or more than a few times," "feeling weak all over," "clogging in my nose," and "feel hot all over." Another item, "personal worries get me down physically," could be included with the psychophysiological group, though it has a more general reference to overall health." Feel somewhat apart even among friends" suggests isolation and inability to relate to others." My memory is not all right" suggests either organic damage or severe preoccupation due to fear, anxiety, or depression. The predominant groups are psychophysiological (11 items), depression (5 or 6 items), and anxiety (3 items). Some psychophysiological items could be attributed to depression (for instance, "appetite poor" is tapping mild anorexia, a typical symptom of depression), or to anxiety (cold sweats and palpitations, trembling). The affective component of depression is clearly represented by only one item ("low spirits"). Since the pool from which all items were drawn was fairly large (120) and contained numbers of anxious, depressed, tense, aggressive, rigid, and other items, it is interesting that these particular ones discriminated between patients and controls, and in the impairment ratings. The antisocial, rigidity suspiciousness, and other a priori dimensions were not represented in the final selection, which was actuarial, rather than based upon specific a priori constructs. The overall content of the score, then, suggests somatization depression-anxiety, in that order. Since these dimensions are hardly orthogonal in real life, it remains to be seen if the score correlates with specific underlying constructs, or social-environmental variables that may emphasize or point to one of these three major content areas.

Correlations with Other Measures

Data from Ware (1979), Dohrenwend et al. (1980), and Radloff (1977), and others allow us to compare the 22-Item Score with other global and with construct-specific measures. This should give us some insight into the underlying construct, even though we do not have an elaborated theoretical framework. Link and Dohrenwend (in Dohrenwend et al., 1980, table 5.2) give the correlations of the 22-Item Score with three other measures, with a correction for the difference in time reference. (The 22-Item Score refers to "ever had," while the CES-D, GWB and SCL-90 usually refer to the "past week"). The correlations given are 22-Item Score with the CES-D (Radloff 1977) = 0.85, with the GWB (General Well Being Schedule) = −0.97, (reported by Mueller, unpublished); with the GWB (Edwards et al., unpublished), = −0.93, and with the SCL-90-Symptom Check List (Edwards et al., unpublished), = 0.80. The correlation with the CES-D scale of 0.85 suggests that depression is a dominant part of what the 22-Item Scale is tapping. The GWB and SCL-90 give us no further specific information on divergent validity, but simply show that these longer measures, when time corrected, are probably part and parcel of some underlying dimension. Link and Dohrenwend conclude that the 22-Item Score, the HOS, and the GWB scales belong in the "demoralization" dimension, while the CES-D and the SCL-90 do not. In view of their time-corrected correlations, this would seem incorrect, and on their face all these scales seem related. The uncorrected correlations show the HOS and 22-Item Score more related to each other than to the CES-D and SCL-90, and apparently for this reason the authors ignored the timecorrected correlations (a conservative interpretation).

Radloff (1977) shows a table with correlations of 0.54 and 0.60 for the Item Score with the CED-Depression scale. These correlations compare favorably with CES-D correlations with other scales purported to measure depression and negative affect, specifically. Correlations are generally higher within the patient sample. These data again seem to favor the interpretation of the 22-Item Scale as heavily depressive in content.

Ware et al. (1977) summarize evidence for a series of measures, citing several studies. The 22-Item Screening Score was found to be related primarily to depression scales, ranging from a validity coefficient of 0.28 to 0.39 (Simpkins & Burke, 1974), in a study based primarily upon black women. Fabrega and McBee (1970) found the 22-Item Score correlated 0.30 with psychiatrists' ratings of general neurotic symptoms, and 0.50 with their ratings of dysphoric affect (anxiety and depression). The subjects were psychiatric outpatients, mostly women, and of low income and education. Here the more general "neurotic" rating is exceeded by the "anxious and depressed" rating. However, the distinction between depression and anxiety is not made. While Dohrenwend found the 22-Item Score related 0.35 to recent life events in a low income Washington Heights sample (1973) this does not help us with identifying content. It does, however, add to the validity, and perhaps suggests a reactive or situational component (recent events).

Simpkins & Burke (1974) found the 22-Item Score correlated 0.36 with seeing a physician about personal, emotional, behavioral, or mental problems, and 0.21 with seeing a therapist for similar problems. The correlation with having been a patient in a mental hospital or clinic was only 0.10, however. They also noted a correlation of 0.38 between the 22-Item Score and the GWB Depressed Scale. In addition, they found the 22-Item Score and the GWB Relaxed vs. Tense Scale (which presumably measures anxiety) were related 0.36. Thus depression and anxiety were about equally related. Correlations with the GWB Satisfying-Interesting Life (Positive Well-Being) and the GWB Emotional/Behavioral Control Scale were 0.28 and 0.29 respectively. The differences between these correlations are negligible, though all are significant at the 0.05 level. Again we are faced with the lack of specificity of many of the findings and the seeming circularity of correlating variously named scales with one another. If anything, the results support *both* anxiety and depression as the content of the 22-Item Score.

An Argument for Demoralization

Dohrenwend et al. (1979) studied 124 community adults and 103 psychiatric patients, using psychiatrists as interviewers. They developed five a priori question groups using a pool of items frequently used in screening, such as the 22-Item, the HOS, the Gurin Mental Status Index (Gurin, Veroff & Feld, 1960) and Bradburn & Caplowitz, (1965). A Structured Interview Schedule (SIS) was used, and the five scales were found to be reliable within community and patient samples, and within ethnic, educational, and sex groups.

The intercorrelations of the five scales, Perceived Physical Health, Psychophysiological Symptoms, Anxiety, Sadness, and Enervation range from 0.42 to 0.61, with an average of 0.51 for the community sample. For the patient-prisoner sample, the range was 0.09 to 0.51, with an average of only 0.36. The correlations between scales are often higher within patient populations, which suggests that this patient group was somewhat different from the usual. The fact that the patient average correlation is only 0.36 might be accepted by some investigators as evidence that the scales are modestly independent. Given the fact that the scales were constructed on an a priori basis, their intercorrelations might be higher than if they were fitted to an orthogonal model. Thus, some aspects of both method and interpretation favor calling the intercorrelations high.

The authors' conclusion, based on their own data and work of other investigators, is that "the five scales measure a single common dimension that is very imperfectly related to clinical psychological disorder. A speculative explanation of the nature of this dimension is offered in terms of Jerome Frank's construct of demoralization."

Given the numerous studies that have factored similar item pools and found independent subscales (for example, the SCL-90, the GWB, the MMPI) it seems premature to lump anxiety, sadness (depressive affect), enervation (a correlate of both depression and various physical illnesses), somatization, and perceived physical health. Evidence from several major surveys would have to be marshalled showing the correlation matrices and carefully explaining the exact factoring procedures or methods of assigning items to dimensions. Tests for latent continua should be made. There should be attempts to obtain divergent validity. Only if these procedures fail, using new data or data from previous large surveys, can we accept the collapsing of five domains that on their face appear quite distinct. "Demoralization" is one of a number of handy ways of thinking about some of the dimensions commonly used in screening instruments, but it must prove itself in future research.

Evidence given by Dohrenwend et al. against screening instruments ignores many of the caveats given by authors of such instruments. For example, the fact that the Gurin Mental Status Index (based on the HOS and 22-Item Score) was only weakly related to the Psychiatric Evaluation Form (Endicott and Spitzer, 1973) and the New Haven Schizophrenia Index (Astrachan et al., 1973) *within a sample of schizophrenics* (0.55 and 0.39 respectively) while these two measures were more related to each other (0.67) ignores the fact, established quite early, that such screening instruments do not tap the extremes of mental disorder, but do rather well in the middle range. Instruments designed as "schizophrenia indices" should indeed work better in samples of schizophrenics than short global measures.

We are also told that eight items, including five from the Gurin scale, were selected by Weissman, Myers and Harding (1978) to measure depression in a community sample of 515 subjects. Only 28% of the highest-scoring 100 respondents were diagnosed as having a major or minor depression by Research Diagnostic Criteria (Endicott & Spitzer, 1978) based on interviews with the SADS instrument (Spitzer, Endicott & Robins, 1978). To estimate the effect size, we would also have to know the proportion of diagnosed depressed cases found in the *lowest*-scoring 100 respondents. It is also not a convincing argument that only 28% were identified as cases of depression, since that would mean that over 5% of the whole community sample were diagnosed depressives. Estimating somewhat lower rates for the next two groups of 100 of 20% and 15%, (a total of 35 cases) there might be at least 63 identified depressives in the community sample, yielding a rate of over 12%. That would appear to be a substantial rate of diagnosed depression, when the usual figure given for all diagnosable cases in the community is around 15% total. Estimates of depressive symptomatology using demoralization and dysphoric mood and sadness approach 25%. "About half of those who are demoralized are also clinically impaired" (Link & Dohrenwend, 1980). By this same logic, there is no reason to throw out a measure that can identify as much as one half of the "true" depressed cases, or to call it something other than a form of subclinical depression.

There is a tradition of dichotomous thinking among those who use the medical model, which would prefer to have diagnosed depression on the ill side, and demoralization or a nonmedical category on the healthy side. Yet of all disorders, depression has a long history of being classified by its *severity* along a continuum. Subclinical depression, "neurotic depression" and "psychotic depression" are generally conceived as lying on a scale of progressive severity. Depressed affect is the central core of this continuum. Longitudinal studies using more sensitive instruments will probably show us in the future that subclinical depressions are constantly going over into clinical depressions, and that diagnosed depressives are "remitting" and becoming subclinical in severity. The moderate relation of anxiety and depression to life events demonstrates that these feeling states respond to changes in the environment. The degree to which depressions of varying severity respond to life events and processes would be crucial information in helping us understand whether a continuum or a dichotomy is appropriate.

Endogenous depressions are believed to respond minimally with changes in the environment. They are looked upon as disturbances in brain function, and may be triggered by toxicity, infection, or injury. Reactive depressions are defined as responses to a specific loss of a loved one, of some material object, or opportunity. Neurotic depressions are defined as exhaustion of adaptation to severe or prolonged stress in an inadequate personality, usually entailing unresolved conflicts, chronic anxiety, fear, or anger. The onset of neurotic depression is gradual, compared with the endogenous and reactive types. The nature, intensity, duration, and symptoms of these depressive types vary, and these definitions and descriptions are neatly set forth by Leonard Cammer (1969) in tabular form. While this seems to argue for a dichotomous model, in fact most of the comparisons are of severity or frequency of various symptoms. That there is differential etiology of several forms of depression can not be doubted. However, the manifestations of depression clearly seem to lie on a continuum. Descriptive categories given by Cammer are: mood, sleep, arising, eating, crying, emotional control, self-esteem, anxiety, expressions of fear, ability to make decisions, ability to concentrate, memory, sense of responsibility, contact with reality and surroundings, delusions, alcoholism, fatigue, reserve of strength, physical symptoms, sexual interest, interpersonal relationships, suicidal thoughts and attempts. Here is the core of so many screening instruments, spelled out for depressed patients. No doubt there will be a time when the extent of these same symptoms can be listed for depressed persons in the community who are not "cases". The degree to which they share these behaviors across different samples is much needed information. This is, in my opinion, a time for slicing, not lumping.

Some Social Correlates of "X" (Depressive Symptoms, Demoralization, etc.)

I am going to call the essence of the screening instruments "X" for the moment, and try to further define X not by its clinical or symptom scale correlates, as we have already done, but by its social correlates. Two consistent findings are mentioned by Dohrenwend et al. (1980). Women and low SES respondents score higher on screening scales of this type. Before going into the correlates of the screening instruments, it is necessary to discuss briefly the prevalence rates yielded by two cutoff scores on the 22-Item Score. A cutoff score of 4 or more symptoms was originally recommended in my 1962 paper, but table 4 of that paper gave proportions of the sample with seven or more symptoms reported. A score of 7+ identified 39.6% of the respondents rated impaired, while a score of 4+ identified 73.5% of the impaired (those rated as showing marked or severe impairment by two psychiatrists, or being incapacitated, on a scale of six points which included Well, Mild, and Moderate symptomatology (the unimpaired). The cutoff of 7+ culled very few false positives (0% Wells, almost 0% Milds, and only 8.5% of the Moderates).

If the sample is dichotomized into impaired and unimpaired, the discriminating power of the screening score is minimized. By using Table 4 of the Screening Score article, the false positives and negatives can be calculated. Since the agreement between psychiatrists was worst at the line between impairment and nonimpairment, the misclassifications will be exaggerated. A score of 4+ on the Screening Instrument identifies 73.5% of all the impaired, but it also selects 18.2% of the unimpaired (false positives). A cutoff score of 7+ selects only 39.6% of the impaired, which is not too satisfactory, but it is very conservative since it selects only 2.5% of the unimpaired (false positives). Table 4 of the Screening Score article shows that if more extreme groups are used, the score does a better job of discrimination. For example, a score of 7+ identifies no "Wells", but 55.5% of the Incapacitated and 53.6% of the Severe group. These are closest to psychiatric inpatients in the severity of their illness. Culling over half of them with no Wells and almost no Milds makes the 7+ cutoff a conservative and fairly safe decision. It would still yield a large group of false negatives, however the total sample of 1660 had 4+ symptoms, and 11.2% had 7+ symptoms. How does that compare with local and national studies? Dohrenwend et al. (1980) report overall rates for seven local and one national study. The median for local studies is 32.9% for a 4+ cutoff, and 14.8% for a 7+ cutoff. The NORC % and the original Midtown % are within a few percentage points of these median figures. However, the range is considerable, being 6% to 23% for the 7+ score.

Sex Differences

Dohrenwend et al. report that in five local community studies, the percentage of women scoring above a cutoff of 7+ symptoms on the 22-Item Screening Score was larger than that of men. The median for men was 22%, for women 32%. The NORC national sample and Dupuy's GWB scale show similar results. Strangely enough, the rates from the Midtown study sample for men and women are not reported by Link. These were contrasted with the rates for men and women in two Mexican communities, one specifically selected because women had achieved high status in that culture relative to their husbands (Langner, 1965, in *Approaches to Cross-Cultural Psychiatry*, edited by Jane Murphy). In that paper, "Psychophysiological Symptoms and Women's Status in Two Mexican Communities," it was hypothesized that in a culture that accords women status nearly equal to that of their men, the mean scores for men and women on the 22-Item instrument would be more nearly equal.

> It is in line with the status hypothesis that women of Midtown as a whole are even closer to men in their level of symptomatology (men 2.38, women 3.11) than those of a comparable metropolis, Mexico City (men 4.21, women 6.06). The women of Midtown, who seem to me to occupy a more favorable position in their society (than those in Mexico City) also report fewer symptoms in relation to Midtown men.
>
> Women in Tehuantepec (who have high status in their community) are closer in their average number of symptoms (4.70) to men of Tehuantepec (3.56) than comparable low income women of Mexico City (7.27) are to low income men of Mexico City (5.18). The mean difference between men and women in Tehuantepec is 1.14 symptoms, while in Mexico City it is 2.09 symptoms. (The difference between these mean differences falls just short of statistical significance at the 5% level, due to the small number of cases in Tehuantepec, 59). The data. . .support the original hypothesis. . .The Tehuanas are one symptom worse off than the Tehuanos, while the women of Mexico City are two symptoms worse off than their men.

These findings suggest that sex differences are based upon more than biology, and that the relative status, power and prestige of the sexes in a culture or community can affect their reported level of symptomatology. This is supported by the study of Sarah Rosenfield (1980) using data from the 1965 Washington Heights survey by the Dohrenwends. Women are classified as showing traditional and nontraditional sex-roles based on whether they were working outside the home. Four scales "relating to depression": psychosomatic symptoms, anxiety ("as a correlate of depression"), immobilization, and sadness, were organized from responses to Structured Interview Schedules. "Because of the high degree of intercorrelation among these scales, they were combined into an overall scale of depressive symptoms (or demoralization, as Dohrenwend et al. have suggested)." Not only were there clear differences between working and nonworking females on the four scales (especially sadness!) but there were conditions under which married women showed lower (not higher) mean scores than married men. This occurred among working women, compared with men whose wives were working. In this nontraditional group, then, women exhibited lower mean scores than men on three out of four scales (all but anxiety). Various interpretations are possible, such as the preselection of depressed men for marriages with working women. However, a more likely candidate is that the loss of power for males with working wives is associated with, and possibly leads to, an increase in depression, feelings of helplessness, etc. Of course, a longitudinal study of mate selection and employment status would help immensely in sorting out directionality. The findings, nevertheless, are quite consistent with the Mexico study cited above and with data from the Family Research Project (using one sample of 1034 women), which will be presented later.

Further suggestions about sex-role socialization and behavior are contained in the Stirling County study of Leighton et al. While 40% of the Depressed Area mothers believe that there is little difference in ideal masculine and feminine behavior in childhood, only 24% of mothers in LaVallée and 17% of those in Fairhaven believe this. The cohesive areas tend to differentiate sex roles to a greater extent than the Depressed Area. This is reflected in later findings, when women in the Depressed Area have rates of alcoholism and antisocial behavior about equal to that of men, a finding not present in the cohesive areas. Early permissiveness for expression of anger may be critical for the reduction of depression in women, and perhaps for an increase in more "masculine" disorders or behaviors (Hughes et al., 1960, page 288).

Social Class Differences

Link and Dohrenwend (in Dohrenwend et al., 1980), cite six local community studies that found a median rate for the lowest social class of 36% vs. a rate of 9% for the highest class. These effects were linear without reversals, and consistent in direction. The national NORC and Dupuy studies support these findings, when education is used as a class measure. Several studies have shown that these effects are not due to response style.

Both the Mexico City sample and the Midtown sample, when broken down by low and high income, show significant differences (Langner, 1965). This low SES predominance of symptomatology has been found consistently across many studies, using many types of instruments. The screening instruments, then, reflect social class results that are very broad in scope.

Relative Ranking of Social Correlates of the 22-Item Screening Score Among Manhattan Mothers

While it seems almost criminal to pile up more data on monolithic screening instruments, our quest is the specification of the underlying construct of the 22-Item or similar instruments. To facilitate this, a linear multiple regression analysis was performed on data from the Family Research Project, with the hope that a rank ordering of the unique contributions to variance in the 22-Item Score would clear out some of the overlapping variables that could be obscuring the meaning of the criterion itself.

Before further analysis, I will briefly describe the methods and sample and refer to more detailed presentations.

Method

Cross-sectional and Welfare samples of 1034 and 1000 families were selected in Manhattan by systematic cluster sampling so that each household contained at least one child aged 6-18. Only the cross-sectional sample will be used in this analysis. The refusal rate was 15.6%, and the families were 56% white, 29% Spanish-speaking, 14% black, and 1% other. Five years later, the samples were followed up, making Time 1 1966-67 and Time 2 1971-72. The followup was made to adhere to the original ethnic proportions, yielding a total of 732 families, or 71% of the Time 1 sample. The age, sex, demographic and global child behavior characteristics did not differ between the two times yielding a reasonably unbiased subsample of the original.

Mothers were interviewed for 2¼ hours with a predominantly structured questionnaire. This elicited material on the development and current behavior of the child, aspects of parental character and the marital relationship, child-rearing practices, and a broad range of demographic variables. The questionnaire was administered in Spanish to Hispanic respondents. Factor analysis was performed on portions of an original pool of 654 child behavior items, yielding 18 behavior dimensions. The same procedure was carried out with 91 items describing the marital relationship and parental character, which yielded eight "parental factors." A factoring of 81 questions on the parent-child relationship and parenting practices yielded five "parent-child" dimensions. These factors were all converted to Z or standard scores. The internal consistency reliabilities for all the factors ranged from moderate (0.40-0.50) to high (0.70-0.94). Elaborate validity checks were made against external sources, such as the child's self-report, school data, police data, and direct psychiatric examination of 25% of the children. These sources are congruent or incongruent, depending upon the construct one wishes to examine. Among other scales, the mothers were also asked the full 22-Item Screening Score at Time 2, and a shorter version at Time 1. (For more details of method, see Langner et al., 1979; Langner, Gersten & Eisenberg, 1977; Gersten et al., 1976; Eisenberg, Langner & Gersten, 1975; and Langner et al., in press.)

Predictor Selection

A series of variables and factors was selected that might be considered potential stressors of the mothers. They were arranged in groups, and these groups were ordered in a hierarchy, so that the most unalterable, the most exogenous, and those closest to the mother were entered as the early sets. There were eight sets capable of being entered using Time 2 data, with the criterion being the 22-Item Score at Time 2. Only six sets were available for prediction from Time 1 data to the Screening Score at Time 2. The two sets (or steps) not available at Time 2 were Step 7 and Step 8. The sets (steps) available were:

Step 1, Demographic Variables

X is Spanish (study child)
Mother's education
Rent
Welfare status
Number of children in the household
Child not continually in natural mother's care
Family income
Father's education
Father's employment status
Mother's employment status
Mother widowed (vs. married)
Mother divorced, separated, abandoned, never married (vs. married)

Step 2, Parental-Marital Factors (PTF)

PTF 1. Isolated parents
PTF 2. Unhappy marriage
PTF 4. Unleisurely parents
PTF 5. Mother's economic dissatisfaction
PTF 6. Parents' quarrels
PTF 7. Husband ill and withdrawn

Step 3, Parental History of Psychiatric Treatment

Mother ever been a psychiatric hospital inpatient or outpatient of any type
Father ever been a psychiatric hospital inpatient or outpatient of any type

Step 4, Parent-Child Factors (PCF)

PCF 1. Parents cold
PCF 2. Mother traditional-restrictive
PCF 3. Parents punitive
PCF 4. Mother excitable-rejecting

Step 5, The Child's Physical Illness Scores (Ill)

Ill-1. Acute physical illnesses
Ill-2. Mild chronic illnesses

Step 6, Child Mental Health (Global Measure TIRZ)

Total impairment rating of child, simulated with age and sex controls (based on regression weights of 18 behavior factors predicting to the five-point psychiatric impairment rating assigned to each child at Time 1 by two psychiatrists).

Step 7, Mother's Unexpressed Violence Factor Scores (MUVFS), Time 2 Only

MUVFS-1. Fatalism-suspiciousness
MUVFS-2. Nontraditionalism

Step 8, Child's Antisocial and School Failure Record, Time 2 Only

DROP. Child dropped out of school (after Time 1)
VIOL 01. Number of charged offenses of child from police and court records

In the interests of brevity, I will not go into all the first-order correlations. It is enough to say that many of them were substantial, and that only variables or factors with reasonably high correlations with the 22-Item Score were selected for the regression analysis. Those correlations ranged from 0.09 to 0.51. Of great interest is the fact that the socioeconomic variables ranged from 0.09 to 0.23, but they virtually disappeared during the partialling process. In other words, *for women, at least,* the social class finding across several studies must be reexamined. Table 1 gives the first order correlation, the partial R for the final step (when all other variables are held constant), and the partial R for the key variables (those accounting for 1% or more of variance in the 22-Item Score in the last set) at the time of their entry.

Since several of the predictors were not on the master tape, their correlation with the Screening Score was not available. The selection of Set 3 variables was based on the assumption that the parents' history of psychiatric treatment would be a good predictor. Alas, there is much previous evidence that treatment is often uncorrelated with measures of psychopathology. This is particularly true when the treatment is not exclusively current, suggesting an emotional crisis. The results cited by Dohrenwend et al. (1979), which found a lack of relationship between the Screening Score and the Psychiatric Status Schedule (PSS) in classifying 55 adults as cases, involved a four-year followup. Given a four-year time gap, one could hardly expect a congruence of "case" identification. Moreover, since the Screening Score probably measures anxiety and depression primarily, one would not expect great stability over time. Similarly H.B.M. Murphy (1974) cited by Dohrenwend, followed 1170 freshmen at the University of Singapore for several years to learn who exhibited abnormal behavior, sought psychiatric aid, and made more than average use of health services. That he found a symptom checklist did not identify vulnerable individuals is not surprising, given his criteria of vulnerability and the time gap. Any prediction greater than a year in length will suffer great attrition in comparison with outcomes within a half year or year. Seeking psychiatric help and health services are just not good criteria for mental disorder, although people who give such services might wish it to be true (see the low correlations with treatment cited by Ware et al., 1979, Table 9). Only current comparisons, using direct examinations or observations and standardized clinical measurements, can be used as hard evidence that there is psychiatric disorder.

The Set 8 variables, Child's School Dropouts and Arrests, was also thought to be a possible stressor of the mother, but first-order correlations were not available. It was felt that variables from another source, community record data, would enhance the final Multiple R. Quite to the contrary, there was no noticeable effect of these rather serious situations or problems of a child on the mother's Screening Score. Perhaps the perspective of a middle-class professor is so out-of-date that he feels school failure and police arrests are serious problems that would depress him if they occurred in his children. So much for the fantasies of the compulsives and worrywarts.

Well, then, what *does* bother Manhattan's mothers enough to show some increment in the psychophysiological-depressed-anxious quotient? In the first set, only mother's employment status made a unique contribution to the Screening Score variance (2.1% at entry, and 1.5% in the final set). This does not mean that the common variance or shared variance accounted for

TABLE 1
Percent of 22-Item Screening Score Variance Accounted for Uniquely (Partial R^2) by Predictor Variables in Final Step 8, and at the Time of Their Entry Into the Regression Hierarchy, with Their First Order Correlations. (All Variables Are Time 2, or Concurrent.)

Set and step	*Variable*	*R^2 at time of entry (% of variance)*	*R^2 at final step (8) (% of variance)*	*First order correlation (R)*	*End of predictor associated with greater mother's 22-item score (more pathology)*
1.	Mother's employment status (MEMS)	2.1	1.5	−0.21	Not employed
	Study child is Spanish (X SPNSH)	†	1.1	0.20	Is Spanish
2.	Unhappy marriage (PTF2)	2.1	1.4	−0.33	Unhappy
	Parents' quarrels (PTF6)	6.0	3.0	0.15	Quarrelsome
3.	Mother had psychiatric treatment (MOPSY)	†	†	0.03[a]	—
	Father had psychiatric treatment (FAPSY)	†	†	0.01[a]	—

TABLE 1 (Continued)

Set and step	*Variable*	*R^2 at time of entry (% of variance)*	*R^2 at final step (8) (% of variance)*	*First order correlation (R)*	*End of predictor associated with greater mother's 22-item score (more pathology)*
4.	Mother traditional-restrictive (PCF2)	1.8	†	−0.25	More restrictive
	Mother excitable-rejecting (PCF5)	3.2	1.4	−0.26	More excitable
5.	Study child's mild chronic physical illness (ILL-2)	2.5	1.3	−0.19	Child sicker
6.	Simulated child's psychiatric total impairment rating (NTIRZ)	3.8	2.2	0.35	Child has more impairment
7.	Mother's unexpressed violence factor Score 1: fatalism-suspiciousness	12.3	12.3	−0.51	Mother has more fatalism

TABLE 1 (Continued)

Set and step	*Variable*	*R^2 at time of entry (% of variance)*	*R^2 at final step (8) (% of variance)*	*First order correlation (R)*	*End of predictor associated with greater mother's 22-item score (more pathology)*
8.	Child's school dropout, last 5 years (DROP)	†	†	0.05[a]	Child dropped out
	Child's number of arrests (VIOL 01)	†	†	0.09[a]	Child arrested

† R^2 = < 1%

[a] Correlations were not available for predictor selection until after regression matrix was run.

by these demographic variables was not considerable (11.6% shown in table 2), but the unique variance is due to that predictor alone, net of all the other predictors in the particular set, and in the final step, net of all the predictors in the entire equation. This means that they are the robust variables, are more likely to have a direct effect on the score, and probably should be the focus of further work.

It is easy to be misled by the first-order correlations. For example, the various social class indicators or class-related variables overlap each other to a great degree. Most of them have fairly high first-order correlations with the Screening Score (Mother's Education 0.21, Rent −0.17, Welfare Status −0.21, Income −0.22, Father's Education −0.17, Father's Employment Status −0.19). How striking it is, then, that all these are essentially partialled out even in the first step, and Mother's Employment Status is the only survivor with a unique contribution. Not only does this question just what social class vs. minority status means to women, (since being Spanish does make a contribution in the final set), it reinforces the findings and interpretation of Rosenfield (1980) that employment status is strongly related to women's depressive and anxious symptoms. I had noted that sadness was the most sensitive of these four scales to working-non-working. This reinforces the hunch that the active ingredient is power and independence of women vs. their feelings of relative helplessness as housewives. The dependence on their husbands probably induces both rage and sadness, and Rosenfield has evidence that anger is greater among nonworking women, though the significance is marginal due to small numbers. Obviously the sex difference in Screening Scores cannot be tested in this sample of mothers, but the *meaning* of sex, or of being a woman, is elucidated, and the widely observed higher rates of treated and untreated depression in women may in part derive from lack of employment and the independence it offers. Future downward trends in women's depression should confirm this hunch.

It was thought that being in a minority group would increase the Screening Score, but while this was true for Hispanic women it was untrue of black women, who showed no increment in their scores. This is a challenging finding and needs further explanation.

Of the Step 2 Parental-Marital variables, Parents' Quarrels showed considerable strength, making a 6% unique contribution at entry, and 3% in the final step. The mother's report of an unhappy marriage (more unhappy than friends' marriages or parents' marriage, husband not ambitious, would like to change her husband, etc.) accounted for 2.1% at entry, and 1.4% in Step 8.

In Step 4, the parenting (both mother and father) variables dropped out, and the mothering factors stayed in. Mother Traditional-Restrictive (Doesn't read books or magazines about children, gives bizarre explanations about sex to child, disapproves of children masturbating, likes quiet well-behaved child, religion and strictness important in upbringing of child, etc.) showed 1.8% at entry, but contributed less than 1% variance in Step 8. (One percent is the level set for a "meaningful" contribution). Mother Excitable-Rejecting (uses screaming a lot; feared pain, a deformed child, and dying in childbirth; changeable with child, fears loss of control with child; scolds; is excitable with child; can't feel warmth toward or get pleasure from child;

etc.) was consistently strong, accounting for 3.2% at entry and 1.4% in Step 8. Here we seem to be tapping the mood swings and irritability of a depressed woman, and her venting of some anger at a relatively powerless target, her child. Some preliminary attempts at cross-lagged and path analysis suggest that the depression is prior to the excitability-rejection of the child more than the other way around. However, the direction of causation does not seem to be clear for any of the other parenting or marital variables, and path models need to be tested before any firm statements can be made. There is in this factor the strong suggestion that the mother has rejected the child since before the birth, with her fears of pain and death during delivery and worries about a deformed child during the pregnancy. A separate factor, Parents' Coldness, emphasized lack of hugging and kissing, and resentment about being a mother. This factor was less related to the Screening Score ($r = 0.15$), and was not included in the regression analysis. There is a consistency to the Coldness dimension, while the Excitable mother swings from warmth to screaming. Again there is reason to distinguish the lability of mild to moderate depression from the consistent icy aloofness, which is less associated with mother's depressive symptoms and complaints.

Step 5 involved four a priori measures of the child's physical illness. Surprisingly, only one of these, and a relatively mild one at that (Mild Chronic Physical Illness) was related to the Screening Score (2.5% at entry, and 1.3% in Step 8). From previous cross-tabulations it was felt that physical illness in the family in almost any form was a serious stressor for the mother, and in order to test that, data on illnesses, operations, accidents, and handicaps were transferred to the master tape for a second set of regression analyses which will be presented briefly later on. That the child's Mild Chronic Illness (bronchitis, ear and eye infections, nose and sinus trouble, colds, etc.) would stress the mother more than Acute Physical Illnesses (fractures, tonsillitis, measles, chicken pox, polio, mumps, etc.) can only be understood in terms of the Screening Score as a measure of reaction to immediate stressful situations. If these are sporadic, as in the case of the usual childhood acute infectious diseases, and there are no serious sequelae, they may not bother her at the time of the interview. The number of mothers with acutely ill children at the time of the survey was probably minimal. However, many mothers had children with continual colds; eye, ear, nose and throat infections; stomach troubles; and allergies; which could be depressing and an immediate continual stressor. The only explanation for the lack of effect of the serious chronic physical illnesses and handicaps (malformed spine, congenital heart disease, cleft palate, deafness, blindness, crippled, etc.) is the relative rarity of the more serious disorders. A cross-tabulation might show the relationship, but with a very skewed distribution, the regression analysis will not pick up the effect, if any.

The child's mental health was represented by the psychiatric Total Impairment Rating. Any number of other measures could have been chosen, but this was global, and it was being related to a semiglobal measure of the mother's impairment. It showed 3.8% at entry, and 2.2% at Step 8. Whether the mother's disturbance triggers the child's, or if her child's disorder depresses her, is a matter which could take much discussion. Suffice it to say that when an array of 18 Time 1 *child* behaviors is related to the Time 2 Screening Score, Regressive Anxiety (0.23), Mentation Problems (speech, memory, concentration 0.19), Isolation (0.16), and Fighting (0.14) show the highest correlations. They suggest that the child's symptoms are somewhat similar to those the mother is showing.

Conversely, looking forward from Time 1 Mother's Physical and Emotional Illness—a factor with three physical health items (general health estimate, number of chronic conditions, and number of serious hospitalizations and illnesses) and with seven of the 22 items in the Screening Score—to Time 2 child behaviors, the Mother's Emotional Illness factor accounts uniquely for 2.1% of Regressive Anxiety. Concurrently at Time 1, the same factor accounts for 2.1% of Regressive Anxiety and for 1.1% of Fighting in the child. Thus anxious mothers are associated with anxious children. Fighting is not a precursor of Delinquency, but is a correlate of childhood depression. Depressed mothers don't seem to breed Delinquents, but rather miniature depressed mirrors of themselves (Langner et al., 1977, page 87).

Step 7 included two factor scores based upon attitude items I had made up for testing criminal offenders at Bellevue prison ward. I was trying to discriminate homicides, drug, assaultive, and suicidal cases. The second factor, Non-Traditionalism, had a first-order correlation of 0.25 with the Screening Score, but fell by the wayside in the partialling. The first factor, labeled Fatalism-Suspiciousness, had the highest first-order correlation (0.51) with the Screening Score of any variable (except for Mother's Physical and Emotional Illness, 0.83, which contained seven of the same items). This set was entered toward the end, since I felt that the Fatalism-Suspiciousness Factor might be simply another dimension of mild depressive disorder, although a very revealing one. This score accounted for 12.3% of Screening Score variance at entry and in the final step. It was by far the strongest predictor. A look at the items that loaded on this factor is very enlightening. The suggestions for face content are added to facilitate discussion.

1. Laws were made to be broken (antisocial).
2. I wish I could get some people off my back (helplessness, loss of control).
3. If there's one thing I hate, it's responsibility (anger, role rejection, fighting control).
4. I often feel people try to pick quarrels with me (projection of anger).
5. I am often bothered by short temper (anger, but "bothered" with guilt or repression).
6. Some people like me are born unlucky (fatalism, externalization of blame).
7. Getting things in life is 1% sweat and 99% luck (fatalism, loss of morale and faith in the system).
8. Getting ahead is a question of good breaks and bad breaks (fatalism, luck).
9. To tell the truth, another person is really running my life (loss of control).

This scale is clearly similar to the axis of internal-external locus of control. Yet it has a lot more to it. The repressed anger and helpless feelings of being manipulated by fate or other people are strongly suggestive of depression. This could be learned helplessness, in the sense that girls are socialized to be helpless or at least act helpless. It could also be the result of chronic helplessness in unchanging situations, such as an unhappy marriage, prolonged care for a chronically ill child (or other person) in the family, or powerlessness due to lack of earning power provided by a job outside the home. There has not been time to relate this factor to the mother's criminal record, but it is our hunch that this violence is *unexpressed*, and the anger repressed. The high correlation with a score containing items that are depressed and anxious in content makes a great deal of sense. While this was not a prediction, in the sense of forecasting from a specified network of connected hypotheses, there appears to be an interesting group of correlates of the Screening Score that point to the dynamics of depression. Helplessness, hopelessness, constriction, anger and inability to express it, the fatalism of people locked into a thankless and powerless role (housewife), the lack of contacts outside the family (which might be available on the job), the unhappy quarrelsome marriage, all seem to paint a familiar picture. Under these conditions, we may see many more women turn to outside work, as over half of the mothers in the sample already have. Many more of them will initiate a divorce or separation, as their situation becomes more intolerable. Outside work and independent income might be a primary preventive for our increasing divorce rates, and for the preponderance of depression among women (usually given as a 3:1 ratio).

Table 2 shows the overall Multiple R (0.66) for the full set of predictors. This figure squared gives the total proportion of variance all the sets accounted for (43.6%), which is a reasonable figure for data of this type. Clearly, the Demographic variables (11.6%), the Marital Factors (11.4%), and Fatalism-Suspiciousness (8.8%) added the greatest amount of variance over previous predictor sets. The school-police set (set 8) and psychiatric treatment history of parents (set 3) added little if any to the prediction of mother's depression.

Six steps could be done both concurrently (Time 2) and prospectively (forecasting from Time 1 variables to Time 2 Screening Score). The Time 2 6th step, as seen in table 2, accounted for 34.7% of Screening Score variance (Multiple R of 0.59). The 6th Step using Time 1 predictors to Time 2 Screening Score (5 years later) showed a great loss of power. Only 16.9% of variance was predicted (Multiple R = 0.41). Less than half the variance was left, after a lapse of five years, showing how great attrition can be, especially in a relatively unstable dimension such as depression-anxiety. This is all the more reason to suspect the score measures reactive or situational depression, and not endogenous depression. If it has much stability, it is due primarily to the stable but stressful conditions and roles of housewife, mother, sick-nurse, and sporadically silent sufferer.

The Role of Physical Health

Special items tapping the physical health of the mother, her husband (most often the child's natural father), and her child were grouped into sets to test the hypothesis that physical illness is one of the most stressful factors in a woman's environment. As the person usually responsible for nursing both her husband and child, she should exhibit more depression and anxiety than her husband, for example. It was necessary to construct a shorter version of the 22-Item Screening Score that would not contain any of the psychophysiological items, since they could easily be confounded with physical illness. This would have made the relationship between the Screening Score and Mother's Physical Illness, in particular, quite elevated and spurious.

The 9-Item Depressed-Anxious (Non-Physiological) Screening Score was composed of the following items, grouped by face content:

		Scored as Pathological
Depressive items	Memory is all right	No
	Nothing turns out the way I want	Agree
	Wonder if anything worthwhile	Agree
	Can't get going	Yes (for days, weeks, months)
	In low, very low spirits	Low, very low
Anxious items	Great restlessness	Yes
	Bothered by nervousness	Often
	Is the worrying type	Yes
Isolated	Feel apart (alone) even among friends	Yes

The presumed pathognomonic responses were simply summed. This 9-Item score correlated 0.90 with the 22-Item Screening Score (Pearson R, both measures at Time 2). It was thus possible to use it as a substitute criterion for the 22-Item Score, and to avoid the potential circularity mentioned.

Table 3 shows the robust variables carried over from the previous analysis, with the addition of health items reported by the mother for herself, her husband, and the study child. The physical illness labels are all self-explanatory, and consist of a health estimate, or "perceived" health (excellent, good, fair, and poor), counts of serious illnesses, chronic conditions and

TABLE 3
Percent of 9-Item Screening Score
(Depressed, Anxious, Non-Physiological)
Variance Accounted for Uniquely (Partial R^2)
by Predictor Variables in Final Step 8,
and at the Time of Their Entry Into the Regression Hierarchy,
with Their First Order Correlations.[a]

Set and step	*Variable*	*R^2 at time of entry (% of variance)*	*R^2 at final step (8) (% of variance)*	*First order correlation R.*	*End of predictor associated with greater mother's 9-item score*
1. Demographic	Mother's employment status (T2 MEMS)	2.8	†	−0.22	Not employed
	Spanish-speaking	2.1	1.4	0.20	Spanish
2. Parental-marital	Parents'quarrels (PTF6)	3.4	†	−0.15	Quarrelsome
	Unhappy marriage (PTF2)	8.3	2.7	−0.31	Unhappy
3. Mother's health	Mother's health estimate	10.1	4.7	0.44	Poor
	Mother's serious illnesses	†	†	0.22	High #
	Mother's chronic conditions	†	†	0.19	High #
4. Father's health	Father's health estimate	†	†	0.18	Poor
	Father's serious illness	†	†	0.09	High #
	Father's chronic conditions	†	†	0.07	High #

TABLE 3 (Continued)

Set and step	*Variable*	*R^2 at time of entry (% of variance)*	*R^2 at final step (8) (% of variance)*	*First order correlation R.*	*End of predictor associated with greater mother's 9-item score*
5. Child's illness*	Total # illnesses (T2)	†	†	0.15	High #
	Total # operations (T2)	†	†	−0.02	High #
	Total # accidents (T2)	†	†	0.00	High #
	Total # hospitalizations (T2)	†	†	0.03	High #
	T2 Mild chronic illness score (2)	†	†	−0.18	Low #
6. Parenting (P-C factors)	Mother exitable—rejecting (PCF5)	5.6	3.5	−0.31	Excitable
7. Child's mental health	Total impairment rating (NTIRZ)	4.1	2.2	0.37	Impaired
8. Mother's attitudes	Fatalism—suspiciousness (MUVFS 1)	13.5	13.5	−0.05	Fatalistic

[a] All variables are Time 2, or concurrent

† R^2 = **<1%**

* Between Time 1 and 2

handicaps, counts of accidents and hospitalizations (for the child only) and the Mild Chronic Illness Score-2 carried over from the previous analysis.

It immediately becomes clear that the Mother's Health Estimate, which accounts for 10.1% of the 9-Item Score at entry, and 4.7% in the final set, is the single most powerful predictor next to Fatalism (13.5%). However, there are three striking facts. First, the father's health estimate contributes nothing, so it is the mother's own health that concerns her. Second, neither of the relatively objective scores of mothers' serious illnesses or chronic conditions and handicaps contribute to criterion variance. This makes us suspect strongly that it is the *subjective* aspect of her health estimate that is related to her depression and anxiety, not her objective illnesses. One could guess that her depression makes for the gloomy *picture* of her own health, not her physical condition. Cross-lagged analysis or path models may help us unravel this causal chain in the future. A third fact is that none of the illness measures of her husband and child (even the Mild Chronic Illness Score) predict her 9-Item Score: well, there's just one less thing to worry about—your family's health.

What is left in the final set? Mother's employment status dropped out, making one wonder if physical health and employment are not linked. Parents' Quarrels also dropped out, though it, like Mother's Employment, showed strength upon entry into the equation. The finalists, (Step 8) in rank order, are *Fatalism-Suspiciousness* (13.5%) *Mother's Health Estimate* (4.7%) *Mother Excitable-Rejecting* (3.5%) *Unhappy Marriage* (2.7%) *The Child's Total Impairment* (2.2%), and being *Spanish-speaking* (1.4%). Objectively, her marriage, her child's mental health, and her minority status may be causal to her depressive tendencies. These are what she may be reacting to, her "situation."

Her fatalism, her negative view of her health, and her labile screaming behavior with her child are, in my opinion, part and parcel of her depression, and *not* the environmental factors she is reacting to. These are more likely to be merely correlates of her depressed anxious state. Her irritability with her child, her angry-fatalistic-hopeless outlook, and her negative perception of her health, are much less likely to be causal factors, or exogenous to her emotional state. Tests of this hypothesis are very difficult to make, but longitudinal analysis can often help.

The Multiple R for the 9-Item Score, given, the predictors in table 3, is 0.69, and the Multiple R^2 (percent of variance accounted for by all the variables in the final step, uniquely and in common) is 47.0%. Increments are large for the Parental-Marital factors, the Mother's Health Estimate, the Mother's Excitability-Rejection, and her Fatalism-Suspiciousness. (The shrunken R^2 is only 1.5% less than the R^2.)

The same set of predictors, used with the 22-Item Screening Score as a criterion, yields a Multiple R of 0.72 and an R^2 of 52.2%. Thus there is not much difference in the total variance accounted for by these sets, using the 22- or 9-Item Score. It is clear, however, that the increment due to the mother's health estimate is exaggerated when using the 22-Item Score as the criterion (17.2% over step 2). This inflation is probably due to the confounding of the physiological complaints and the mother's perception of her health as bad.

Summary

At this point it probably makes little difference whether we refer to the "X" in the global screening instruments as demoralization, mild reactive depression, dysphoric states, or unhappiness, among the many possibilities. The further investigation of persons or groups who are in special acute social situations, such as disasters, as contrasted with chronic situations, may uncover different reactive patterns. Greater sensitivity to the nuances of these reactions is required now, with hypotheses about the specificity of situation and behavior carefully drawn, i.e., divergent validity. The mechanisms by which these behaviors are learned and perpetuated must be documented over many years of research. For example, an insight into the perpetuation of depression in women was given by Lenore Radloff at a meeting of the Society for Life History Research in Psychopathology. In discussing a paper on the Buffalo Creek disaster (Gleser et al., 1978), she pointed out that during the flood, the women were forced to sit in a building minding the children, while the men were encouraged to get out into the storm and use their muscles to rescue people and possessions. The physiological repercussions of being immobile in a frightening situation must be measurable. The idea of Walter Cannon that the human body and the autonomic system are adapted for fight or flight (but not for sitting quietly in the face of severe threat) is the basis for most of psychosomatic medicine and stress-reaction research. The overlap of the psychophysiological items with the depression and anxiety items in screening instruments, and the higher scores of women, are quite likely tied to the early training of women for indirect coping responses, for inaction, and the reinforcement of this tendency throughout their lives. Helpless people (many patients, cripples, prisoners) should all show some of these reactions. Loss of morale (second cousin to Bruce Dohrenwend's and Frank's "demoralization"), seems subtly different and may be likened to the wartime phenomenon of combat fatigue, which was often widespread due to excessive loss of life. This was described as a breaking of a psychodynamic bargain between the leader and those he led, a loss of faith in the system. The symptoms were primarily psychosomatic and often involved hysterical paralyses. It would be interesting to see if screening scale items of a depressed-anxious and psychosomatic nature also correlated highly with scales tapping loss of faith in our social system, marriage, child-rearing, work, politics, the economy, and religion.

There is evidence that the loss of faith in the social system is moderately correlated with depressive symptoms in our own data set. The second factor of "Mother's Unexpressed Violence" turned out to be made up of disagreement with stable middle-class values and the Protestant work ethic. The items were scored for anti-traditional responses as follows:

1. Trial by jury is fair (False).
2. Policemen are mostly people who want to be criminals but didn't have the nerve (True).
3. You are more likely to get beaten up by the police than by criminals (True).

4. Policemen are more crooked and criminal than the average man they arrest (True).
5. Having children or a family should never keep a person from doing what he wants to do (True).
6. When a girl gets old enough, she should get herself a man, by hook or crook, any way she can (True).
7. It's not what you know, but whom you know that counts (True).
8. Sometimes the only way to get ahead is to cheat just a little, but not so much that it hurts somebody else (True).
9. When you can't beat the system, the best thing to do is to change it (True).
10. You can't win at the game the way things are, so it's better to change the rules of the game (True).

This factor score, "Anti-Protestant Ethic," correlated −0.25 with the 22-Item Screening score (both Time 2 measures). (This is a direct, not an inverse relationship, the minus sign being an artifact of scoring. This means that the nontraditional mothers are more depressed. They are also more like R. K. Merton's "innovators" who would bend the rules [means] although they may agree with the goals.) This compares with a correlation of −0.51 with the first factor, Fatalism. The nontraditional factor (Anti-Protestant Ethic) is not only weaker in its relation to depression-anxiety (22-Item) than Fatalism, but it loses its unique power during the partialling. The loss of morale or faith in the system is apparently not so intrinsic to depression as the fatalism element in the first factor.

Years of rewarding research can be done on the relation between social attitudes and social states or situations. How these relate to behavioral dimensions, and to diagnostic types, is the core of social psychiatry. I hope this paper, describing the correlates of one belabored screening instrument, can refocus attention away from establishing rates based on models of known "cases," and encourage research into the explanatory mechanisms that link subjective and objective position with feeling states and behavior.

Acknowledgments

The Family Research Project (a series of interconnected studies) is administered from the Division of Epidemiology, Columbia University School of Public Health, and the Department of Psychiatry. The investigations were supported principally by U. S. Public Health Service Project Grant MH11545 and MH 18260 of the National Institute of Mental Health, Center for Epidemiologic Studies; and also by the U.S. Department of Health, Education and Welfare, Social and Rehabilitation Service, Cooperative Research and Demonstration Grants Branch, grant SRS-CRD-348 (SRS-56006); by the Office of Child Development, grants OCD-CB-348 and OCD-CB-480; and by the National Institute of Mental Health, Center for Studies of Crime and Delinquency, grant MH 28182. The principal investigator was supported by Career Scientist Awards I-338 and I-640, Health Research Council of the

City of New York, and is currently supported in part by a Research Scientist Award MH20868 from the ADAMHA awarding institute, NIMH. Key professionals involved in the Family Research Project were the director, Thomas S. Langner, Ph.D.; Joanne C. Gersten, Ph.D.; Jeanne G. Eisenberg, M. A.; Elizabeth D. McCarthy, Ph.D.; Ora Simcha-Fagan, D.S.W.; Thomas A. Wills, Ph.D; Edward L. Greene, M.D.; Joseph H. Herson, M.D.; Jean D. Jameson, M.D.; and Clifford York, M.A., among many others. The principal supporting staff (among many) were Gerda Burina-Cordova and Dorothy A. Stephens.

References

Astrachan, B. M., Harrow, M., Adler, D., Brauer, L., Schwartz, A., Schwartz, C. & Tucker, G. (1973). A checklist for the diagnosis of schizophrenia. *Br J Psychiatr* 121:529-539.

Bradburn, N. M. & Caplowitz, D. (1965) *Reports on happiness.* Chicago: Aldine.

Buros, O. I. (ed.) (1959), *The Fifth Mental Measurements Yearbook*, Highland Park, N.J.: Gryphon.

Cammer L., (1969), *Up From Depression*, New York: Simon and Schuster.

Dohrenwend, B. S. (1973), Life events as stresssors: A methodological inquiry, *J Health Social Behav* 14:167-175.

Dohrenwend, B. P., Dohrenwend, B. S., Gould, M. S., Link B., Neugebauer, R. & Wunsch-Hitzig, R. (1980) *Mental Illness in the United States, Epidemiological Estimates.* Chap. 5, Formulation of Hypotheses About the True Prevalence of Demoralization in the United States, by Bruce Link and Bruce P. Dohrenwend. Praeger.

Dohrenwend, B. P., Oksenberg, L., Shrout P. E., Dohrenwend, B. S. & Cook, D. (1979), What brief psychiatric screening scales measure. In (ed.) Sudman, S., *Proceedings of the Third Biennial Conference on Health Survey Methods*, Washington, D.C.: National Center for Health Services Statistics.

Dupuy, H. J. (1973) Developmental rationale, substantive, derivative, and conceptual relevance of general well-being, Washington, D.C.: National Center for Health Statistics. (Draft working paper).

Edgerton, J. W., Bentz, W. & Hollister, W. (1970) Demographic factors and responses to stress among rural people. *Am J Public Health* 60:1965-1971.

Edwards, D., Yarvis, R., Mueller, D., Zingale, H. & Wagman, W. Test-taking and the stability of adjustment scales: Can we assess patient deterioration? Unpublished manuscript. Available from Dr. Daniel Edwards. Sacramento Medical Center, 4430 U. Street, Sacramento, CA 95817.

Eisenberg, J. G., Langner, T. S. & Gersten, J. C. (1975) Differences in the behavior of welfare and non-welfare children in relation to parental characteristics. *J Commun Psychol*, Monograph Supplement No. 48, 33pp.

Endicott, J. & Spitzer, R. L. (1978) A diagnostic interview. *Arch Gen Psychiatr* 35:837-844.

Fabrega, H., Jr. & McBee, G. (1970) Validity features of a mental health questionnaire. *Soc Sci Med* 4:669-673.

Gaitz, O. M. & Scott, J. (1972) Age and the measurement of mental health. *J Health Social Behav* 13:55-67.

Gersten, J. C., Langner, T. S., Eisenberg, J. G., Simcha-Fagan, O. & McCarthy, E. D. (1976) Stability and change in types of behavioral disturbance of children and adolescents, *J Abnormal Child Psychol* 4:111-127.

Gleser, Goldine, et al., paper on Buffalo Creek Disaster, delivered April 7-8, 1978, at meeting of Society for Life History Research in Psychopathology, Cincinnati, Ohio. To be published in a volume edited by David Ricks and Barbara Dohrenwend.

Gurin, G., Veroff, J. & Feld, S. (1960) Americans View Their Mental Health. New York: Basic Books.

Haberman, P. W. (1964). Psychological test score changes for wives of alcoholics during periods of drinking and sobriety, *J Clinical Psychology.* 20:230-232.

Haese, P. N. & Meile, R. L. (1967) The relative effectiveness of two models for scoring the Midtown Psychological Index, *Commun Mental Health J,* 3:335-342.

Hughes, Charles, C., Tremblay, M., Rapoport, R. N. & Leighton, A. H. (1960) *People of Cove and Woodlot,* New York: Basic Books.

Langner, T. S. (1962) A twenty-two item screening score of psychiatric symptoms indicating impairment. *J Health Human Behav* 3:269-276.

Langner, T. S. (1965) Psychophysiological symptoms and the status of women in two Mexican communities. In: *Approaches to Cross-Cultural Psychiatry,* eds. Murphy, J. M. & Alexander H. Leighton. Ithaca, NY: Cornell University Press.

Langner, T. S. Gersten, J. C. & Eisenberg, J. G. (1977). The epidemiology of mental disorder in children: Implications for community psychiatry. In: *New Trends of Psychiatry in the Community,* ed. Serban, G. Cambridge, Mass: Ballinger Publishing Co., pp. 69-109.

Langner, T. S, Gersten, J. C., Eisenberg, J. G., Greene, E. L. & Herson, J. H. (in press) *Children Under Stress: Family and Social Factors in the Behavior of Urban Children and Adolescents.* New York: Columbia University Press.

Langner, T. S., Gersten, J. C., McCarthy, E. D., Eisenberg, J. G., Greene, E. L., Herson, J. H. & Jameson, J. D. (1976) A screening inventory for assessing psychiatric impairment in children six to eighteen. *J Consult Clin Psychol.* 44:286-296.

Langner, T. S., McCarthy, E. D., Gersten, J. C., Simcha-Fagan, O. & Eisenberg, J. G. (1979) Factors in children's behavior and mental health over time: The Family Research Project, In *Research in Community and Mental Health* - An Annual Compilation of Research, ed. Simmons, R.G., Part II, pp. 127-181.

Link, B. & Dohrenwend, B. P. (1980), Formulation of hypotheses about the true prevalence of demoralization in the U.S. In *Mental Illness in the United States: Epidemiologic Estimates,* ed. Dohrenwend, B. P.

Macmillan, A. M. (1957) The health opinion survey: Technique for estimating prevalence of psychoneurotic and related types of disorder in communities. *Psychol Rep.* 3:325-329.

Manis, J. G., Brawer, M. J., Hunt, C. L. & Kercher, I. C. (1964) Estimating the prevalence of mental illness. *Am Sociol Review.* 29:84-89.

Meile, R. L. & Haese, P. N. (1969) Social status, status incongruence and symptoms of stress. *J Health Social Behav* 10:237-244.

Mueller, D. (1980) Personal communication, cited by B. Dohrenwend, et al., 1980. (Link & Dohrenwend.)

Murphy, H. B. M. Two stress measures in three cultures-their prognostic efficiency, significance and incongruities. In: *International Symposium on Epidemiological Studies in Psychiatry,* Tehran. Eds. Leigh, D., Noorbakhsh, J. & Isadi, C. Available from Dr. Murphy.

Phillips, D. L. (1966) Deferred gratification in a college setting: Some costs and gains. *Soc Prob* 13:333-343.

Phillips, D. L. & Segal, B. H. (1965) Sexual status and psychiatric illness. *Am Soc Rev* 34:58-72.

Radloff, L. S. (1977) The CES-D Scale: A self-report depression scale for research in the general population. *App Psychol Meas* 1:385-401.

Rosenfield, S. (1980) Sex differences in depression: Do women always have higher rates? *J Health Social Behav* 21:33-42.

Simpkins, C. & Burke, F. F. (1974) *Comparative Analyses of the NCHS General Well-Being Schedule: Response Distributions, Community vs. Patient Status Discriminations, and Content Relationships.* Center for Community Studies, John F. Kennedy Center, George Peabody College, Nashville, Tenn., Contract #HRA 106-74-13.

Spitzer, R. L., Endicott, J. & Robbins, E. (1978) Research diagnostic criteria: Rationale and reliability. *Arch Gen Psychiatr,* 35:773-782.

Summers, G. F., Seiler, L. H. & Hough, R. L. (1971) Psychiatric symptoms: Cross-validation with a rural sample, *Rural Sociol* 36:367-378.

Ware, J. E. Jr., Johnston, S. A., Davies-Avery, A. & Brook, R. H. (1979) *Conceptualization and Measurement of Health for Adults in the Health Insurance Study: Vol. III, Mental Health.* Santa Monica, CA: The Rand Corporation.

Weissman, M., Myers, J. K. & Harding, P. S. (1978) Psychiatric disorders in a United States urban community: 1975-76. *Am J Psychiatr* 4:459-462.

Weissman, M., Sholomskas, D., Dottemer, M., Prusoff, B. & Locke, B. (1977) Assessing depressive symptoms in five psychiatric populations: A validation study. *Am J Epidemiol* 106:203-214.

Woodworth, R. S. (1917) *Personal Data Sheet.* Chicago: C.H. Stoelting.

Yancy, W. I., Rigsby, I. & McCarthy, E. D. (1972) Social position and self-evaluation: The relative importance of race. *Am J Sociol* 78:338-359.

Chapter 16

Screening Scales From the Psychiatric Epidemiology Research Interview (PERI)

BRUCE P. DOHRENWEND
ITZHAK LEVAV
PATRICK E. SHROUT

The Psychiatric Epidemiology Research Interview (PERI) is a new instrument for investigating dimensions of psychopathology and for psychiatric screening in the general population. It is based on our previous research on problems of case identification and diagnosis in psychiatric epidemiology (B. P. Dohrenwend, Yager, Egri and Mendelsohn, 1978; B. P. Dohrenwend, Oksenberg, Shrout, B. S. Dohrenwend and Cook, 1979; B. S. Dohrenwend, B. P. Dohrenwend and Cook, 1973;) and, while some aspects of it are still being tested and refined, work is far enough along for much of it to be useful now.

PERI was designed for investigations of demographically complex samples of adults from the general population where only small portions of "cases" have ever been in treatment with members of the mental health professions (Link and Dohrenwend, 1980). It has three main components:

1. A set of symptom scales to measure various dimensions of psychopathology.
2. A set of measures of social functioning.
3. A schedule of questions about recent life events as a basis for measuring potential stressors.

The measures of stressful life events have been described in considerable detail elsewhere (B. P. Dohrenwend, 1974); (B. S. Dohrenwend, Krasnoff, Askenasy, and B. P. Dohrenwend, 1978; B. S. Dohrenwend, 1977; B. S. Dohrenwend and Martin, 1979). They will not be discussed further here. The PERI measures of role functioning (B. S. Dohrenwend, B. P. Dohrenwend and Cook, 1981), and most of the symptom scales (Dohrenwend, Shrout, Egri, and Mendelsohn, 1980), have also been presented in other reports. Our purpose in this paper will be to describe a subset of PERI symptom scales that we have found to be highly promising for identifying likely cases of a variety of types of functional psychiatric disorder in the general population, regardless of whether the individuals have ever been in treatment with members of the mental health profession. The data on which we will rely come from several different studies:

1. *The general population sample of 200 New York City adults on which PERI was originally developed.* This sample was designed to consist of substantial proportions of blacks and Puerto Ricans, as well as non-Puerto Rican whites, and to contain roughly equal representation of three educational levels—less than high school graduation, high school graduation, and college graduation. Because the sample was derived from a four-year old enumeration of subjects, and because the interview completion rates were poor (about 60% on the first of these interviews), it cannot be considered representative of household heads in New York City despite the fact that full probability procedures were used. More details of the sampling are presented elsewhere (Dohrenwend, Shrout, Egri, and Mendelsohn, 1980). Suffice it to say here that this small New York City sample economically provided general population respondents from contrasting social and cultural backgrounds for testing the new measures contained in PERI.
2. *An investigation by Stokes (1976) of a sample of 91 patients in treatment for drug addiction in Pennsylvania and New Jersey.* Over 70 percent of these subjects were, as nearly as possible, consecutive admissions to methadone outpatient clinics in Philadelphia and Norristown, Pennsylvania and Mercer County and Camden County, New Jersey. The remainder were consecutive admissions to the inpatient program of the Eagleville Hospital and Rehabilitation Center, a residential, abstinence oriented therapeutic community that treats drug and alcohol addicts together in a combined treatment program. The PERI interview was administered approximately 10 days after the patient entered treatment. Completed interviews were obtained from about 60% of the patients. The high rate of refusals was due to the fact that the subjects were part of a larger study that required other tests and questionnaires, which were given higher priority than the PERI. The majority of this sample, about 55 percent, were black, and only 2 subjects were Puerto Rican. As might be expected, males outnumbered females by about 4:1.
3. *A study by Tessler (1977) of 146 nearly consecutive admissions to the three largest units of Northampton State Hospital, located in Western Massachusetts.* Patients were included in this study if they were between 18 and 65 years of age, if at the time of admission mental retardation was not the primary diagnosis, if they spoke English, and if they were not admitted to the hospital under the jurisdiction of a court. Approximately 67% of those approached agreed to participate and provided complete or nearly complete data in a subset of PERI symptom scales. The large majority were interviewed during the first week of hospitalization.

The sample was homogeneously white and almost equally distributed between males and females. Most of the subjects had been previously admitted either to Northampton State Hospital or to other institutions; the average number of prior admissions was 3.5. The sample consists, therefore, predominately of persons whose problems are chronic and recurrent. Slightly more than 70% were diagnosed by a hospital physician as psychotic, and the majority of these as schizophrenic.

4. *A pilot study of a sample of 205 residents of six neighborhoods in Jerusalem, Israel, and 216 psychiatric inpatients and outpatients in that city.* This study represents a collaboration between the Dohrenwends, Shrout, and their group at Columbia University, and Levav at the Hadassah University Hospital in Jerusalem. The objective of the pilot research has been to determine the feasibility of using an instrument such as PERI which was developed in the United States for an epidemiological study of contrasting sex, ethnic, and social class groups in Israel. For this reason, PERI, translated into Hebrew, was administered during the past year to such diverse ethnic groups in the Jerusalem samples as Jews of European, Iraqi and Moroccan background, with care to include immigrants as well as Israeli-born. These three groups are almost equidistant from each other on a continuum ranging from social advantage (Jews of European background) to social disadvantage (Jews of Moroccan background) (Peres, 1977).

Full probability sampling procedures were used in the general population sample, with a completion rate of 84%. The patients were drawn on the basis of convenience from all psychiatric hospitals, outpatient clinics, welfare offices, and a probation office for adults in Jerusalem as well as from all other relevant facilities such as a halfway house, rehabilitation club, drug addict clinic, and center for alcoholics. Most hospitalized patients were readmissions rather than first admissions, and were interviewed during the first week of hospitalization whenever possible. The main criterion for selection of patients was diagnosis; the aim was to select 60 schizophrenics; 60 with severe affective disorders; 60 neurotics; and 60 who in the aggregate were antisocial personalities, drug addicts, and/or alcoholics. To this end, records were reviewed and the patient's psychiatrist frequently was interviewed by Levav or his team to establish the current diagnosis by the treatment agent or agency. Where the information about current diagnosis was vague, the case was passed over. A subsample of about a quarter of the patients was interviewed by our research psychiatrists who applied Research Diagnostic Criteria (Spitzer, Endicott, and Robins, 1978) on the basis of interviews with the lifetime version of the Schedule for Affective Disorders and Schizophrenia (SADS-L) (Endicott and Spitzer, 1978). The treatment diagnoses were made according to ICD-8 (Eighth Revision Conference, 1968); the research diagnoses have more in common with the criteria developed by Feighner et al. (1972) and with DSM-III (Task Force on Nomenclature and Statistics, 1980).

Development of PERI Symptom Scales

The item pool for PERI symptom scales came for the most part from two sources. One consisted of the StructuredInterview Schedule (SIS) that we used in a previous study (Dohrenwend, Oksenberg, Shrout, Dohrenwend, and Cook, 1979). The SIS relied mainly on questions from brief, self-report screening scales that have been used widely since World War II. The other consisted of items taken from the Psychiatric Status Schedule (PSS) (Spitzer, Endicott, Fleiss, and Cohen, 1970) but rewritten in self-report formats on the basis of our experience with that instrument (Dohrenwend, Yager, Egri, and Mendelsohn, 1978). Although PSS items were previously scored in terms of clinical judgments of whether the symptom was true or false of the respondent, we rewrote the items that we selected so that they became closed questions using, as a rule, either one of the following fixed alternative response formats that were employed for almost all of the PERI symptom items:

— Very often, fairly often, sometimes, almost never or never.
— Very much like you, much like you, somewhat like you, very little like you, not at all like you.

The time period referred to in the frequency format was the past year.

These symptom items were sorted by three board-certified psychiatrists into groupings that they judged to be homogenous in clinical content. These were labeled with such terms as "anxiety," "suspiciousness," "false beliefs and perceptions" and so on. After the items were grouped, their psychometric characteristics were investigated using data from the sample of New York City adults described above. As a result of preliminary analyses, some modifications were made in some of the item groupings. The resulting scales were considered reliable. As our test of the latter, we required that each scale be reliable in the 8 subdivisions of the sample, i.e., three ethnic groups, three educational levels, two sexes. We applied this standard by calling a scale reliable for research purposes in the subsample if it had a value of Cronback's alpha (Cronback, 1951), a measure of internal consistency, of 0.50 or better (Nunnally, 1967).

The sorting procedure by the clinicians enabled us to start with 33-item groupings; we ended up with 25 that survived clinical and psychometric scrutiny. The most usual reason for dropping item groupings was because they did not meet our reliability standards. Content areas of these unreliable scales included: boredom, withdrawal, flat affect, speech disorganization, and hysteria. The 25 remaining scales nevertheless covered a wide range and variety of types of psychiatric symptomatology and were given the following names:

Dread
Anxiety
Sadness
Helplessness
Hopelessness
Psychophysiological Symptoms
Perceived Physical Health
Poor Self Esteem
Somatic Problems (likely to be related to physical illness)
Confused Thinking
Guilt
Enervation
False Beliefs and Perceptions
Manic Characteristics
Suicide: Ideation and Behavior
Insomnia
Distrust
Perceived Hostility from Others
Rigidity
Passive Aggressive Behavior
Active Expression of Hostility
Approval of Rule Breaking
Antisocial History
Sex Problems
Reasons for Drinking
Problems Due to Drinking

In general, the reliabilities were rarely below 0.70 in the New York City sample as a whole and they held quite well in the subgroups (Dohrenwend and Shrout, in press). This seems satisfactory given the fact that the internal consistency reliability tends to increase with the number of items in a scale and only 5 of these 25 scales contain as many as 10 items each.

We also tested the internal consistency reliability scales in the samples of the general population and of psychiatric patients in Jerusalem. Each of these samples includes the following Jewish ethnic groups: Israeli-born, immigrants of European origin, immigrants from Iraq and immigrants from Morocco. By and large, the reliabilities were at least as good as in the New York City sample. The same was true of the scales tested with the New Hampshire inpatients and the sample of drug addicts from Pennsylvania. However, we learned in the New York City study that, despite the fact that all 25 scales had different names and were designed to measure different phenomena, some of them proved to be extremely highly correlated with each other. Were they in fact measuring different phenomena, or were at least some of them measures of the same thing?

Eight Scales Measuring Nonspecific Psychological Distress and Their Relation to Jerome Frank's Construct of "Demoralization"

One way to assess the extent to which two scales measure the same dimension of psychopathology is to examine the reliability of a score obtained from the difference between the scores on the two scales (Cohen and Cohen, 1975). This tells us whether we can accurately classify subjects scoring high on, say, a scale called "anxiety" and low on another scale such as "sadness." If we can classify at least some of our subjects in this way, we have an indication that, however much the two scales share, there is something different that each is measuring. To the extent that we cannot, the two scales for all practical purposes are measures of the same thing. Eight of our 25 symptom scales turned out to have difference score reliabilities that were less than .50 half or more of the time in the New York City sample from the general population. Furthermore, all 8 of these scales load highly on the same factor and correlate with each other about as highly as their reliabilities permit. The 8 scales are Poor Self Esteem, Hopelessness-Helplessness, Dread, Confused Thinking, Sadness, Anxiety, Psychophysiological Symptoms, and Perceived Physical Health. The evidence indicates that they are all measures of the same thing. Whatever it is, moreover, cannot be accounted for by acquiescence, need for approval, or differences in desirability ratings of the items in these by contrast with the other scales (Dohrenwend, Shrout, Egri, and Mendelsohn, 1980.)

Three of the 8 scales, Anxiety, Sadness, and Psychophysiological Symptoms, contain a substantial number of items commonly used in the brief psychiatric screening scales that have been developed since World War II. For example, fully half of the 20 items in these three scales come from the 22-item Screening scale developed by Langner (1962). On the basis of our previous experience with scales similar to these, (Dohrenwend, Oksenberg, Shrout, Dohrenwend, and Cook, 1979), we found that they correlate as highly as their reliabilities permit with the Langner scale. The Langner scale, in turn, correlates as highly as reliabilities permit with most of the other brief screening scales in wide use (Link and Dohrenwend, 1980). It follows that the screening scales and our 8 most highly intercorrelated PERI scales are all measures of the same dimension of psychopathology.

Previous review and analysis of relevant research with these screening scales by our research group (Dohrenwend, Oksenberg, Shrout, Dohrenwend, and Cook, 1979) suggest that the scales measure a dimension of nonspecific psychological distress that seems analogous in some ways to measures of body temperature. The reason for this conclusion is that elevated scores on these scales have been observed in such a wide variety of circumstances: for example, in combat troops by contrast with other soldiers (Star, 1949); in persons with more episodes of physical illness by contrast with persons with less (Eastwood, 1975); in psychiatric patients by contrast with nonpatients (Star, 1950; Langner, 1962; Macmillan, 1977; Dohrenwend and Crandell, 1970; and Manis, Brawer, Hunt, and Kercher, 1963); in college students by contrast with their peers in the general population (Mechanic and Greenley, 1976); in persons from lower classes by contrast with persons from higher classes (Abramson, 1966; Dohrenwend and Dohrenwend, 1969; Meile and Haese, 1969); and in suburban housewives by contrast with inner city housewives (Murphy, 1978). Clearly, an elevated score on these scales, like elevated body temperature, is an indication that something is wrong; however, as with fever, it does not tell you what is wrong.

The psychiatric conception that seems to us to best describe this type of distress is Jerome Frank's (1973) formulation of "demoralization." In Frank's formulation, ". . . a person becomes demoralized when he finds that he can-

TABLE 2
Multiple R and Multiple R^2, with Increments in % of Variance Explained (R^2) for Each of Eight Steps in a Stepwise Hierarchical Multiple Regression Analysis with the 22-Item Screening Score as the Criterion Variable.

Step	*Set description*	*Multiple R**	*Multiple R^2 (% of variance)*	*Increment over previous set†*
1.	Demographic	0.34	11.6%	—
2.	Parental-marital factors	0.50	23.0%	+11.4%
3.	Parents had psychiatric help	0.50[a]	25.2%	+ 2.2%
4.	Parent-child factors (parenting)	0.54	29.4%	+ 4.2%
5.	Child's physical illness	0.57	32.1%	+ 2.7%
6.	Child's total impairment rating	0.59	34.7%	+ 2.6%
7.	Mother's fatalism-suspiciousness (unexpressed violence scores)	.66	43.5%	+ 8.8%
8.	Child's school dropout and arrests	0.66	43.6%	+ 0.1%

*Shrunken R^2 approximately 2% less than R^2
†Increments not tested for significance

not meet the demands placed on him by the environment, and cannot extricate himself from his predicament" (1973: p. 316). In this view, demoralization may or may not accompany clinical psychiatric disorders (p. 315). More often, it, like the screening scale scores, is related to a large variety of other things such as situations of extreme environmental stress (p. 316); physical illnesses especially those that are chronic (pp. 46-47); or "existential despair" (p. 317).

Table 1 presents the content of all 8 PERI scales juxtaposed with various of Frank's descriptions of demoralization. It is evident that our latent dimension of nonspecific psychological distress is remarkably similar in content to the construct of demoralization as Frank has described it.

It was possible to construct a composite scale of demoralization by standardizing each of the eight subscales in table 1 to control for differences in the number of items and then adding these adjusted scores. The resulting scale has a possible range of 0 to 32 and, in our New York City sample from the general population, a mean of 7.59, and a standard deviation of 4.72. The internal consistency reliability of the composite is 0.90 in the sample as a whole, and is highly reliable as well in all subgroups. An equally satisfactory alternative would be to use the 27 asterisked items in table 1 since they form a scale of face valid items with similarly high reliability. On the possibility that some aspects of demoralization have temporal priority over others and successive measures over short periods of time are planned, the subscales can be scored separately. For purposes of further analyses of the remaining PERI scales in the data sets from New York City and Jerusalem, we have used either the 8 scale composite or the 27 asterisked items as a single scale measuring demoralization.

Symptom Scales that are Distinct from Demoralization

Unlike the eight scales measuring demoralization, the remaining symptom scales tested in New York City and Jerusalem are generally distinct from each other (i.e., the reliabilities of the difference scores are above 0.50) and from the demoralization scales, although a number are significantly correlated with demoralization. For example, in the New York City data, we found that 8 scales share more than 15% of their variance with the demoralization composite. These are Enervation, Somatic Problems, Guilt, Perceived Hostility from Others, Insomnia, Suicidal Ideation and Behavior, Manic Characteristics, and False Beliefs and Perceptions. Six other scales were significantly correlated with demoralization, but shared less than 11% of their variance: Active Expression of Hostility, Sex Problems, Distrust, Rigidity, Reasons for Drinking, and Problems Due to Drinking. Finally, three scales were not significantly related to the demoralization composite scale: Passive-Agressive Behavior, Anti-Social History and Approval of Rule Breaking. In table 2 we list short descriptions of all of the PERI scales, other than those in the demoralization composite, that were tested and found reliable in the New York and Jerusalem studies.

TABLE 1
Frank's Descriptions of Demoralization in Relation to the Eight Most Highly Intercorrelated PERI Symptom Scales.

The 8 most highly intercorrelated PERI scales	*Frank's description of the symptom content of demoralization*
Poor self esteem	
* 1. Since__________, how often have you felt confident? (0 very often; 1 fairly often; 2 sometimes; 3 almost never; 4 never)	"Insofar as the patient's symptoms are expressions of his demoralized state, restoration of his *self esteem* by whatever means causes them to subside" (p. 316).
* 2. Since__________, how often have you felt useless? (4 very often; 3 fairly often; 2 sometimes; 1 almost never; 0 never)	
* 3. Think of a person who feels that he is a failure generally in life. Is this person (4 very much like you; 3 much like you; 2 somewhat like you; 1 very little like you; 0 not at all like you)	
* 4. Think of a person who feels he has much to be proud of. Is this person (0 very much like you; 2 somewhat like you; 3 very little like you; 4 not at all like you)	
5. Think of a person who feels he has a number of good qualities. Is this person (0 very much like you; 1 much like you; 2 somewhat like you; 3 very little like you; 4 not at all like you)	
* 6. In general, if you had to compare yourself with the average (man/woman) your age, what grade would you give yourself? (0 excellent; 1 good; 2 average; 3 below average; 4 a lot below average)	

TABLE 1 (Continued)

* 7. In general, how satisfied are you with yourself? (0 very satisfied; 1 somewhat satisfied; 3 somewhat dissatisfied; 4 very dissatisfied)	
8. In general, how satisfied are you with your body? (0 very satisfied; 1 somewhat satisfied; 3 somewhat dissatisfied; 4 very dissatisfied)	
Hopelessness-helplessness	
* 1. How often have you had times when you couldn't help wondering if any thing was worthwhile any more? (4 very often; 3 fairly often; 2 sometimes; 1 almost never; 0 never)	"In other terms, to various degrees the demoralized person feels. . .hopeless and helpless" (p. 314).
* 2. Since __________, how often have you felt that nothing turns out for you the way you want it to, would you say (4 very often; 3 fairly often; 2 sometimes; 1 almost never; 0 never)	
* 3. Since __________, how often have you felt completely helpless? (4 very often; 3 fairly often; 2 sometimes; 1 almost never; 0 never)	
* 4. Since __________, how often have you felt completely hopeless about everything, would you say (4 very often; 3 fairly often; 2 sometimes; 1 almost never; 0 never)	

TABLE 1 (Continued)

Item	Source
Dread	
* 1. Since ________, how often have you feared going crazy; losing your mind? (4 very often; fairly often; 2 sometimes; 1 almost never; 0 never)	"In severe cases they [the demoralized] fear that they cannot even control their own feelings, giving rise to fear of going crazy..." (p. 314)
* 2. Since ________, how often have you had attacks of sudden fear or panic? (4 very often; 3 fairly often; 2 sometimes; 1 almost never; 0 never)	
* 3. Since ________, how often have you feared something terrible would happen to you? (4 very often; 3 fairly often; 2 sometimes; 1 almost never; 0 never)	
4a. Since ________, how often have you feared travelling? (1 very often or fairly often; 0 sometimes, almost never or never)	
4b. Since ________, how often have you feared crowds? (1 very often or fairly often; 0 sometimes, almost never, or never)	
4c. Since ________, how often have you feared being in a special place like up high or in an enclosed or dark place? (1 very often or fairly often; 0 sometimes, almost never, or never)	

Scoring notes: Questions 1 through 3 are scored in the same direction on a five-point scale. Question 4 is a composite item made up of three parts. Scoring for question 4 is as follows: subjects receiving all 0's on parts a, b & c are assigned 0. Subjects receiving one 1 and two 0's are assigned "1." Subjects receiving two 1's and one 0 are assigned "3," and subjects receiving all 1's on parts a, b & c are assigned "4."

TABLE 1 (Continued)

Confused thinking	
* 1. Since __________ , how often have you felt confused and had trouble thinking? (4 very often; 3 fairly often; 2 sometimes; 1 almost never; 0 never)	"...to demoralize..[is] to...bewilder, to throw... into disorder or confusion" (p. 314).
2. Since __________ , how often have you kept losing your train of thought, would you say (4 very often; 3 fairly often; 2 sometimes; 1 almost never; 0 never)	
* 3. Since __________ , how often have you had trouble concentrating or keeping your mind on what you were doing? (4 very often; 3 fairly often; 2 sometimes; 1 almost never; 0 never)	
4. Since __________ , how often have you had trouble remembering things? (4 very often; 3 fairly often; 2 sometimes; 1 almost never; 0 never)	
Sadness	
* 1. Since __________ , how often have you been been bothered by feelings of sadness or depression—feeling blue? (4 very often; 3 fairly often; 2 sometimes; 1 almost never; 0 never)	"...the demoralized person is prey to...depression as well as...other dysphoric emotions" (pp. 314-315).
2. Since __________ , how often have you been in very low or low spirits? (4 very often; 3 fairly often; 2 sometimes; 1 almost never; 0 never)	

TABLE 1 (Continued)

3. Since ________, how often have you felt like crying? (4 very often; 3 fairly often; 2 sometimes; 1 almost never; 0 never)	
* 4. Since ________, how often have you felt lonely? (4 very often; 3 fairly often; 2 sometimes; 1 almost never; 0 never)	
Anxiety	
1. Since ________, how often have you had frightening dreams? (4 very often; 3 fairly often; 2 sometimes; 1 almost never; 0 never)	"...the demoralized person is prey to anxiety...as well as...other dysphoric emotions" (pp. 314-315).
2. Since ________, how often have you had personal worries that get you down physically, that is, make you physically ill? (4 very often; 3 fairly often; 2 sometimes; 1 almost never; 0 never)	
3. Since ________, how often have you feared getting physically sick? (4 very often; 3 fairly often; 2 sometimes; 1 almost never; 0 never)	
* 4. Since ________, how often have you felt anxious? (4 very often; 3 fairly often; 2 sometimes; 1 almost never; 0 never)	
* 5. Since ________, how often have you been bothered by nervousness, being fidgety or tense? (4 very often; 3 fairly often; 2 sometimes; 1 almost never; 0 never)	

TABLE 1 (Continued)

* 6. Since __________, how often have you been bothered by feelings of restlessness? (4 very often; 3 fairly often; 2 sometimes; 1 almost never; 0 never)	
* 7. Since __________, how often have you feared being left all alone or abandoned? (4 very often; 3 fairly often; 2 sometimes; 1 almost never; 0 never)	
8. Since __________, how often have you feared being robbed, attacked, or physically injured? (4 very often; 3 fairly often; 2 sometimes; 1 almost never; 0 never)	
* 9. Think of a person who is the worrying type—you know, a worrier. Is this person—(4 very much like you; 3 much like you; 2 somewhat like you; 1 very little like you; 0 not at all like you)	
*10. When you get angry, how often do you feel uncomfortable, like getting headaches, stomach pains, cold sweats and things like that? (4 very often; 3 fairly often; 2 sometimes; 1 almost never; 0 never)	
Psychophysiological symptoms	
1. Since __________, how often have you been bothered by acid or sour stomach *several times a week,* would you say (4 very often; 3 fairly often; 2 sometimes; 1 almost never; 0 never)	"...anxiety...or its somatic manifestations are expressions of a feeling of helplessness" (p. 236)

TABLE 1 (Continued)

* 2. Since __________, how often has your appetite been poor? (4 very often; 3 fairly often; 2 sometimes; 1 almost never; 0 never)	
* 3. Since __________, how often have you been bothered by cold sweats? (4 very often; 3 fairly often; 2 sometimes; 1 almost never; 0 never)	
4. Since __________, how often did your hands ever tremble enough to bother you, would you say (4 very often; 3 fairly often; 2 sometimes; 1 almost never; 0 never)	
* 5. Since __________, how often have you had trouble with headaches or pains in the head? (4 very often; 3 fairly often; 2 sometimes; 1 almost never; 0 never)	
6. Since __________, how often have you had trouble with constipation? (4 very often; 3 fairly often; 2 sometimes; 1 almost never; 0 never)	
Perceived physical health	
* 1. Since __________, how often have you felt you were bothered by all different kinds of ailments in different parts of your body? (4 very often; 3 fairly often; 2 sometimes; 1 almost never; 0 never)	"...anxiety...or its somatic manifestations are expressions of a feeling of helplessness" (p. 236)
2. Would you say your physical health in general has been (0 excellent; 1 good; 2 fair; 3 poor; 4 very poor	

* One of 27 items that can be used to form a highly reliable (alpha close to .90 in all subgroups) short scale of demoralization.

TABLE 2
Description of PERI Symptom Scales
Other Than Those in the Demoralization Composite.

False beliefs and perceptions

This scale attempts to measure perceptions outside of the ordinary and beliefs not shared by western culture. It usually indicates presence of a disorder, most likely but not exclusively schizophrenia.

Manic characteristics

Persons with large scores on this scale are reporting a feeling of "high." This state can be induced by chemicals (e.g., alcohol, amphetamines) and it is also the typical affect present during a manic episode of a bipolar disorder.

Suicide: ideation and behavior

Persons scoring high on this item report having thoughts of committing suicide or having actually attempted suicide. It is likely to indicate depression, either major or minor.

Guilt

This scale attempts to measure feelings of guilt. It might or might not indicate psychopathology, depending on the apparent presence or absence of a rational basis of such feeling. Whenever irrational, it is probably accompanying depression.

Enervation

This scale attempts to measure lack of energy, anhedonia or listlessness often associated with depression, some types of schizophrenia or certain character disorders. It could also be indicative of poor physical condition.

Insomnia

This scale attempts to measure difficulty in falling asleep, staying asleep and early waking. It is frequently found in a number of psychiatric disorders, including anxiety states, depression and psychosis.

Perceived hostility from others

This scale attempts to measure the respondent's suspicion that he or she is treated with hostility. It might or might not indicate paranoid characteristics (paranoid personality, paranoid schizophrenia or paranoid disorders). It is similar to DISTRUST except that it refers to hostile behavior from others.

Distrust

This scale attempts to measure lack of trust in others. Similar to PERCEIVED HOSTILITY FROM OTHERS, it might or might not indicate paranoid characteristics.

**Rigidity*

This scale attempts to measure rigid personality characteristics. It is not meant to be interpreted necessarily as symptomatic of psychopathology, but only as a personality characteristic.

**Passive aggressive behavior*

Persons scoring high on this scale report that when angry they try to hurt others by passive rather than by active means. The items listed are not symptoms, but descriptions of behaviors that might indicate passive aggressive personality.

TABLE 2 (Continued)

Active expression of hostility

Persons scoring high on this scale report that when angry they express their feelings through active hostile behavior. None of the items are descriptions of symptoms and many persons scoring on the scale might not have any psychiatric disorder. However, the scale is consistent with personality disorder (explosive type) or an acute psychotic episode. This scale is the opposite of passive aggressive behavior.

Approval of rule breaking

This scale attempts to measure the respondent's attitudes towards rule breaking. Respondents express an opinion about a person breaking certain rules. Many of the rules are not typically enforced by officers of the law and all the rules (if crimes) are typically not felonies.

Antisocial history

This scale contains items about the past only; no present behavior is examined. Those who score highly on this scale admit to having engaged in behavior that does not conform with the usual values of society, or that is actually against the law. The behaviors reported have occurred at various times of their lives. This type of past history might indicate antisocial personality.

Reasons for drinking

This scale attempts to measure the degree to which respondents drink to escape unpleasant states of mind. The items are derived from D. Cahalan, I. H. Cisin, and H. M. Crossley's scale of escape reasons for drinking *(American Drinking Practices,* New Brunswick, N.J.: Rutgers Center of Alcohol Studies, 1969).

Problems due to drinking

This scale attempts to measure impairment in some areas of life due to drinking. High scores probably indicate either problem drinkers or alcoholics.

Sex problems

This scale attempts to describe sex problems related to inhibited sexual desire, excitement (impotence, frigidity) or orgasm.

Somatic problems of possible psychogenic origin

These include such symptoms as heart beating hard, asthma attacks, fainting spells, weight loss, and weight gain.

***Schizoid personality*

This scale attempts to measure a defect in the capacity to form social relationships characteristic of but not specific to the schizoid personality. It includes items that measure withdrawal from close personal contacts; excessive shyness; tendency to solitary activities such as daydreaming.

TABLE 2 (Continued)

***Derealization—depersonalization*
This scale attempts to measure the respondent's feelings that the world around is unreal or that he himself is unreal. Though oftentimes those feelings appear in normal adolescents, in adults they are frequently indicative of any one of a variety of psychiatric disorders such as schizophrenia or anxiety neurosis or substance abuse.
***Conversion symptoms*
This scale is composed of items which tap the presence of disorders of the special senses or of the voluntary nervous system, e.g. aphonia, paralysis. This scale is not specific to hysteria since conversion symptoms are found in other disorders such as depression or schizophrenia.

* Tested in U.S. research only.
** Tested in Israel research only.

Evidence of Validity of the PERI Symptom Scales

As was shown in the research during World War II and other studies, including our own (Dohrenwend, Oksenberg, Shrout, Dohrenwend, and Cook, 1979), measures of nonspecific psychological distress discriminate quite sharply between samples of psychiatric patients and samples drawn from the general population. We will concentrate, therefore, on the PERI scales that are distinct from these measures of nonspecific psychological distress.

Tessler (1977) included five of the PERI symptom scales in the study of psychiatric inpatients at Northampton State Hospital in Massachusetts. As table 3 shows, these scales discriminate sharply between our community sample and Tessler's inpatients. Note the especially strong contrast on False Beliefs and Perceptions; it is just the difference one would expect if the scale were sensitive to delusions and hallucinations, given that the large majority of Tessler's patients had been diagnosed as psychotic.

In addition, Stokes (1976) used most of PERI in the study of samples of drug addicts conducted at Eagleville Hospital in Pennsylvania. Table 4 shows that there is far less difference between the scores of the addict sample and our community sample on False Beliefs and Perceptions than there was between our sample and the inpatients in table 3. The largest contrast in table 4, as we would expect, is on the scale of Antisocial History. Note also the contrast on two other scales designed to measure antisocial tendencies and symptoms—Attitude Toward Rule Breaking and Expression of Hostility. These differences are again what we would expect in two samples that contrast as markedly as these in actual rates of antisocial behavior.

TABLE 3
Comparisons of Means From Massachusetts Clinical Sample to New York Community Sample.

	Massachusetts clinical sample		*New York community sample*	
	Mean	***SD***	***Mean***	***SD***
False beliefs and perceptions	1.42	1.05	0.148	0.30
Guilt	1.52	1.11	0.742	0.67
Components of demoralization				
Sadness	2.47	0.96	1.33	0.94
Confused thinking	2.07	1.22	1.04	0.84
Perceived physical health	1.54	1.26	1.09	0.90
Average	2.03	—	1.15	—

N's for New York sample range from 168-110
N's for Massachusetts clinical sample is 147
All differences are significantly different from zero, p 0.01

PERI as a Screening Instrument: Evidence from the Jerusalem Pilot Study

One of the research objectives of the pilot study conducted in Israel was the development of PERI as a screening instrument for several diagnostic types from the general community. These types are Schizophrenia, Affective Disorders including Neurotic Depression, other Neuroses, and Antisocial Personality Disorders. As mentioned above, in the pilot study we were able to administer PERI to samples from the general community and to samples of psychiatric patients in Israel. Using these data in a discriminant analysis (Lachenbruch, 1975), we have obtained preliminary evidence of PERI's efficacy as a screening instrument, not only screening "cases" from "non-cases," but also gaining some indication of the specific type of disorder present.

In proceeding with the discriminant analysis, it was necessary that the diagnostic groups be as pure as possible. While the four diagnostic groups could be purified using institutional records, we were concerned that the no-disorder group might include community members with unrecognized psychiatric disorders. To minimize this possibility, we eliminated those persons in the community whom our interviewers (all of whom were experienced mental health professionals) judged to be possible cases.

After eliminating these community members, as well as respondents with excessive missing data, we had for calibration purposes 61 Community Non-Cases, and, based on the treatment diagnoses, 55 Schizophrenics, 44 Affec-

TABLE 4
Comparison of Means From New York Community Sample and Eagleville Sample.

Scale	New York sample Mean	New York sample Standard deviation	Eagleville sample Mean	Eagleville sample Standard deviation
1. False beliefs and perceptions	0.148	0.302	0.323**	0.569
2. Manic	0.903	0.762	1.304**	0.728
3. Suicide: ideation and behavior	0.157	0.534	2.323**	3.654
4. Guilt	0.742	0.676	0.978*	1.114
5. Enervation	0.067	0.757	1.701**	0.866
6. Insomnia	1.138	1.062	1.364	0.888
7. Distrust	1.265	0.818	2.089**	0.804
8. Perception of hostility	0.609	0.681	1.258**	0.773
9. Rigidity	1.753	0.683	2.224**	0.536
10. Passive aggressive behavior	1.487	0.868	2.039**	0.913
11. Expression of hostility	1.274	0.528	1.666**	0.618
12. Antisocial history	0.218	0.411	1.770**	0.894
13. Attitude toward rulebreaking	0.752	0.640	1.639**	1.034
14. Sex problems	0.809	0.754	0.979	1.021
15. Reasons for drinking	0.228	0.428	0.598**	0.836
16. Problems due to drinking	0.161	0.473	0.220	0.576
17. Demoralization	0.915	0.572	1.291**	0.593

N's for New York sample range from 168 to 110
N's for Eagleville sample range from 77 to 68
*Eagleville mean significantly larger than NY mean $p < .05$.
**Eagleville mean significantly larger than NY mean $p < .01$.

tive Disorders including Neurotics, 52 other Neurotics, and 40 Antisocial Personality Disorders. As we reported above, a subsample of about a quarter of the patients was interviewed with SADS-L by research psychiatrists who made diagnoses according to Research Diagnostic Criteria (RDC) (Spitzer, Endicott, and Robins, 1978). Since more than one diagnosis is permitted according to RDC, we used the following procedure for comparing the research (RDC) and clinical diagnosis:

Where there was more than one current RDC diagnosis, the priority for forming the four groups of cases was in the order of Schizophrenia, Affective Disorder, Antisocial Personality Disorder, and Neurosis. There proved to be more correspondence between the current treatment diagnoses and the current research diagnoses than might have been expected, given the fact that not only did diagnostician and nomenclature vary, but also the way the data on signs and symptoms were collected. The correspondence for Schizophrenia and Affective Disorder was considerably greater than for the other two broad types of disorder. Of the 15 patients who had treatment diagnoses of Schizophrenia, 10 met RDC criteria for current disorder of this type on the basis of SADS-L interviews. Only one patient receiving an RDC diagnosis of current Schizophrenia did not have a similar treatment diagnosis. Of the 15 patients in the subsample with treatment diagnoses of Affective Disorder, 14 received a research diagnosis for current Affective Disorder; however, the research diagnosis was far more inclusive, placing 33 patients in this category in all. The correspondence for Antisocial and Neurosis was far worse, with the treatment diagnosis far more inclusive than the research diagnosis.

Since, except for affective disorder, the treatment diagnoses were the more inclusive, and since we had larger numbers for the purpose, we used the treatment diagnoses to test the screening ability of the PERI scales. It seemed unlikely that all of the PERI scales would be needed to screen respondents into the four broad diagnostic groups and the community non-cases. We were reluctant, however, to let a statistical routine select the best scales since such selection procedures capitalize on chance sampling fluctuations. Instead, we used the following procedure: Based on the consensus of our research group, we selected on conceptual grounds the best candidate scales for discriminating between the five groups: (a) Demoralization, (b) False Beliefs and Perceptions, (c) Manic, (d) Enervation, (e) Antisocial History, (f) Drinking Problems, and (g) Suicide. When the means of these scales were compared across the five groups, we discovered a validity problem for the Manic Scale. The problem was that the Antisocial Personality group scored the highest on this scale, and the Affective Disorder group was not different from the Schizophrenic nor the Neurotic groups. In view of these results, the Manic scale was dropped from consideration.

The remaining six scales all showed appropriate group differences and were thus used as a basis for the discriminant analysis. When this set of scales was held constant, only one of the other PERI scales showed significant group differences, i.e., only one other scale reflected differences in the five groups that were not already accounted for by the six scales the research team had chosen. This other scale was Schizoid Personality, a new scale developed for the Israeli project. Thus, for purposes of screening the four diagnostic types in Israel, seven PERI scales seem to be sufficient.

Table 5 gives an indication of how well these seven scales discriminate between the groups. The discriminant function analysis produced four significant functions that can be used to classify respondents. Using the conservative jackknife-like classification procedure described by Lachenbruch (1975), the original respondents used to estimate the discriminant functions are "reclassified" to estimate the expected classification error rates. Since the classification system is to be used to screen respondents, the analysis was asymmetrically designed so that it would treat misclassifications of cases as non-cases (false negatives) as twice as undesirable as misclassifications of non-cases (false positives).

From table 5 it can be seen that about 76% of the non-cases were correctly classified. Moreover, if the four pathological groups are collapsed into one group needing followup, 93% of the cases would be correctly classified into that group. In addition, it is clear that the Antisocial Personality group was well separated from the others, and the majority of the Schizophrenics were correctly classified. The separation of Affective Disorders from Neurotics, however, was not so good. Overall, 62% of the respondents were correctly classified using the five diagnostic categories.

Since the sensitivity and specificity estimates from a discriminant function tend to be biased upward (even when the conservative jackknife-like procedure is used), it is desirable to compare these results to some standard. It has been argued (Dohrenwend, Oksenberg, Shrout, Dohrenwend and Cook, 1979; Link and Dohrenwend, 1980; and Dohrenwend, Shrout, Egri, and Mendelsohn, 1980), that traditional screening scales, such as Langner's 22 items (Langner, 1962), are identical to measures of Demoralization (see above); thus we might expect our measure of Demoralization to give screening results like what we would get if we used a traditional scale. Using only Demoralization and again requiring that relatively fewer false negatives be made than false positives, it was found that only 40% of the non-cases were correctly classified. Again grouping the four pathological groups together, we found that the sensitivity of this rule was high—90% of the persons from the pathological groups would have been designated for an eventual followup—but it is obvious that this high sensitivity was obtained at the expense of the specificity. Perhaps the most striking difference between the seven scale classification rule and Demoralization alone is the misclassification among the various diagnostic groups: on the average, only 23% of the respondents were correctly classified. Thus, for our purposes, we find the seven scale classification rule far superior, especially with regard to screening for Schizophrenics and Antisocial Personality. This increased discrimination is achieved at the expense of a relatively minor burden; 46 items need to be added to the 27-item Demoralization scale in order to considerably improve the results.

It should be noted that it cannot be guaranteed that these seven scales are the most appropriate for screening in other populations. If the populations differ or the diagnostic categories to be identified are altered or expanded, or if the diagnostic criteria differ sharply from those used by the treating agencies in Israel, some of the reliable PERI scales listed in table 2 may prove to be useful additions to or substitutions for the present seven scales we have discussed. Furthermore, the estimates of sensitivities and specificities that we obtained from the discriminant analyses must be treated as preliminary. For a more rigorous design for the estimation of these statistics, see Dohrenwend and Shrout (1981).

Conclusions

We have presented evidence of the internal consistency reliability of PERI symptom scales in groups of individuals with vastly different social and cultural backgrounds, evidence of their criterion-oriented validity, and evidence of the sensitivity and specificity with which seven of them

TABLE 5
Estimates of Classification Error of Discriminant Functions*
Using Jackknife-like Estimation Procedure.

		Predicted group				
Actual group	*N*	*Community*	*Schizophrenics*	*Affective*	*Neurotic*	*Antisocial personality*
Community	62	47(75.8%)	4	5	3	3
Schizophrenic	55	4	35(63.6%)	9	5	2
Affective disorders	44	4	10	17(38.6%)	11	2
Neurotic	52	5	7	13	25(48.1%)	2
Antisocial personality	40	1	2	2	2	33(82.5%)

* The functions utilize the following scales: demoralization, false beliefs and perceptions, enervation, antisocial history, drinking problems, suicide, and schizoid personality

discriminate psychiatric patients with a variety of types of functional psychiatric disorder from a sample of non-cases drawn from the general population. To date, other potentially promising and to some extent similar approaches to constructing conceptually meaningful measures of the dimensions of psychopathology (e.g., Derogatis, 1977; Jackson and Messick, 1971) have not been subjected to such tests of their possible usefulness in epidemiological research in the general population.

PERI symptom scales were not developed, however, to yield specific diagnoses according to DSM-III (Task Force on Nomenclature and Statistics, 1980) or ICD-9 (Ninth Revision Conference and the Twenty-Ninth World Health Assembly, 1977). PERI in fact contrasts with research interviews that are explicitly articulated with one or the other of these two most current and most influential nosologies. Unlike PERI which relies on self-reports, the diagnostic interviews come from a rating scale tradition in psychiatry. In this tradition, clinical judgment is relied upon to provide scorable evidence of psychopathology. The most widely used of these diagnostic instruments are the Present State Examination (PSE) (Wing, Cooper, Sartorius, 1974) and the Schedule for Affective Disorders and Schizophrenia (SADS) (Endicott and Spitzer, 1978).

Both SADS and the PSE have been developed mainly on the basis of research with psychiatric patients rather than in research with samples from the general population. Results from our research with the Psychiatric Status Schedule (PSS) (Spitzer, Endicott, Fleiss, Cohen, 1970) a precursor of SADS, suggest that such clinical instruments may not give reliable measurements over the range of scores observed in the general population (Dohrenwend, Yager, Egri and Mendelsohn, 1978). We encountered problems in trying to use the PSS in research with the general population. For example, a computer program for diagnosing schizophrenia that was developed on the basis of PSS research with patients (Spitzer and Endicott, 1968), grossly overrepresented schizophrenia in a sample of general population subjects that we studied with the same instrument (Dohrenwend, Shrout, Egri and Mendelsohn, 1980). Nor are such problems limited to the PSS, as some recent results reported by Wing and his colleagues (1978, p. 213) show. These researchers found marked differences between "cases" of depression identified by their own computer program in a sample from the general population and cases of depression in samples of psychiatric patients. As with the PSS program, the PSE computer program was developed on the basis of research with patients.

An instrument such as PERI, then, which was developed through research with samples from the general population, can yield reliable measures of a wide variety of dimensions of psychopathology and can be used to screen samples from the general population for likely cases of psychiatric disorders in general and even for likely subtypes. The classifications of subtypes are somewhat gross, however, and the resulting groups will not be as homogeneous in diagnostic type as we would like. On the other hand, diagnostic interviews such as SADS and PSE that were developed with psychiatric patients and provide reliable diagnoses in patient groups are likely to prove problematic when applied to the general population. The SADS and the PSE, especially in the hands of skilled clinicians for whom they were designed, are also expensive to administer with large samples from the general population.

Against this background, consider the possibility of using the two types of interviews together in epidemiological research. According to this plan, an interview such as PERI, which uses a self-report format rather than clinical ratings, would be used to screen members of the general population economically, yielding subsamples with high rates of severe symptomatology in general and/or high rates of particular types of disorder. The screened individuals would then be followed up and interviewed by skilled clinicians with diagnostic instruments such as SADS or the PSE to provide rates for particular types of disorders in the general population. While potential advantages of such two-stage procedures have long been evident (Cooper and Morgan, 1973), they have only rarely been used in psychiatric epidemiology (Duncan-Jones and Henderson, 1978). Not the least of the advantages of this procedure is that it brings two tests (self-report and clinical rating interviews) to bear in a situation where each has different strengths and weaknesses. It seems to us that exploration of the possibilities of two-stage procedures is the next logical step to take toward an improved solution of the key methodological problem in psychiatric epidemiology: How to identify and diagnose psychiatric disorders in the general population.

Acknowledgments

This research has been supported by Research Grants MH-10328, MN-30710, and Research Scientist Award K05-MH14663 from the National Institute of Mental Health, U.S. Public Health Services, and by the Foundations' Fund for Research in Psychiatry. We thank especially Donald F. Klein for suggesting the relevance of Frank's concept of demoralization to some of our findings. We would also like to acknowledge the valuable contributions of Alexander R. Askenasy, Diana Cook, Barbara Dohrenwend, Gladys Egri, Lawrence Krasnoff, Frederick S. Mendelsohn, and Thomas Yager to the development of the instrument PERI. Thanks go as well to Richard Tessler and Janet Stokes, who used many of the PERI symptom scales in their research with psychiatric inpatients and drug addicts respectively, and generously provided us with the data for the comparisons with our community sample. Finally, we express our gratitude to staff members of many institutions in Israel whose ready cooperation made the pilot study in that country possible.

References

Abramson, J. H. (1966), Emotional disorder, status inconsistency and migration: A health questionnaire survey in Jerusalem, *Milbank Memorial Fund Quarterly*, 44:23-48.

Cohen, J. & Cohen, P. (1975), *Applied Multiple Regression/Correlation Analysis for the Behavioral Sciences.* New York: John Wiley & Sons.

Cooper, B. & Morgan, H. G. (1973), *Epidemiological Psychiatry*. Springfield, Illinois: C.C. Thomas.

Cronback, L. J. (1951), Coefficient alpha and the internal structure of tests, *Psychometrics*, 16:297.

Derogatis, L. R. (1977), *SCL-90.R. (Revised) Version Manual I*. Baltimore: Clinical Psychometrics Research Unit, Johns Hopkins University School of Medicine.

Dohrenwend, B. P. (1974), Problems in defining and sampling the relevant population of stressful life events. In: *Stressful Life Events: Their Nature and Effects*, ed. Dohrenwend, B. S. & Dohrenwend, B. P. New York: Wiley pp. 275-310.

Dohrenwend, B. P. & Crandell, D. L. (1970), Psychiatric symptoms in community, clinic, and mental hospital groups, *American Journal of Psychiatry*, 126:1611-1621.

Dohrenwend, B. P. & Dohrenwend, B. S. (1969), *Social Status and Psychological Disorders*. New York: John Wiley & Sons.

Dohrenwend, B. P., Oksenberg, L., Shrout, P. E., Dohrenwend, B. S. & Cook, D. (1979), What brief psychiatric screening scales measure. In: *Health Survey Research Methods: Third Biennial Research Conference*. National Center for Health Services Research. Washington, D.C., U.S. Department of Health and Human Services DHHS Publication No. (PHS), 81-3268, pp. 188-198.

Dohrenwend, B. P. & Shrout, P. E. (1981), Toward the development of a two-stage procedure for case identification and classification in psychiatric epidemiology. In: *Research in Community and Mental Health, Vol. 2*, ed. Simmons, R. G. Greenwich, Connecticut: Jai Press, pp. 292-323.

Dohrenwend, B. P., Shrout, P. E., Egri, G. & Mendelsohn, F. S. (1980), Measures of nonspecific psychological distress and other dimensions of psychopathology in the general population, *Arch Gen Psychiat* 37:1229-1236.

Dohrenwend, B. P., Yager, T. J., Egri, G. & Mendelsohn, F. C. (1978), The psychiatric status schedule (PSS) as a measure of dimensions of psychopathology in the general population, *Arch Gen Psychiat* 35:731-739.

Dohrenwend, B. S. (1977), Anticipation and control of life events: An exploratory analysis. In: *Origins and Course of Psychopathology*, ed. Strauss, J. S., Babigian, M. & Roff, M. New York: Plenum Press, pp. 135-186.

Dohrenwend, B. S., Dohrenwend, B.P. & Cook, D. (1981), Measurement of social functioning in community populations. In: *What is a Case? Problems of Definition in Psychiatric Community Surveys*, ed. Wing, J. K., Bebbington, P. & Robins, L. N. London: Grant, McIntyre, pp. 183-201.

Dohrenwend, B. S., Dohrenwend, B.P. & Cook, D. (1973), Ability and disability in role functioning in psychiatric patient and non-patient groups. In: *Roots of Evaluation, ed.* Wing, J. K. & Hafner, H. London: Oxford University Press, pp. 337-360.

Dohrenwend, B. S., Krasnoff, L., Askenasy, A. & Dohrenwend, B. P. (1978), Exemplification of a method for scaling life events: The PERI Life Events Scale, *J Health Soc Beh* 19:205-229.

Dohrenwend, B. S. & Martin, J. S. (1979), Personal versus situational determination of anticipation and control of the occurrence of stressful life events, *Am J Community Psychol,* 7:453-468.

Duncan-Jones, P. & Henderson, S. (1978), The use of a two-stage procedure in a prevalence survey, *Social Psychiatry* 13:231-237.

Eastwood, M. R. (1975), *The Relation Between Physical and Mental Illness,* Buffalo: University of Toronto Press.

Eighth Revision Conference (1968), *Manual of the International Statistical Classifications of Diseases, Injuries, and Causes of Mental Disorders.* Geneva: World Health Organization.

Endicott, J. & Spitzer, R. L. (1978), A diagnostic interview: The Schedule for Affective Disorders and Schizophrenia, *Arch Gen Psychiatr,* 35:837-844.

Feighner, J. P., Robins, E., Guze, S. B., Woodruff, R. A., Winokur, G. & Munoz, R. (1972), Diagnostic criteria for use in psychiatric research, *Arch Gen Psychiatr* 26:57-63.

Frank, J. D. (1973), *Persuasion and Healing,* Baltimore: Johns Hopkins University Press (originally published, 1961).

Jackson, D. N. & Messick, S. (1971), *Differential Personality Inventory.* London, Ontario: Authors.

Lachenbruch, P. A. (1975), *Discriminant Analysis,* New York: Hafner Press.

Langner, T. S. (1962), A twenty-two item screening score of psychiatric symptoms indicating impairment, *J Health Human Behav,* 3:269-276.

Link, B. & Dohrenwend, B. P. (1980), Formulation of hypotheses about the true prevalence of demoralization in the United States. In: *Mental Illness in the United States: Epidemiologic Estimates,* eds. Dohrenwend, B. P., Dohrenwend, B. S., Gould, M. S., Link, B., Neugebauer, R. & Wunsch-Hitzig, R. New York: Praeger, pp. 114-132.

Macmillan, A. M. (1977), "The health opinion survey: Technique for estimating prevalence of psychoneurotic and related types of disorder in communities," *Psychol Rep,* 3:325-329.

Manis, J. G., Brawer, M. H., Hunt, C. L. & Kercher, L. C. (1963), Validating a mental health scale, *Amer Sociol Review,* 28:108-116.

Mechanic, D. & Greeley, J. R. (1976), The prevalence of psychological distress and help seeking in a college student population, *Social Psychiatry,* 11:1-14.

Meile, R. L. & Haese, P. N. (1969), Social status, status incongruence and symptoms of stress, *J Health Soc Behav,* 10:237-244.

Murphy, H. B. M. (1978), The meaning of symptom checklist scores in mental health surveys: A testing of multiple hypotheses, *Soc Sci Med,* 12:67-75.

Ninth Revision Conference (1977), *Manual of the International Statistical Classifications of Diseases, Injuries, and Causes of Mental Disorders,* Geneva: World Health Organization.

Nunnally, J. C. (1967), *Psychometric Theory.* New York: McGraw-Hill.

Peres, Y. (1977), *Ethnic Relations in Israel,* Tel Aviv: Sifriat Hapoalim (in Hebrew).

Spitzer, R. L., Endicott, J., Fleiss, J. L. & Cohen, J. (1970), The Psychiatric Status Schedule: A technique for evaluating psychopathology and impairment in role functioning, *Arch Gen Psychiatr,* 23:41.

Spitzer, R. L., Endicott, J. & Robins, E. (1978), Research Diagnostic Criteria: Rationale and reliability. *Arch Gen Psychiatr* 35:773-782.

Star, S. A. (1949), Psychoneurotic symptoms in the army. In: *Studies in Social Psychology in World War II. The American Soldier: Combat and Its Aftermath,* ed. Stouffer, S. A., Guttman, L. A., Suchman, E. A., Lazarsfeld, P. F., Star, S. A. & Clausen, J. A. Princeton: Princeton University Press, pp. 411-455.

Star, S. A. (1950), The screening of psychoneurotics in the army: Technical development of tests, In: *Measurement and Prediction,* eds. Stouffer, S., Guttman, L., Suchman, E. A., Lazarsfeld, P. F., Star, S. A. S. & Clausen, J. A. Princeton: Princeton University Press, pp. 486-547.

Stokes, J. (1976), *The Psychological Symptoms of Drug Addicts,* mimeographed, Eagleville Hospital and Rehabilitation Center, P.O. Box 45, Eagleville, Pennsylvania 19408.

Task Force on Nomenclature and Statistics (1980), *Diagnostic and Statistical Manual of Mental Disorders,* Third Edition. Washington, D.C.: American Psychiatric Association.

Tessler, R. (1977), *Reliability of Selected Measures Derived from the Psychiatric Epidemiology Research Interview: A Preliminary Report Based upon a Study of Psychiatric Patients,* mimeographed. Department of Sociology: University of Massachusetts, Amherst, Massachusetts 01002.

Wing, J. K., Cooper, J. E. & Sartorius, H. (1974), *The Measurement and Classification of Psychiatric Symptoms: An Instruction Manual for the PSE and CATEGO Program,* London: Cambridge University Press.

Wing, J. K., Mann, S. A., Leff, J. P. & Nixon, J. M. (1978), The concept of a "case" in psychiatric population surveys, *Psycholog Med,* 8:203-217.

Chapter 17

Some Biometrics Contributions to Assessment: PSS, CAPPS, SADS-L/RDC, and DSM III

JANET B. W. WILLIAMS
JEAN ENDICOTT
ROBERT L. SPITZER

Current psychiatric epidemiologic research attempts to assess the prevalence in the community of specific mental disorders (treated and untreated). Unfortunately, this attempt is often hampered by the lack of a suitable assessment procedure that is appropriate to the task. Ideally such a procedure should cover a wide range of psychopathology, have evidence of acceptable reliability and validity and, in order to minimize costs in large-scale surveys, be suitable for administration by personnel without graduate-level education. This chapter describes some of the instruments for the assessment of psychopathology and diagnosis that have been developed over the last fifteen years by the Biometrics Research Department at the New York State Psychiatric Institute, and that may be particularly useful in epidemiologic studies. The instruments described include the Psychiatric Status Schedule (PSS), the Current and Past Psychopathology Scales (CAPPS), and the lifetime version of the Schedule for Affective Disorders and Schizophrenia (SADS-L). (Although the PSS and CAPPS have largely been supplanted by the more recently developed SADS-L, their development is discussed to give the reader an historical perspective.) The chapter concludes with a discussion of the Third Edition of the Diagnostic and Statistical Manual of Mental Disorders (DSM-III), whose development was coordinated by Dr. Spitzer.

Methodological Considerations

An assessment of psychopathology is usually made during a clinical interview. In addition to information collected during the interview, a clinician may consult other sources of information, such as referral notes, a previous case record, or another informant. During the interview, the clinician asks a series of questions which are, in part, guided by what areas of functioning the clinician deems most relevant, the clinician's observations, and the interpretation that the clinician makes of the person's responses and other behavior during the interview. Finally, the clinician may summarize these clinical judgments into a diagnosis. In epidemiologic studies, trained "raters" are given the task of approximating these clinical assessments.

The usefulness of the specific evaluation procedures used is determined to a great extent by their interrater reliability; that is, the extent to which two or more raters, assessing the same subjects, can make independent ratings that agree with each other. To the extent that a procedure for evaluating psychopathology or making diagnostic judgments is unreliable, a limit is placed on its validity for any use. The four major sources of unreliability that lead to disagreement among clinicians or raters are (1) information variance, (2) observation and interpretation variance, (3) criterion variance, and (4) occasion variance (Spitzer and Williams, 1980).

Information Variance

This source of unreliability is present when clinicians or raters have different amounts and kinds of information. For example, one rater may speak with a family member who indicates that the subject has problems with alcohol; another clinician may not be told of those problems, and during the interview the subject may deny them. Or a subject may give different responses because of different interviewing techniques and different questions being asked, as when one clinician elicits delusional material after intensive questioning about psychotic symptoms, whereas another clinician in a separate evaluation interview does not elicit such material because he or she made only a perfunctory inquiry into the presence of psychotic symptoms.

Observation and Interpretation Variance

This source of unreliability is present when clinicians or raters who are presented with the same stimuli, differ in what they notice and remember (observation variance). For example, one rater may notice that a subject showed signs of psychomotor retardation, whereas another rater might not notice the signs. This type of variance also includes differences in the threshold for attaching clinical significance to certain observations; in other words, raters may interpret what they see differently (interpretation variance). For example, two raters may hear the same account of how a subject believes he is being harassed by neighbors. One rater may conclude that the context of the belief makes it uncertain whether or not a delusion is present; the other rater may conclude that, without doubt, it is a delusion.

Criterion Variance

This source of unreliability is present when there are differences in the definitions raters use to determine the presence or absence (or degree present) of a symptom, or when clinicians use different sets of criteria to summarize data into diagnoses. When clinicians or raters make ratings or diagnoses without explicit definitions or criteria, they are forced to use their own idiosyncratic definitions or criteria, basing these on their own personal concepts. For example, there may be disagreements as to the definition of "disorganized behavior," or whether or not some degree of chronicity is necessary for a diagnosis of schizophrenia.

Occasion Variance

Occasion variance is present when a subject's condition is actually different at different times. Thus, if one rater conducts an evaluation on one day, and a second rater conducts a similar evaluation on another day, the subject may have developed some new symptoms in between, or some symptoms may have resolved in the interim. Although occasion variance reduces reliability, since it reflects facts it is not a source of error variance.

Procedures are available to minimize the effect of each type of error variance that contributes to interjudge unreliability. Information variance can be minimized by making sure that all raters have available the same body of information, such as reviewing the same case material or observing the same interview. It can also be minimized by using structured interview schedules, so that each rater asks similar questions. Observation and interpretation variance is best minimized by adequate training in observation skills and the interpretation of behavior. Differences in interpreting the significance of specific behaviors can be minimized by using guidelines that specify thresholds for significance, such as a statement specifying that a symptom must cause some impairment in social or occupational functioning to be considered clinically significant. Criterion variance is best minimized by each rater using the same specific symptom definitions or criteria for diagnosis.

Psychiatric Status Schedule

The Psychiatric Status Schedule (PSS) (Spitzer et al., 1970) was developed in the late 1960s at a time when almost all available rating scales and evaluation procedures were limited to the evaluation of psychopathology elicited during a mental status examination. Social role functioning (e.g., as mate, parent, worker, student) as well as alcoholism, drug use, and antisocial behavior were generally not covered at all, or in any depth, yet these areas are necessary to assess in community surveys. The main purpose of the PSS was to provide an assessment measure that included mental status as well as these other areas of psychopathology.

The PSS includes a standardized interview schedule which the interviewer uses to elicit information needed to judge a matching inventory of dichotomous (true-false) items, most of which are brief nontechnical descriptions of small units of overt behavior. A sample of the PSS is presented in table 1. As can be seen, the interview schedule is only semi-structured, allowing the interviewer to clarify or probe areas that remain unclear, and to maintain good rapport with the subject. The specificity of the questions helps minimize information variance as it provides some assurance that each rater will use the same questions to inquire about the same areas of behavior. In addition, raters are expected to gather, judge, and record all the data during the interview so the interview and evaluation are completed simultaneously. The detailed descriptions of the items help minimize criterion variance, since all the raters have the same explicit guidelines for interpreting responses of the subjects. The basic scoring system of the PSS uses the items to yield scale scores of dimensions of psychopathology and social functioning (although not diagnoses). The time period covered is the week prior to and including the interview. Because only a cross-sectional evaluation of a subject is obtained, episodes of psychopathology that occurred prior to the week before the evaluation are not recorded.

An evaluation using the PSS takes from 30 to 50 minutes, depending on the amount of psychopathology of the subject, the number of applicable occupational and life roles to be inquired about, and the subject's verbal abilities and cooperation. It can be administered by interviewers who have not had a great deal of prior clinical experience and professional training. A training manual, teaching tapes and suggested procedures for training interviewers are available.

In addition to several studies in which relatively high interjudge reliability was obtained, the validity of the PSS has been partially established by the instrument's ability to discriminate among samples of subjects such as inpatient vs. outpatient vs. community samples, and patients with different diagnoses, such as organic brain syndromes, schizophrenia, and neurosis. For the most part, the use of the PSS has been limited to studies of treatment response in groups of psychiatric patients (Herz et al., 1971; Herz et al., 1975; Washburn et al., 1976; Piper et al., 1977) and descriptions of the psychopathology of selected samples (Spitzer et al., 1969; Silberfarb et al., 1980). The PSS has had only limited use in epidemiology as an evaluation procedure for nonpatients (Dohrenwend et al., 1978).

The Use of Rating Scales in Diagnostic Assessment

In the past 15 years, as interest increased in improving the validity and reliability of diagnosis, a need arose for procedures to minimize various sources of error variance involved in routine clinical diagnosis. Epidemiologic studies had generally employed symptom rating scales that merely indicated some degree of "caseness" rather than specific diagnoses.

The unreliability of routine clinical diagnosis has been well documented (Spitzer and Fleiss 1974; Beitchman et al., 1978) and shown to be mainly due to information variance and criterion variance. The PSS was originally

TABLE 1
Part of the Psychiatric Status Schedule.

Interview schedule		*Inventory*
	Dressing	
How long does it take you to get dressed? (Why does it take that long?)		13 Indicates he spends an excessive amount of time dressing or grooming himself because of rituals, indecision, perfectionism, dawdling or lethargy.
	Mood	
What kind of moods have you been in recently?		14 Says he has felt elated or "high" (do not include mere good spirits).
	Worries	
What kind of things do you worry about? If admits to worries: (How much do you worry?)		15 Mentions he worries a lot or that he can't stop worrying.
	Fears	
What kind of fears do you have? (Are there things or situations you are afraid of?) (Anything else?)		16 Admits to three or more different fears OR says that he keeps feeling afraid of different things. 17 Indicates he is fearful of losing his mind or losing control of his emotions.
People sometimes have fears they know don't make sense — like crowds or certain activities. What kinds of fears do you have like this? If says he does not like or worries about an object or situation ask: (But are you afraid of _______ ?) If indicates any fear: (Does this fear of _______ prevent you from doing something you want to do?)		18 Indicates a morbid fear that something terrible will happen to him. 19 Indicates he has an irrational fear of a particular object or situation (e.g., crowds, heights) [phobia]. 20 Says he gets attacks of sudden fear or panic. 21 Indicates his fear prevents him from participating in some activity.

TABLE 1 (Continued)

Interview schedule		Inventory
	Anxiety	
How often do you feel anxious or tense?		22 Admits that he is often anxious.
If unclear: (Nervous) (How much of the time do you feel this way?)		23 Admits he feels anxious most of the time.
	Restlessness	
What about feeling restless? If unclear: (Can't stay still.)		24 Mentions he is often restless or unable to stay still.
	Depression	
How often do you feel sad, depressed or blue? (How much of the time do you feel this way?)		25 Admits he is often sad or depressed. 26 Admits he feels depressed most of the time.
	Crying	
When was the last time you felt like crying?		27 Admits he felt like crying.
	Self-appraisal	
How do you feel about yourself? Do you like yourself?		28 Accuses himself of being unworthy, sinful or evil.
If unclear: (When you compare yourself with other people, how do you come out?) (Do you feel that you are a particularly important person or that you have certain special powers or abilities?)		29 Indicates he is bothered by feelings of inadequacy or that he doesn't like himself. 30 Indicates he is bothered by feelings of having done something terrible (guilt). 31 In appraising himself he indicates an inflated view of his value or worth (grandiosity).

developed to help minimize information variance by providing a standard way to gather clinical information. One of the earliest attempts to standardize the rules by which clinicians summarized their clinical observations into diagnoses (criterion variance) was the development of a computer program (DIAGNO I) (Spitzer and Endicott, 1968) which uses data collected with the PSS to arrive at one of 25 DSM-I (American Psychiatric Association, 1952) diagnoses. A computer program is potentially useful in that it will always arrive at the same diagnosis when given the same raw data describing a subject, and by eliminating this source of variance (criterion variance), achieves perfect reliability. Another advantage of computerderived diagnoses over those of clinicians is that computers can store and utilize a very large number of complex rules for arriving at diagnoses.

DIAGNO I was designed to use a logical decision tree approach rather than mathematically-based rules to arrive at diagnoses, on the assumption that this model would have the greatest flexibility and would not be tied to the base rates of a specific population (Fleiss et al., 1972). Thus the rules for making the diagnoses could be changed as diagnostic concepts changed.

When the validity of the DIAGNO I program was tested by comparing its diagnoses with those of pairs of clinicians who also used data from the PSS, the agreement between the computer and clinical diagnoses was as good as that between the diagnoses of the pairs of clinicians, although both were only fair. Although used in a study of cross-national differences in diagnostic practice (Cooper et al., 1972), the PSS and DIAGNO I have had limited value in diagnostic research, probably because the information gathered and used to make diagnoses is limited to the past week.

Current and Past Psychopathology Scales (CAPPS)

Despite the advance of minimizing criterion variance by standardizing the rules for diagnosis in the PSS/DIAGNO I program, it was recognized that accurate diagnosis often requires not only information about an entire current episode (often longer than a week), but also about past psychopathology and functioning. The Current and Past Psychopathology Scales (CAPPS) was developed in an effort to obtain a broader sampling of behavior, including historical data, for a number of purposes including diagnosis (Endicott and Spitzer, 1972). The coverage of the CAPPS includes items of importance in the evaluation of severity of illness and prognosis, dimensions of psychopathology and functioning, and diagnosis. Current status is evaluated for the one month prior to the interview, and the past section covers the period from age 12 up to the month prior to the interview. An interview guide ensures coverage of areas in which judgments are required, although the interviewer may ask supplementary questions for clarification when necessary. Most of the judgments are recorded on six-point scales of severity, ranging from "none" to "extreme." Summary scale scores of dimensions of current and past psychopathology and functioning are available. A sample of the CAPPS is presented in table 2.

TABLE 2
Part of the CAPPS.

Antisocial traits in childhood	
Determine presence, severity, and duration of antisocial traits. Did you get into many fights? Did you lie much? Did you ever steal things?. . .break windows?. . .set fires?. . .or anything like that? What about being cruel to animals?	315 Prior to age 12 he exhibited antisocial traits such as excessive aggression, destructiveness, firesetting, stealing, sadism, or chronic lying (consider number and intensity). ? 1 2 3 4 5 6
Adolescent friendship pattern	
Determine presence of special friends, amount of contact, who initiated contact, enjoyment in being with friends, and participation in group activities with probes. When you were in your teens, how much time did you spend with friends? What kinds of things did you do together? How popular were you? How many special or close friends did you usually have? Whose idea was it when you got together? Would you often get together with a group of friends? (Did you usually enjoy being with them?)	316 Adolescent Friendship Pattern (Ages 12-18) ?. 1. Superior. Spent a good deal of time with many special friends and groups of friends he enjoyed being with. He often initiated the interaction and was asked to join social activities by others. 2. Very good. 3. Good. 4. Fair. Had a few special friends but either avoided or did not enjoy group activities. 5. Poor. Had no special friends and preferred to be by himself most of the time or was actively avoided by peers. 6. Grossly inadequate. Had practically no social contact.

TABLE 2 (Continued)

	School
Determine highest completed school grade and academic performances at each level beginning with junior high school. (How far did you get in school?)	317 Highest completed school grade? 1. Professional (MA, MS, ME, BMs, MD, PhD, LLB) 2. Four years college graduate (BA, BS) 3. 1 to 3 years college or business school 4. High school graduate 5. 10 to 11 years of school (part high school) 6. 7 to 9 years of school 7. Under 7 years of school

Adequate interjudge reliability has been established using raters with a wide range of prior clinical experience. Concurrent validity in the discrimination of contrasting populations of subjects and contrasting diagnostic groups has also been demonstrated. A computer program, DIAGNO II (Spitzer and Endicott, 1969), was developed to use data from the CAPPS to make diagnoses according to DSM-II (American Psychiatric Association, 1968). This program also uses a logical decision tree approach. When compared with the diagnoses made by patients' therapists and those of two psychiatrists who examined CAPPS protocols, DIAGNO II diagnoses on the average agreed with the diagnoses of the clinicians as well as the clinicians agreed with each other.

The CAPPS and DIAGNO II have had more use than the PSS and DIAGNO I with subjects living in the community who were not identified as psychiatric patients. These studies have included subjects considered to be at risk for mental disorder, subjects who scored high on a screening questionnaire, medical patients and others (Auerbach and Marcus, 1978; Garrison, 1978; Holland and Plumb, 1978; Waldron, 1976; Wender et al., 1977).

The CAPPS and DIAGNO II are not considered appropriate for making lifetime diagnoses. The computer program focuses on the current symptoms and uses past symptoms only to establish the chronicity of the current condition. If a subject does not have symptoms at the time of the interview he or she will be diagnosed as "not ill" or, if only mild symptoms are present, given a "nonspecific" diagnosis. This may be the case even if the subject previously met criteria for a diagnosis for schizophrenia and currently has residual symptoms only.

The work in the area of computerized diagnosis continued with the development of DIAGNO III (Spitzer and Endicott, 1974). This computer program for diagnosis was designed to be used with psychiatric patients. Diagnoses were derived from systematic ratings made by the patient's primary therapist of detailed items about mental status and psychiatric anamnesis. This program became part of the Multistate Information System for Psychiatric Patients (Spitzer and Endicott, 1974; Spitzer et al., 1974) and is thought to have been an aid to the differential diagnosis of patients in hospitals participating in the MSIS system.

Dissatisfaction with computerized diagnosis and a desire to improve clinical diagnosis eventually led to a focus on the development of criteria to be used by clinicians rather than computers. (Some of the problems and constraints on the validity of computerized diagnosis are described in detail elsewhere [Spitzer et al., 1974].)

The Development of Diagnostic Criteria for Clinicians

Somewhat parallel to the development of standardized and computerized methods for making diagnoses was the development of specified clinical criteria for guiding diagnostic judgments. Research investigators have generally found standard diagnostic glossaries of little help in identifying relatively homogeneous groups of subjects for study because of the lack of specificity of guidelines for making the diagnoses. They therefore began to develop explicit criteria and classification schemes.

One of the first sets of specified criteria for the diagnosis of a number of major mental disorders was developed by a group of investigators at Washington University in St. Louis, and is often referred to as the "Feighner criteria," after the senior author of the article in which they were first reported (Feighner et al., 1972). These criteria contained specific inclusion and exclusion criteria for sixteen major psychiatric disorders.

Shortly after the Feighner criteria were published, Drs. Spitzer, Endicott, Eli Robins and colleagues developed a set of diagnostic criteria for a selected group of functional disorders, called the Research Diagnostic Criteria (RDC) (Spitzer et al., 1978). The RDC were developed as part of a collaborative project on the psychobiology of the depressive disorders sponsored by the Clinical Research Branch of the NIMH. The RDC is an expansion, elaboration and modification of the Feighner criteria and includes specified criteria for 25 major psychiatric conditions. In addition, many different nonmutually exclusive ways of subcategorizing some of the conditions, such as major depressive disorder and schizo-affective disorder, are included. The diagnostic categories included in the RDC are listed in table 3.

TABLE 3
Research Diagnostic Criteria Diagnoses.

Schizophrenia
Acute—chronic
Schizo-affective disorder—manic
Acute—chronic
Schizo-affective disorder—depressed
Acute—chronic
Depressive syndrome superimposed on residual schizophrenia
Manic disorder
Hypomanic disorder
Bipolar with mania (bipolar I)
Bipolar with hypomania (bipolar II)
Major depressive disorder
Primary
Secondary
Recurrent unipolar
Psychotic
Incapacitating
Minor depressive disorder with significant anxiety
Intermittent depressive disorder
Panic disorder
Generalized anxiety disorder with significant depression
Cyclothymic personality
Labile personality
Briquet's disorder (somatization disorder)
Antisocial personality
Alcoholism
Drug use disorder
Obsessive compulsive disorder
Phobic disorder
Unspecified functional psychosis
Other psychiatric disorder
Schizotypal features
Currently not mentally ill
Never mentally ill

Schedule for Affective Disorders and Schizophrenia

The Schedule for Affective Disorders and Schizophrenia (SADS) (Endicott and Spitzer, 1978) was developed in order to reduce information variance during clinical interviews used to gather data needed to make RDC diagnoses. The SADS is an interview schedule that interviewers use to ensure adequate coverage of critical areas of psychopathology and functioning. The organization of the interview and the item coverage is designed to elicit information necessary for making diagnoses using the RDC, as well as to describe the subjects' symptoms and levels of functioning.

There are three versions of the Schedule for Affective Disorders and Schizophrenia: the regular version (SADS), a lifetime version (SADS-L), and a very brief version for measuring change (SADS-C). The SADS-L is the version most useful for epidemiologic studies in which there is less of a need for an extremely detailed description of a subject's current condition because most subjects are not currently ill, and there is more of a focus on current and lifetime diagnosis, prognosis, and overall severity of illness. The SADS-L is similar to the past section of the regular SADS in that it covers psychiatric disturbances throughout the lifetime of the individual, but it also includes assessment of any current disturbance.

The organization of the SADS-L is similar to that of a clinical interview focused on differential diagnosis. The interview schedule provides a progression of questions and items that systematically rule in and rule out specific RDC diagnoses. To give the reader a sense of the coverage and format of the SADS-L table 4 represents a sample of the interview. The items usually refer to symptoms, duration or course of illness or severity of impairment. Each item is accompanied by questions suggested for use to elicit the specific information called for.

The most suitable personnel for administering the SADS-L and using the RDC are individuals with prior clinical experience in interviewing psychiatric patients and in making judgments about manifest psychopathology. Although questions are provided to assist in collecting the information and all of the items are defined to assure uniform criteria for all raters, the types of judgments called for require more knowledge of psychiatric concepts than is required for the PSS and CAPPS. For this reason, raters should generally be limited to psychiatrists, clinical psychologists, and psychiatric social workers. If other personnel are used, usually much more training is necessary.

An experienced and well-trained interviewer who is familiar with the SADS-L and RDC should usually be able to complete an evaluation of a subject in the community in 45 minutes to an hour, depending on the degree of any current psychiatric disturbance and the complexity of the subject's psychiatric history.

The reliability of the RDC categories, derived from SADS-L interviews of relatives of patients with Affective Disorders is presented in table 5. For virtually all of the categories the reliability is very high, and with only a few exceptions, higher than have generally been reported in other research studies. In those few instances in which the coefficients of reliability are low for major diagnostic categories, they are accounted for by disagreements on a small number of cases for diagnoses infrequently given by either rater.

The SADS-L has several advantages over the CAPPS. Firstly, diagnoses derived from CAPPS data were available only after the data were analyzed by the DIAGNO II computer program. The computer algorithms use complicated indices that cannot easily be translated into rules that are clinically understandable and useful. With the SADS-L/RDC system, diagnoses are made by the clinician after examination of the subject's responses to the various SADS-L items. Also, the logic of the decision-making process is not reflected in the organization of the CAPPS interview, as it is in the SADS-L. Furthermore, as previously mentioned, the data for the subject's current condition are limited to the past month in the CAPPS, rather than the entire lifetime of the subject, as with the SADS-L. In addition, of course, much more up-to-date diagnostic criteria are inquired about in the SADS-L interview and used to make RDC diagnoses, while the DIAGNO II program makes DSM-II diagnoses. Finally, since many of the diagnostic criteria contained in the RDC are very similar to those included in DSM-III, information gathered during a SADS-L interview is much more useful for making diagnoses according to DSM-III.

The SADS-L and RDC have been used as the diagnostic instruments in a wide variety of research projects. Most notably, the SADS-L was used to gather diagnostic and descriptive information by Weissman and colleagues in their recent community survey (Weissman & Myers, 1978). This is the first time that a structured interview schedule designed to elicit information necessary to make a diagnosis according to specified criteria was used in a community survey. This study has had a tremendous impact on epidemiologic work, and the current NIMH Epidemiological Catchment Area program relies on the NIMH Diagnostic Interview Schedule (DIS) (Robins et al., 1981) which was heavily influenced by the methodology used in the development of the SADS-L and RDC.

DSM-III

The American Psychiatric Association in 1952 developed its first Diagnostic and Statistical Manual of Mental Disorders (DSM-I). For the first time an official classification of mental disorders was accompanied by a glossary that contained descriptions of the various diagnostic categories. Although by current standards these descriptions are quite inadequate for research because of their lack of specificity, at the time they represented a significant advance. The second edition (DSM-II) was published in 1968, and differed only in relatively minor ways from its predecessor.

Work on the third edition, DSM-III (American Psychiatric Association, 1980), began in 1974, guided by the American Psychiatric Association's Task Force on Nomenclature and Statistics chaired by Dr. Spitzer. The Task Force decided to incorporate into DSM-III, diagnostic criteria for each of the specific mental disorders in order to increase the reliability with which the diagnoses could be made. This was judged of paramount importance since

TABLE 4
Part of the SADS-L.

Criteria for major depressive syndrome

There are 3 criteria listed consecutively so that failure to meet any 1 of them permits the rater to skip the entire section. However, with subjects who may minimize the disturbance in mood during a depressive episode, it may be advisable to explore all 3 criteria before making a final judgment on the first. An episode that meets the first 2 criteria, but not the third, may be recorded later in another section.

	Criterion	Code	Rating
I.	Has had 1 or more distinct periods lasting *at least 1 week* during which he was bothered depressive or irritable mood or had pervasive loss of interest or pleasure. *Did you ever have a period that lasted at least 1 week were bothered by feeling depressed, sad, blue, hopeless, down in the dumps, that you didn't care anymore, or didn't enjoy anything?* *What about feeling irritable or easily annoyed?*	0 1 2	No information or not sure or part of simple grief reaction No Yes
II.	Sought or was referred for help from someone during *dysphoric* period(s), took medication, or had impaired functioning socially, with family, at home, at work, or at school. *During that time did you seek help from anyone, like a doctor, or minister or even a friend, or did anyone suggest that you seek help? Did you take any medication? Did you act differently with people, your family, at work, or at school?*	0 1 2	No information No Yes

(Codes 0 or 1 on I or II:) Skip to Non-affective Non-organic Psychosis page 13.

TABLE 4 (Continued)

Criteria for major depressive syndrome			
III. Had at least 3 (if past episode) or 4 (if current episode) symptoms associated with the most severe period of depressed or irritable mood or pervasive loss of interest or pleasure. (Inquire all symptoms.)			
During the most severe period were you bothered by	No Info	No	Yes
..*poor appetite or weight loss, or increased appetite or weight gain?*	X	1	2
..*trouble sleeping or sleeping too much?*	X	1	2
..*loss of energy, easily fatigued, or feeling tired?*	X	1	2
..*loss of interest or pleasure in your usual activities or sex (may or may not be pervasive)?*	X	1	2
..*feeling guilty or down on yourself?*	X	1	2
..*trouble concentrating, thinking, or making decisions?*	X	1	2
..*thinking about death or suicide? (Did you attempt suicide?)*	X	1	2
..*being unable to sit still and have to keep moving or the opposite—feeling slowed down and have trouble moving?*	X	1	2

Number of definite symptoms______ . Criterion = 4 if current only; 3 if past.

TABLE 5
Reliability of Research Diagnostic Criteria Based On Use of the Lifetime Version of the Schedule for Affective Disorders and Schizophrenia with Relatives (N = 49).[a]

Diagnosis	*No. of subjects given diagnosis by interviewer*	*Kappa*
Manic disorder	3	0.79
Bipolar with mania	2	0.66
Hypomanic disorder	1	0.66
Major depressive disorder	7	0.85
Primary	6	0.76
Secondary	1	1.00
Recurrent	5	1.00
Psychotic	1	1.00
Incapacitating	2	0.79
Minor depressive disorder	6	0.90
Generalized anxiety disorder	3	0.85
Cyclothymic personality	2	1.00
Briquet's disorder	1	1.00
Phobic disorder	3	1.00
Other psychiatric disorder	4	0.46
Borderline features	1	1.00
Currently not mentally ill	40	0.62
Never mentally ill	28	0.87

[a]Spitzer et al., 1978

TABLE 6
Reliability of Routine Psychiatric Diagnosis Using DSM-11.[a]

Diagnostic category	*Reliability*
Mental deficiency Organic brain syndrome Alcoholism	Satisfactory (Kappa 0.71-0.77)
Psychosis Schizophrenia	Fair (Kappa 0.55-0.57)
Affective disorder Neurosis Personality disorder	Poor (Kappa 0.26-0.41)

[a]Spitzer & Fleiss, 1974

numerous studies with DSM-I and -II had shown those classifications to be generally quite unreliable (Spitzer and Fleiss, 1974). Table 6 summarizes the reliability obtained across several studies using DSM-II.

In initial drafts of DSM-III the RDC criteria, either unchanged or with slight modifications, were used for the corresponding categories in DSM-III, and diagnostic criteria were developed for the more than 150 DSM-III categories not included in the RDC. In successive drafts of DSM-III, many of the RDC criteria underwent further modification based on critiques by clinicians and researchers, and on experience with their use. For example, the RDC category of schizophrenia only requires a duration of illness of at least 2 weeks. After much controversy a decision was made not to have an acute subtype of schizophrenia in DSM-III; instead, schizophrenia is defined as requiring at least six months' duration of illness. Thus, the final DSM-III definition of schizophrenia differs considerably from the RDC. For other categories, such as panic disorder, the criteria are virtually the same in both systems.

Another major feature of DSM-III is the inclusion of a multiaxial system for evaluation. The basic principle of a multiaxial evaluation is that the clinician is expected to evaluate each subject according to each of several different areas of information, or axes. The DSM-III multiaxial system contains five axes, the first three of which are diagnostic. Axes I and II comprise the mental disorders, with Axis II reserved for personality disorders (generally in adults) and specific developmental disorders (generally in children). All of the other mental disorders are noted on Axis I. The Axis II conditions are assigned to a separate axis since they are frequently overlooked when attention is drawn to the usually more florid Axis I disorders. Axis III is used to record any physical disorder or condition that the clinician judges to be important in the management or treatment of the subject. Axis IV is used to rate the severity of psychosocial stressors that are judged significant to the initiation or exacerbation of the Axis I and II disorders. Axis V also provides a rating scale for rating the highest level of adaptive functioning that the subject was able to sustain for at least a few months during the past year. Presumably this has prognostic significance in that an individual who develops a mental disorder after maintaining a relatively high level of functioning is more likely to return to that level of functioning than an individual who has always functioned poorly.

During the development of DSM-III, drafts of the manual were used in a series of field trials by more than 500 clinicians from a wide variety of clinical settings. A major purpose of these field trials was to establish the reliability of the various DSM-III categories to determine if the use of diagnostic criteria and the multiaxial system would in fact result in improved reliability. This was done by having over 350 clinicians in pairs evaluate a total of 670 adult and 126 child and adolescent patients. The results of this study are presented in Tables 7 and 8. As can be seen, the reliability obtained using DSM-III is in most cases considerably above that obtained using DSM-I and -II.

Note that the reliabilities of the DSM-III are generally lower than those of the RDC categories. This is probably due to two main factors. The raters

TABLE 7
Kappa Coefficients of Agreement for Axes I and II DSM-III Diagnostic Classes for Adults (18 and Older).*

	Phase One (N = 339)		*% of Sample*	*Phase Two (N = 331)*		*% of Sample*
Axis I						
Disorders usually first evident in infancy, childhood or adolescence	.65		5.3	.73		3.6
Mental retardation		.80	1.8		.83	2.1
Attention deficit disorder					-.003	0.6
Conduct disorder					.003	0.6
Other disorders of infancy, childhood or adolescence		.66	1.2		.002	0.3
Eating disorders		.59	2.1			
Stereotyped movement disorders		-.001	0.3			
Other disorders with physical manifestations					1.00	0.6
Organic mental disorders	.79	11.8	.76			10.0
Dementias arising in the senium and presenium		.85	2.4		.91	1.8
Substance-induced		.63	7.4		.58	3.6
OBS of other or unknown etiology	.66	4.1			.65	5.4
Substance use disorders	.86		21.2	.80		21.2
Schizophrenic disorders	.81		17.7	.81		23.3

TABLE 7 (Continued)

	Phase One (N = 339)		% of Sample	Phase Two (N = 331)		% of Sample
Paranoid disorders	.66		1.2	.75		1.5
Psychotic disorders not elsewhere classified	.64		11.2	.69		6.7
Affective disorders	.69		43.1	.83		38.7
Major affective disorders		.68	28.9		.80	26.9
Other specific affective disorders		.49	18.3		.69	12.4
Atypical affective disorders		.29	3.2		.49	3.6
Anxiety disorders	.63		9.1	.72		8.8
Somatoform disorders	.54		3.8	.42		3.3
Dissociative disorders	.80		0.9	-.003		0.6
Psychosexual disorders	.92		2.1	.75		1.5
Gender identity disorders		-.001	0.3		-.002	0.3
Paraphilias		1.0	0.6			
Psychosexual dysfunctions		1.0	1.5		.86	1.2
Factitious disorders	.66		1.2	-.005		0.9
Disorders of impulse control not elsewhere classified	.28		1.8	.80		1.8
Adjustment disorder	.67		12.1	.68		8.5

TABLE 7 (Continued)

	Phase One (N = 339)	*% of Sample*	*Phase Two (N = 331)*	*% of Sample*
Psychological factors affecting physical condition	.62	3.2	.44	2.1
V codes	.56	3.0	.66	3.0
Additional codes	−.003	0.6	.28	1.8
Overall kappa for Axis I	.68		.72	
Axis II				
Specific developmental disorders			.40	1.2
Personality disorders	.56	59.9	.65	49.8
Overall kappa for Axis II	.56		.64	

*Taken from Appendix F of DSM-III: DSM-III Field Trials: Interrater Reliability and List of Project Staff and Participants

TABLE 8
Kappa Coefficients of Agreement for Axes I and II DSM-III Diagnostic Classes for Children and Adolescents (Under 18).*

	Phase One (N = 71)	*% of Sample*	*Phase Two (N = 55)*	*% of Sample*
Axis I				
Disorders usually first evident in infancy, childhood or adolescence	.69	54.9	.63	67.3
Mental retardation	1.0	8.5	1.0	3.6
Attention deficit disorder	.58	15.5	.50	14.6
Conduct disorder	.61	26.8	.61	38.2
Anxiety disorders of childhood or adolescence	.25	8.5	.44	16.4
Other disorders of infancy, childhood or adolescence	.79	8.5	.73	9.1
Eating disorders	.66	2.8	1.0	3.6
Stereotyped movement disorders	1.0	1.4		
Other disorders with physical manifestations			.48	5.5
Pervasive developmental disorders	.85	5.6	-.01	1.8
Organic mental disorders			.66	3.6
Substance-induced			-.01	1.8
OBS of other or unknown etiology			1.0	1.8

TABLE 8 (Continued)

	Phase One (N = 71)		*% of Sample*	*Phase Two (N = 55)*		*% of Sample*
Substance use disorders	1.0		5.6	.54		9.1
Schizophrenic disorders	1.0		5.6	.66		3.6
Psychotic disorders not elsewhere classified	.85		5.6			
Affective disorders	.53		16.9	.30		9.1
Major affective disorders		.36	11.3		-.02	3.6
Other specific affective disorders		.38	5.6		-.02	3.6
Atypical affective disorders		-.01	2.8		1.0	1.8
Anxiety disorders	1.0		2.8	1.0		1.8
Somatoform disorders	1.0		1.4	-.009		1.8
Psychosexual disorders	1.0		1.4			
Paraphilias		1.0	1.4			
Disorders of impulse control not elsewhere classified	.66		2.8			
Adjustment disorder	.66		31.0	.36		32.7
Psychological factors affecting physical condition	-.01		1.4	-.02		3.6
V codes	-.02		4.2	.54		9.1

TABLE 8 (Continued)

	Phase One (N = 71)		*% of Sample*	*Phase Two (N = 55)*		*% of Sample*
Additional codes	1.0		1.4	-.03		5.5
Overall kappa for Axis I	.68			.52		
Axis II						
Specific developmental disorders		.77	22.5		.51	29.1
Personality Disorders	.56		26.8	.61		18.2
Overall kappa for Axis II	.66			.55		

*Taken from Appendix F of DSM-III: DSM-III Field Trials: Interrater Reliability and List of Project Staff and Participants in the RDC reliability study were specially trained and were using a standardized interview schedule to obtain the information. In contrast, in the DSM-III field trials, the clinicians participating had no special training in use of the criteria, and did not have the advantage of a standardized interview.

It is expected that the DSM-III criteria will be widely adopted in epidemiologic research since for the first time they provide explicit criteria for diagnosing mental disorders that are generally accepted by clinicians and researchers alike. Evidence of this is the recent incorporation into the DIS of the DSM-III criteria for those categories thought to be most important for community surveys.

References

American Psychiatric Association, (1952), *Diagnostic and Statistical Manual of Mental Disorders,* first ed., Washington, D.C.: American Psychiatric Association.

American Psychiatric Association, (1968), *Diagnostic and Statistical Manual of Mental Disorders,* second ed., Washington, D.C.: American Psychiatric Association.

American Psychiatric Association, (1980), *Diagnostic and Statistical Manual of Mental Disorders,* third ed., Washington, D.C.: American Psychiatric Association.

Auerbach, J. & Marcus, J. (1978), *Neonatal and Environmental Factors in Serious Mental Disorder,* final research report to the U.S. Israel Binational Science Foundation. Unpublished manuscript.

Beitchman, J. H., Dielman, T. E., Landis, J. R. , Benson, R. M. & Kemp, P. L. (1978), Reliability of group for advancement of psychiatry diagnostic categories in child psychiatry. *Arch Gen Psychiatr* 35:1461-1466.

Cooper, J. E., Kendell, R. E., Gurland, B. J. , Sharpe, L., Copeland, J. R. M. & Simon, R. (1972), *Psychiatric Diagnosis in New York and London.* London: Oxford University Press.

Dohrenwend, B. P., Yager, T. J., Egri, G. & Mendelsohn, F. S. (1978), The Psychiatric Status Schedule as a measure of dimensions of psychopathology in the general population. *Arch Gen Psychiatr* 35:731-737.

Endicott, J. & Spitzer, R. L. (1972), Current and Past Psychopathology Scales (CAPPS): Rationale, reliability, and validity. *Arch Gen Psychiatr* 27:678-687.

Endicott, J. & Spitzer, R. L. (1978), A diagnostic interview: The Schedule for Affective Disorders and Schizophrenia. *Arch Gen Psychiatr* 35:837-844.

Feighner, J. P., Robins, E., Guze, S. B., Woodruff, R. A., Winokur, G. & Munoz, R. (1972), Diagnostic Criteria for use in psychiatric research. *Arch Gen Psychiatr* 38:57-63.

Fleiss, J. L., Spitzer, R. L., Endicott, J. & Cohen, J. (1972), Quantification of agreement in multiple psychiatric diagnosis. *Arch Gen Psychiatr* 26:168-171.

Garrison, V. (1978), Support systems of schizophrenic and nonschizophrenic Puerto Rican migrant women in New York City. *Schiz Bull* 4:561-596.
Herz, M. I., Endicott, J., Spitzer, R. L. & Mesnikoff, A. (1971), Day versus inpatient hospitalization: A controlled study. *Am J Psychiatr* 132:413-418.
Herz, M. I., Endicott, J. & Spitzer, R. L. (1975), Brief hospitalization of patients with families: Initial Results. *Am J Psychiatr* 132:413-418.
Holland, J. & Plumb, M. (1978), Current and past psychologic adjustment. *Am Soc Clin Oncol* 19:14-28.
Piper, W. E., Debbane, E. G. & Garant, J. (1977), An outcome study of group therapy. *Arch Gen Psychiatr* 34:1027-1032.
Robins, L. N., Helzer, J. E., Croughan, J. & Ratcliff, K. S. (1981) National Institute of Mental Health Diagnostic Interview Schedule. Its history, characteristics, and validity. *Arch Gen Psychiatr* 38:381-389.
Silberfarb, P. M., Maurer, L. H. & Crouthamel, C. S. (1980), Psychosocial aspects of neoplastic disease: I. Functional status of breast cancer patients during different treatment regimens. *Am J Psychiatr* 137:450-455.
Spitzer, R. L., Cohen, G., Miller, J. D. & Endicott, J. (1969), The psychiatric status of 100 men on skid row. *Intl J Soc Psychiatr* 15:230-234.
Spitzer, R. L. & Endicott, J. (1968), DIAGNO: A computer program for psychiatric diagnosis utilizing the differential diagnostic procedure. *Arch Gen Psychiatr* 18:746-756.
Spitzer, R. L. & Endicott, J. (1969), DIAGNO II: Further developments in a computer program for psychiatric diagnosis. *Am J Psychiatr* 1125:12-21 (Jan. Suppl.).
Spitzer, R. L. & Endicott, J. (1974), Can the computer assist clinicians in psychiatric diagnosis? *Am J Psychiatr* 131:523-530.
Spitzer, R. L. & Endicott, J. (1974), Computer diagnosis in automated record-keeping systems: A study of clinical acceptability. In: *Progress in Mental Health Information Systems: Computer Applications*, ed. J. Crawford, D. Morgan & D. Gianturco. Cambridge: Ballinger Publishing Company pp. 73-105.
Spitzer, R. L., Endicott, J. & Robins, E. (1978), Research diagnostic criteria: Rationale and reliability. *Arch Gen Psychiatr* 35:773-782.
Spitzer, R. L., Endicott, J., Cohen, J. & Fleiss, J. L. (1974), Constraints on the validity of computer diagnosis. *Arch Gen Psychiatr* 31:197-203.
Spitzer, R. L., Endicott, J., Fleiss, J. L. & Cohen, J. (1970), The Psychiatric Status Schedule: A technique for evaluating psychopathology and impairment in role functioning. *Arch Gen Psychiatr* 23:41-55.
Spitzer, R. L. & Fleiss, J. L. (1974), A re-analysis of the reliability of psychiatric diagnosis. *Br J Psychiatr* 125:341-347.
Spitzer, R. L. & Williams, J. B. W. (1980), Classification of mental disorders and DSM-III. In: *Comprehensive Textbook of Psychiatry*, third ed., vol. 1, ed. H. Kaplan, A. Freedman, & B. Sadock. Baltimore: Williams & Wilkins pp. 1035-1072.
Waldron, S. (1976), Significance of childhood neurosis for adult mental health. *Am J Psychiatr* 133:532-538.
Washburn, S., Vannicelli, M., Longabaugh, R. & Scheff, B. (1976), A controlled comparison of psychiatric day treatment and inpatient hospitalization. *J Consult Clin Psychol* 44:665-675.

Weissman, M. M. & Myers, J. K. (1978), Affective disorders in a U.S. urban community. The use of research diagnostic criteria in an epidemiological survey. *Arch Gen Psychiatr* 35:1304-1311.
Wender, P., Rosenthal, D., Rainer, J., Greenhill, L. & Sarlin, B. (1977), Schizophrenics' adopting parents: Psychiatric status. *Arch Gen Psychiatr* 34:777-784.

Chapter 18

The Development and Characteristics of the NIMH Diagnostic Interview Schedule

LEE N. ROBINS

In 1967, Rema Lapouse roundly criticized the current state of psychiatric epidemiology. Her criticisms were directed at the Stirling County (Leighton et al., 1963) and Midtown Manhattan (Srole et al., 1962) studies, which were the first large-scale surveys of mental health in the western hemisphere. The criticisms of Lapouse must be still reckoned with when we plan studies that hope to understand the distribution and cause of psychiatric disorder through surveys of the general population.

One of Lapouse's criticisms concerned the use of prevalence rather than incidence data in the search for causes. She said:

> Prevalence rates measure the size of the disease problem and as such are useful in planning services. They are, however, a fallible indicator of the risk of acquiring any chronic disease including psychiatric disorder. Since prevalence is a function of incidence and duration, any factors affecting duration of disease will similarly influence its prevalence rate. . . . [These factors] may in turn be associated with demographic factors. Consequently, an association between these factors and prevalence may occur even though demographic factors bear no relationship to the genesis of the disease. The only suitable measure applicable to the search for possible causes of disease is the incidence rate.

This criticism was in response to the Midtown Manhattan study's cross-sectional assessment of the current prevalence of each symptom, with no provision for a follow-up to assess the rate at which new symptoms emerge.

Lapouse also criticized the methods by which evaluations of mental health or illness were made. Psychiatrists assigned each subject to a "caseness" category on the basis of a global impression after reviewing summaries of answers to interviews, administered in the Midtown Manhattan study by social workers and psychologists. Lapouse said:

> Bias is a serious hazard when respondents are questioned by psychiatrically sophisticated interviewers with a preconception of psychopathology. The risk is increased when these interviewers are permitted to probe the respondents' answers at will, and is further heightened when the probes, impressions, and summaries of the interviewers serve as the basis upon which the psychiatrist classifies the respondent as well or ill.

She complained about the absence of uniformity in data collection resulting from the psychiatrists' being given information from treatment records and opinions of key informants when available, since these sources were not routinely available for all subjects. The freedom of interviewers to decide when and how much to probe further increased the unevenness of the quantity of information collected for different subjects:

> There can be no doubt that different kinds and amounts of information are produced by interviews of varying length and by the use of variable materials from variable sources. . . . [T]he lack of uniform data collection renders the rates unreliable.

Lapouse cited the failure of these studies to distinguish ordinary human discomfort from psychiatric symptoms:

> There may well exist in any community a high level of signs and symptoms which reflect physical and emotional discomfort and are associated with a greater or lesser degree of impairment in efficiency of living. If this is true, does it signify a high level of psychiatric disorder? This question poses the fundamental issue of what is a case.

Interviews in both studies contained questions about feelings that are shared from time to time by a majority of the normal population. Interviewers could count these feelings as symptoms without determining whether the frequency or severity of these feelings removed them from the level of ordinary experience to the level of symptoms. Nor was there any provision for distinguishing symptoms due to psychiatric disorders from those due to physical illness.

Lapouse was particularly concerned about the inclusion of the so-called psychosomatic disorders as psychiatric disease:

> D. C. Leighton also points out that the presence of many psychophysiologic complaints may have influenced the evaluators to regard. . . person(s) as psychoneurotic even in the absence of marked psychoneurotic symptoms. . . . Although theoretical grounds are often advanced for including the so-called diseases of adaptation within the spectrum of psychiatric disorder, there is little if any firm evidence as yet available from well-controlled experimental, clinical or epidemiologic studies to substantiate the hypothesis that stress or any other psychogenic agency is the sole or primary cause of these diseases.

Finally, there was the issue of an absence of specific diagnoses. Both studies made only a determination of "caseness" rather than using the traditional psychiatric nomenclature. Srole argued that psychiatric diagnosis was so unreliable that it could not be used in the Midtown Manhattan Study, and Dr. Lapouse seemed to agree that psychiatric diagnosis was in such a sad state that ascertaining the prevalence and incidence of specific psychiatric disorders was a futile exercise:

> Psychiatric diagnosis. . .rests on a highly nonobjective method, the clinical judgment of the psychiatrist. . . .Absence of uniform classification and diagnostic criteria reduces the utility of diagnosis as an indicator of the prevalence of mental disease.

This indictment of the state of psychiatric epidemiology as practiced in the 1950s and 1960s has challenged researchers to solve problems both of study design and diagnostic instruments. Had Rema Lapouse lived to see how far the series of studies planned and supported by the NIMH under the title "The NIMH Epidemiological Catchment Area Project" has come in answering these criticisms, she would have been pleased. The study design for this project was constructed by the Division of Biometry and Epidemiology, and is reported in some detail in another chapter (Eaton et al., 1983). Principal contributors to that design were Ben Locke, Carl Taube, Darrel Regier, Irving Goldberg, John Bartko, Karen Pettigrew, William Eaton, and Martha Munson-Little. The design allows obtaining incidence as well as prevalence data because it provides for reassessment after one year. It applies consistent methods and levels of data collection to large samples of both household and institutional populations in five geographical areas of the United States.

The instrument used to assess the mental health of respondents, the NIMH Diagnostic Interview Schedule (Robins et al., 1979) was specially developed for this project. It overcomes many of the deficiencies of earlier instruments pointed out by Rema Lapouse. It provides approximately equivalent amounts of data for each subject because it specifies the degree of probing and content of the probes. Evaluation is based on interview alone, without the addition of information from hospital records or informants for respondents capable of responding to it. The interview attempts to distinguish psychiatric symptoms both from everyday worries and from symptoms of physical illness and from side effects of alcohol, medication, or other drugs. It applies uniform diagnostic criteria of standard classification systems so as to obtain reliable specific diagnoses, and these systems do *not* include the psychosomatic illnesses. Because questions and probes are spelled out, the interview can be administered by both lay interviewers and clinicians, and even when given by clinicians, the clear specifications of questions, probes, and rules under which questions should be asked or omitted allow little scope for bias due to interviewer's preconceptions. Furthermore, the application of computer algorithms for diagnosis directly to answers to specific symptom questions eliminates the "global impression" of the clinician and thus greatly reduces the risks of biased evaluation.

This paper recounts the history of the development of this instrument and attempts to show how it fits into the development of thinking about diagnosis and its ascertainment.

Two Psychiatric Survey Traditions

The NIMH Diagnostic Interview Schedule (DIS) draws on two separate interview traditions. One is a tradition of surveys using interviews developed from paper and pencil tests, particularly the Minnesota Multiphasic Personality Inventory and its offspring, the Army Neuropsychiatric Screening Adjunct and the Cornell Medical Index. The second tradition attempts to formalize the clinical interview given by psychiatrists. Both traditions produced interviews known by their acronyms.

The interviews that grew out of paper-and-pencil tests were designed for use on large samples. Interviews based on these tests include the Home Interview Survey (HIS) used in the Midtown Manhattan study, initiated by Thomas Rennie and published by Leo Srole et al. (1962), and the Health Opinion Survey (HOS), first used in the Stirling County Study in Nova Scotia, Leighton et al. (1963). These interviews counted the "mentally disordered," but did not provide specific diagnoses. Later developments in this tradition were the two interviews written by Dohrenwend, the Structured Interview Schedule (SIS), and the Psychiatric Epidemiological Research Interview (PERI), which provide neither a count of the mentally ill *nor* diagnoses, but instead give scores on symptom scales (Dohrenwend & Shrout, 1978).

The second tradition is one of increasingly formalized clinical interviews. This tradition began with epidemiologic studies carried out by German and Scandinavian psychiatrists. These studies were carried out either by a single psychiatrist or by a group of psychiatrists working closely together in a small community well known to them personally. Studies by Klemperer (1933), Stromgren (1950), Fremming (1951), Helgason (1964), and Essen-Moller (1956), who then turned his research over to Hagnell (1966), are of this type. The psychiatrist himself either interviewed key informants (Helgason) or tried to interview every community member in order to judge who were psychiatrically disordered and what their diagnoses might be. Questions were not spelled out ahead of time. Instead, Hagnell, for instance, carried with him a single card of mnemonic notations to remind him of the topics to be covered. The psychiatrist spoke with relatives and the local doctor instead of, or as well as, the subject and collected records from the police, social agencies, temperance boards, and hospitals. The psychiatrist-investigator had often himself been the responsible physician for those most seriously affected. He thus had greatly varying levels of information about different subjects—from reports by a relative or doctor to an extensive history based on having himself cared for the subject over a period of years.

Information from these various sources was pooled to reach a diagnostic decision, but the rules for combining information to make diagnoses were not spelled out. Problems with reliability were minimal, since typically one clinician-interviewer made all the judgments. Whatever criteria he used presumably remained reasonably constant throughout. The problems were instead consistency with criteria used by other psychiatrists and comparability across studies (Dohrenwend & Dohrenwend, 1969). One solution was to submit the sum of collected data to psychiatrists who did not know the subject or his family for a consensus diagnosis (Helgason, 1964).

To increase comparability across studies, more standardized instruments were developed, also known by their acronyms. These included the Present State Examination (PSE) devised by John Wing and others (1974) and the Psychiatric Status Schedule (PSS) devised by Robert Spitzer and Jean Endicott (Spitzer et al., 1970).

The development of instruments in both traditions were responses to a concern that psychiatrists were notoriously unreliable and idiosyncratic diagnosticians. The authors of the HIS, HOS, and PERI were so pessimistic about diagnostic reliability that no attempt was made to diagnose at all. The PSS and PSE had their own pessimism. They assumed recall was so poor that information about events and feelings prior to a month earlier was unreliable. They asked only about current symptoms, and thus diagnoses that required a history could not be made. These instruments achieved reliability by careful training of interviewers, by providing suggested questions that served to guide the psychiatrist's inquiry, and by computerizing the combination of symptoms into syndromes.

While interview schedules that grew out of paper-and-pencil tests were designed for epidemiological studies in large samples from the general population, interview schedules that grew out of the surveys done by individual psychiatrists were initially used primarily for diagnosing current psychiatric patients. The PSS and PSE were developed for the US-UK study of diagnosis in two mental hospitals, one in Brooklyn and one in London. It was known that schizophrenia was a common diagnosis in the United States and rare in the United Kingdom, while a diagnosis of depression was much more common in the United Kingdom than in the United States. The purpose of the study was to learn whether British patients differed sufficiently from American patients to explain these very different prevalence figures, or whether the difference in prevalence merely reflected a difference in the diagnostic styles of psychiatrists in the two countries. Because these interviews required the psychiatrists to record the presence or absence of individual symptoms, as well as make a global diagnosis, they made it possible to discover whether patients' *symptoms* differed in the two locales or only the relative *weights* given the same symptoms by physicians from different diagnostic traditions. The answer was that it was indeed a difference in diagnostic style, not in symptoms, that explained the different prevalences (Gurland et al., 1972).

The PSE was used again in the International Pilot Study of Schizophrenia (WHO, 1973). For this study, psychiatrists in nine different countries were trained to make comparable diagnoses using the PSE. Since both the US-UK study and the International Pilot Study of Schizophrenia concerned the diagnosis of severely ill psychiatric patients, the PSE is most detailed with respect to schizophrenia and the affective disorders. Currently, the PSE has been used to some extent in general populations, when given by carefully trained lay interviewers (Wing, 1977). While these interviews, like the RDI,

HIS, HOS, and the PERI, include specific questions, they differ in that the questions are often open-ended or cover only some aspects of the item to be scored from the answers, with no rules specified for moving from responses to the question to scoring the symptom item to which it refers. As Spitzer (1968) put it, "The interviewer uses the interview schedule to elicit information needed to judge the items of the inventory." The need for such judgment means that interviewers must be clinically trained. Furthermore, it is recommended that clinicians substitute for and add to these questions as they see fit, and that they seek external sources of information as well as information from the respondent himself.

Both these traditions originally required psychiatric manpower. The PSE and PSS used psychiatrists as interviewers. The HIS and HOS relied on psychiatrists to judge whether or not a person was a "case" after reviewing a summary of the interview. More recently, lay interviewers have been trained to give the PSE, and the psychiatrist's global judgment in the HIS has been replaced by a computer program designed to approximate from symptom scores the judgments the psychiatrists would have made (Srole, 1975).

The Renard Diagnostic Tradition

In addition to these two traditions, a third line of development of psychiatric interviews took place, first in Boston and then at Washington University in St. Louis and at the New York Psychiatric Institute. This tradition began with case-control studies of anxiety neurosis (Wheeler at al., 1950) and hysteria (Cohen et al., 1953). Interviews were designed to provide a better understanding of specific diagnosis entities, covering symptoms over the patient's whole lifetime. They began with an open-ended inquiry about the chief complaint, followed by a list of symptoms thought to characterize the disorder which the psychiatrist had to affirm as positive (ever present) or negative (always absent), inventing questions for this purpose when sufficient information had not been volunteered during the initial open-ended questioning. In addition, the psychiatrist scored a set of observations as positive or negative, based on his judgment of the quality and manner of the patient's presentation of the psychiatric history. These observations tested the view that hysterics were seductive, dramatic, and vague in their presentation of symptoms. Since the whole lifetime was covered, the interview provided lifetime prevalence, which is logically equivalent to lifetime incidence. However, this use of "prevalence" and "incidence" differs from traditional epidemiologic usage, where both are defined by a fixed unit of calendar time, not by variable ages. Although these interviews were not designed for epidemiological surveys, the study of hysteria (E. Robins et al., 1952) not only described the disorder in women, but noted its near absence in men, an epidemiologic result that has stood the test of many replications.

When Eli Robins joined the Washington University faculty in 1951, his first clinical research was a followup of patients diagnosed "hysteric" in childhood (Robins & O'Neal, 1953). Because he wanted to learn not only whether these child patients were hysterics as adults but *which* disorders they developed, he expanded the symptom lists from the Boston hysteria and anxiety neurosis studies to include symptoms of psychopathic personality, schizophrenia, and the manic depressive psychoses. He also grouped symptoms of each diagnosis by content, and required that a minimum number of these groups be represented among the positive symptoms. While diagnosis remained a global judgment made by a psychiatrist, the psychiatrist's freedom to select a diagnosis was now restricted by these rules. An undiagnosed category was also provided for persons who had symptoms but whose symptoms fit none of the diagnoses provided.

In Robins' next study, of suicide attempters (Robins et al., 1957), symptoms of alcoholism, drug dependence, homosexuality, dementia, psychoneurotic depressive reaction, mental retardation, and obsessive compulsive neurosis were added, completing the standard list of symptoms that was to appear in departmental studies from then on. He also added the first hierarchical rules for preemptive diagnoses: psychoneurotic depression should yield to *any* preexisting illness, and alcoholism should give way to psychopathy and manic depressive disorder. These rules further limited the psychiatrist's freedom to follow his global impressions.

Shortly after the suicide attempt study began, Drs. Patricia O'Neal and Lee Robins began a 30-year follow-up of child guidance clinic patients (Robins, 1966), using this set of symptoms and diagnostic rules. At first psychiatrists gave the diagnostic section of the interview, while lay interviewers gave the remainder. As subjects who had moved to other cities were located, however, a single lay interviewer was used, both to reduce travel costs and because psychiatrists were unavailable for extensive travel. The lay interviewer was trained by a psychiatrist, and the psychiatrist reviewed each interview with the lay interviewer shortly after its completion. Following this review, the psychiatrist made a single diagnosis, based on his global impression subject to the constraints mentioned above. When it was found that lay interviewers could provide adequate data for diagnosis (Robins & Braroe, 1964), they were allowed to give the psychiatric section to local subjects as well, to avoid losing cases by refusal between the lay interviewer's and psychiatrist's interviews.

In Eli Robins' next study, on completed suicides (Robins et al., 1959), medical students were included among the interviewers, following the pattern of training, review, and psychiatrist's diagnosis used in the Child Guidance Clinic study. In this study, the criteria for symptom severity that had been used in earlier studies were first made explicit: to be counted as positive a symptom had to result in seeking medical advice, taking medication, or limiting occupational or social functioning, unless the symptom was specifically designated as so clinically significant (e.g., a suicide attempt) that no such severity criteria need be applied. With this addition, the form and content of what came to be called "The Department Interview" was set.

In the next 20 years, that interview or a close approximation to it was used by many members of the Department in cross-sectional and longitudinal studies of remarkably varied populations: professional women, felons, members of homophile organizations, psychiatric clinic patients, psychiatric inpatients, referrals for psychiatric consultation from medical and surgical services, medically ill subjects, drug addicts, the recently divorced, vomiters, pain patients, and many subjects unselected for medical or psychiatric disturbance or behavior problems who were studied either in their own right, as relatives of patients, or as control subjects for the groups mentioned above. Toward the end of that period, in a study of emergency room patients (Robins et al., 1977), patients were first allowed multiple diagnoses, as long as the preemptive rules were followed.

This Department Interview was never formally published, although parts of it were reproduced in the many papers written from these studies. Indeed it was not truly a single interview: in each new study, diagnoses covered were selected to fit that study's needs.

In each of these studies, diagnostic decisions were made by the consensus of two or more psychiatrists who had independently reviewed the total list of symptoms scored as present and met to resolve disagreements. Although the Washington University psychiatrists prided themselves on basing their diagnostic decisions on a set of well-defined, specific criteria, it was not until 1972 that the criteria used to make these diagnoses were published as what have come to be called the Feighner criteria (Feighner et al., 1972). Feighner was the chief resident who persuaded his professors to meet weekly to write a paper describing the Departmental criteria. He thus first earned his place in the psychiatric literature by successfully nagging the Department to publish an article that has since become a landmark in psychiatric nosology (Blashfield, 1982).

The Development of the RDC and SADS

At the time the Feighner criteria were being published, NIMH began planning a collaborative study of the psychobiology of depression. Eli Robins, Robert Spitzer, and Jean Endicott were members of the committee responsible for defining criteria for selecting study cases with depressive disorders. Together they elaborated and modified the Feighner criteria to form the Research Diagnostic Criteria (RDC) (Spitzer et al., 1978). Their modifications consisted primarily of subdividing the diagnoses of depression and schizophrenia, reflecting a central interest of the collaborative study in deciding whether depression was one or many disorders. Spitzer and Endicott (1977a) then wrote an interview, the Schedule for Affective Disorder and Schizophrenia (SADS) to be used to collect the information necessary to score the RDC.

Because the SADS was designed to be used to select inpatients for the Collaborative Study of Depression, questions about depression, mania, and schizophrenia concentrate on current or recent symptoms, while questions about other diagnoses are asked on a lifetime basis in Part II. Part II was later published separately as the SADS-L, or SADS Lifetime (Spitzer & Endicott, 1977b). A modified version of the SADS-L has been used in a general population study in New Haven (Weissman & Myers, 1978) and in a study of a general practice population (Hoeper et al., 1979).

Like the PSE and the PSS, the SADS and SADS-L were designed to be given by psychiatrists. However, problems recruiting enough psychiatric manpower led to intensive training of a few nonpsychiatrist interviewers for 2 to 3 months, after which they were able to score the RDC reliably, and equivalently to a psychiatrist.

The Development of the Renard Diagnostic Interview

At the time the SADS was being developed, but quite independently of it, a multidisciplinary group at Washington University—including psychiatrists, a sociologist, a psychologist and a mathematician—were devising brief diagnostic modules that produced results similar to asking the corresponding full sets of criterion items from the Department Interview. The goal was a brief, accurate diagnostic interview that covered all the diagnoses in the Departmental Interview and that could be administered by lay interviewers.

To choose symptoms for the screening interview, the investigators used protocols collected during a study of 500 consecutive psychiatric outpatients given the Department Interview (Woodruff et al., 1969, 1972). The first diagnosis tackled was hysteria, because it had the largest number of criteria. From the 60 hysteria items, 14 were selected by computer and combined into a decision tree able to discriminate every patient in The Clinic 500 Study with the diagnosis of hysteria from those without it. Most patients were allocated as meriting or not meriting the diagnosis after ascertaining the presence of only four or five symptoms. After questions to represent each of the 14 selected symptoms were constructed, this diagnosis-specific screening interview was applied to new samples, and its results compared with interviews using all 60 items from the Department Interview. When results for hysteria were excellent (Woodruff et al., 1973), a screening interview for alcoholism was constructed in the same way (Reich et al., 1975). That worked well too. The next diagnosis attempted was antisocial personality. Here problems arose. Because the traditional Department Interview had not included some of the Feighner criteria for antisocial personality, the data set provided no basis on which to select among Feighner antisocial symptoms. It was also noted that two steps were being taken at once: to select a minimum set of symptoms and to convert the selected symptoms into fully specified questions. As a result, if diagnoses made by the screening interview failed to agree with diagnoses based on the Department Interview, it was not clear whether the wrong items had been selected or whether questions designed for the right items had been poorly worded.

To solve both problems, it was decided to first create a complete diagnostic instrument in question form that contained all the Feighner criterion symptoms and show that it was equivalent to the Department Interview. Then questions could be selected from it for a short interview, with the knowledge that the selected questions effectively elicited the intended symptoms. This interview was named the Renard Diagnostic Interview (RDI). It covers all the Feighner criterion symptoms, except for the diagnosis of mental retardation, in fully specified questions, and provides specified probes to ascertain whether severity criteria are met. Its equivalence to the Department

Interview was tested in 120 inpatients by comparing its results when given to an unselected sample of patients with results of the traditional Department Interview format given to the same patients by psychiatrists who improvised questions and probes to cover Feighner symptoms. Its reliability was tested by comparing its results when given to the same patients by two psychiatrists, two lay interviewers, or a psychiatrist and lay interviewer combination (Helzer et al., 1981). Results were highly satisfactory. Furthermore, the RDI was found to be teachable to lay interviewers in a short time and acceptable to psychiatrists, who began using it for evaluating consultation cases. However, the next step, using the RDI as the parent interview from which we could then select questions of proven effectiveness for our screening interview, did not take place because DSM-III appeared on the scene, making the Feighner criteria obsolete.

The History of DSM-III

In 1974, while creating the RDC, Dr. Spitzer became head of the Task Force to develop the third edition of the Diagnostic and Statistical Manual (DSM-III) of the American Psychiatric Association (1980). His work with the Research Diagnostic Criteria inspired him to try to give DSM-III the same kind of rigor that the RDC provided, so diagnoses would be comparable across centers and, as much as possible, based on research results rather than clinical impressions. The APA Task Force included some psychiatrists and psychologists who were unfamiliar with or unsympathetic with the view that criteria should be operationalized and it sought the views or received the opinions of many clinicians with widely differing experiences and views. DSM-III reflects this diverse input, but it still shows its debt to its Feighner criteria heritage. Table 1 compares the DSM-III diagnostic criteria for panic disorder with Feighner criteria for anxiety neurosis. Although there are some differences, the overall resemblance is striking.

In addition to showing the resemblance between DSM-III and the Feighner criteria, Table 1 illustrates the elements of the diagnostic process, and consequently the tasks a diagnostic interview must accomplish. It must not only determine whether a given symptom has occurred, but also whether it has occurred with sufficient regularity to be significant and whether it has occurred outside of circumstances under which it would be a normal response (in this case physical exertion or an objectively frightening situation). Measures of severity must be included to be certain the symptoms are clinically significant. If a symptom is sufficiently severe, the interview must ascertain whether it has occurred in the absence of physical illness that might explain it. Furthermore, the interview must determine whether a sufficient number of the characteristic symptoms occurred both *together* and *transiently*, so that they could be said to constitute a discrete episode or "attack." Persons meeting all these criteria can be said to have experienced panic attacks, but they do not necessarily suffer from panic disorder. The final task of the interview is to rule out other psychiatric disorders in which panic attacks also occur. To summarize, the interview must determine the

TABLE 1
DSM-III Roots: The Feighner Criteria.

DSM-III	*Feighner*
Panic disorder	***Anxiety neurosis***
Frequent and "abnormal"	
At least 3 panic attacks within a three-week period in circumstances other than during marked physical exertion or in a life-threatening situation. Not due to a physical disorder.	At least 6 anxiety attacks, each separated by at least a week from the others. They must occur at times other than during marked physical exertion or in life-threatening situations, and in the absence of a medical illness that *could* account for symptoms of anxiety.
Required symptoms	
Panic attacks are manifested by discrete periods of apprehension or fear.	Anxiety attacks are manifested by apprehension, fearfulness or sense of impending doom.
At least 4 of the following symptoms appear during each attack:	At least 4 of the following symptoms are present during the majority of attacks:
Dyspnea Palpitations Chest pain or discomfort Choking or smothering sensation Dizziness, vertigo, unsteady feelings Paresthesias Feelings of unreality Hot and cold flashes Sweating	Dyspnea Palpitations Chest pain or discomfort Choking or smothering sensation Dizziness Paresthesias

TABLE 1 (Continued)

DSM-III	*Feighner*
Panic disorder	***Anxiety neurosis***
Faintness Trembling or shaking Fear of dying, going crazy, or doing something uncontrolled	
Exclusion criteria	
Not due to another mental disorder such as major depression, somatization disorder, or schizophrenia.	In the presence of other psychiatric illness(es) this diagnosis is made only if the criteria . . . antedate the onset of the other psychiatric illness by at least 2 years.
Age	
No age criterion.	Age of onset prior to 40.

presence of symptoms, their frequency and severity, their clustering in time, and be able to distinguish them from normal reactions to stress, from the effects of physical disease or side effects of the intake of alcohol, medications, or other drugs, and from the effects of other psychiatric disorders.

Needs of the ECA Project

A major goal of the NIMH Division of Biometry and Epidemiology's Epidemiology Catchment Area Program (ECA) was to carry out population surveys in various parts of the country that would, for the first time, ascertain the prevalence and incidence of specific psychiatric disorders in the general population. Since many psychiatric disorders are rare, large samples were required to provide accurate estimates. Large samples meant relying on lay interviewers. Since DSM-III was to be the official diagnostic system for the country, it would obviously be desirable for DSM-III criteria to be at least one of the bases for prevalence counts.

As a first step in choosing an instrument for this enterprise, the Division asked Dr. David Goldberg to review the appropriateness of four existing instruments, the PSE, the PERI, the SADS-L, and the RDI. A meeting was then called with authors and users of these four instruments to allow them to describe these instruments.

At that meeting, it was noted that the PERI did not provide specific diagnoses, and that its scales were based on internal consistency rather than approximating traditional clinical syndromes. The remaining three instruments produced measures closer to DSM-III diagnostic categories, and all applied severity criteria and excluded symptoms entirely explained by physical disease and ingestion of substances. The SADS-L and the RDI had two advantages over the PSE. First, because they shared roots in the Feighner Criteria with DSM-III, many DSM-III criterion symptoms already appeared in these two instruments. Second, they both reviewed the history of symptoms over the lifetime, thus allowing making true diagnoses, while the PSE, which asked about symptoms only in the last month, could be used only at the level of recent syndromes, not diagnoses. However, the SADS, like the PSE, provided only screening questions for some diagnoses, while the RDI covered the full set of symptoms. Nor did the RDI permit interviewers to skip out of a diagnostic section before a positive or negative diagnosis was established, while the SADS and PSE directed interviewers to use "cutoffs". Sometimes these cutoffs served as screening questions, i.e., if the first questions were negative, it was assumed that most of the remainder would be as well and the diagnostic criteria would not be met. Sometimes they reflected diagnostic hierarchies, i.e., if previous questions had indicated the presence of a diagnosis that would preempt another diagnosis, all questions related to the second diagnosis should be skipped. The absence of screening questions and cutoffs in the RDI made it less likely than the SADS-L or PSE to produce false negatives in a general population survey.

Most importantly, only the RDI spelled out every question and most probes to make it easy for lay interviewers to use. The SADS-L and PSE were both interview guides, which left it up to a skilled interviewer to improvise some questions and to devise most probes before deciding whether a problem was serious enough to consider it a symptom. Finally, only the RDI directly coded each answer and coded *reasons* a symptom was negative (not present, not severe enough, explained by physical disorder, explained by drug or alcohol use) so that strictness of diagnostic criteria would be varied by easy modifications of computer programs.

However, the RDI had one important drawback: it did not distinguish current from past diagnoses. In the tradition of the Washington University Department Interview, it asked all questions on a lifetime basis.

After comparing the available instruments, the Division of Biometry and Epidemiology decided the RDI was closest to meeting their needs, and asked the Washington University group—Lee Robins, John Helzer, and Jack Croughan, with the help of Robert Spitzer and Janet Williams—to develop a new instrument that would preserve the specific questions and probes of the RDI and its completeness of coverage and coding, but would add a distinction between current and past diagnoses and add questions as necessary to allow making DSM-III diagnoses and to score RDC criteria. (Since several important studies had used RDC criteria, it would be advantageous to be able to compare their prevalence rates with rates in ECA samples of the general population.)

Creating the DIS

To create the new interview, questions were taken from a variety of sources. Many were questions from the Renard Diagnostic Interview that had survived the tests for reliability and validity described above. Some questions came from the SADS-L. This first draft was Version I.

This version was tested by researchers at various centers*, and suggestions for changes were offered. Revisions were made and the revisions tested with patients and nonpatient volunteers, and modified as necessary. Questions from the Mini-Mental State Examination (Folstein et al., 1975) were incorporated to assess cognitive deficit. Questions were then reordered to improve the conversational flow, and the new order was again tested. The instrument was then used in training sessions for lay interviewers and psychiatrists in preparation for a test of its validity (Robins et al., 1981, 1982) and questions found difficult for respondents to understand were revised. During this training, a Probe Flow chart was added to specify precisely when probes necessary to decide whether criteria for psychiatric symptoms are met should be used, how they should be phrased, and how scored. This revised instrument, tested for validity and used by Yale in its Wave I ECA interview, was known as Version II.

*Those helping to test it include Darrel Regier, Rachel Gittelman, Shirley Hill, Harvey Stancer, Victory Hesselbrock, Eli Robins, Paula Clayton, Myrna Weissman, Helen Orvaschel, Pam Harding, James Stabenau, Michie Hesselbrock, Kathryn Ratcliff, Celia Homans, Martha Munson, Fern Burnett, and Ben Locke.

Following analysis of the validity data, questions responsible for a disproportionate number of disagreements were revised. Suggestions were accepted for clarifications of questions based on early experiences of the Yale group in the field, and questions were added to respond to last minute revisions of DSM-III. Instructions to interviewers were incorporated into the body of the interview when possible. The Probe Flow Chart was improved. The interview thus modified was published as Version III, and used in Wave I of all subsequent ECA projects.

The DIS, Version III

In many ways, the DIS brings together the two major interview traditions described earlier. It resembles the HIS, HOS, and PERI in that it requires relatively little judgment from the interviewer and scores answers to questions directly without requiring an interpretive leap to clinical concepts. On the other hand, like the SADS, PSE, and other clinical interviews, it emphasizes distinguishing significant symptoms from the ordinary worries and concerns of daily life by setting minimum severity requirements, and it attempts to distinguish psychiatric symptoms from symptoms caused by physical illness or the side effects of drugs or alcohol. In addition, it has moved farther than any previous instrument to free itself from the need for psychiatric manpower. Once interviewers code answers to specified questions and probes, diagnosis is done entirely by computer.

The DIS makes 36 of the adult diagnoses in DSM-III (table 2), as well as all Feighner diagnoses (except undiagnosed) and 27 RDC diagnoses.

Table 3 summarizes some of the features that make the DIS particularly useful for general population surveys. It is economical because it does not require clinical manpower either to administer the interview or to make diagnoses. Because it covers all necessary symptoms, rather than screening for illness, it is self-contained, requiring neither follow-up examination with a more detailed instrument nor hospital record data before diagnoses can be made. With the exception of a few open-ended questions, the interview is completely precoded so answers can be directly entered into the computer after editing. The few open-ended questions are not necessary to diagnosis and may be left uncoded, to be used only to resolve questions about the correctness of the coding decisions. Because questions and probes are fully specified, interviewers can be trained to behave in very similar ways. The absence of cutoffs and screening sections increases the precision of diagnosis. The DIS takes no longer than similar interviews that lack these features—about an hour for patients and a bit less for nonpatients.

The interview has been used with both patients and members of the general population and seems acceptable to both. Breakoff rates in the ECA project were less than 1%. Although there are questions about sex, drinking, drug use, and police trouble necessary to make diagnoses of alcohol abuse, drug abuse, antisocial personality, and psychosexual dysfunction, subjects rarely refused to answer these questions. Thus the interview covers psychiatrically

TABLE 2
Diagnoses Covered by the DIS.

DSM-III	*RDC*	*Feighner*
Cognitive Impairment	RDC does not provide criteria.	Organic brain syndromes (criterion A only)
Severe		
Mild		
Affective disorders		
Manic episode[a]	Manic disorder[a]	Mania[a]
With impairment[a]	Hypomanic disorder[a]	
Without impairment[a]		
Major depressive episode	Major depressive disorder[a]	Depression[a,b]
With impairment[a]		
Without impairment[a]		
Dysthymia[a]		
Bipolar[a]		
Major depression		
Single episode		
Recurrent		
Atypical bipolar		
Grief reaction		

TABLE 2 (Continued)

DSM-III	*RDC*	*Feighner*
Schizophrenic disorders		
Schizophrenia	Schizophrenia[a,b]	Schizophrenia[a,b]
Problems in current year[a]	Schizo-affective disorder, manic type	
Earlier symptoms only[a]	Schizo-affective disorder, depressed type	
Schizophreniform[a]		
Substance use disorders	Alcoholism	Alcoholism[b]
Alcohol abuse		
Alcohol dependence		
Barbiturate, hypnotic abuse	Sedatives, hynotics, tranquilizers abuse	Drug dependence[b]
Barbiturate, hypnotic dependence	Sedatives, hypnotics, tranquilizers dependence	
Opioid abuse	Narcotics abuse	
Opioid dependence	Narcotics dependence	
Amphetamine abuse	Amphetamine-like stimulants abuse	
Amphetamine dependence	Amphetamine-like stimulants dependence	
Cocaine abuse	Cocaine abuse	
Hallucinogen abuse	LSD or other hallucinogens abuse	
Cannabis abuse	Marijuana, hashish, THC abuse	
Cannabis dependence	Marijuana, hashish, THC dependence	
	Poly-drug abuse	
	With impairment	
	Without impairment	

TABLE 2 (Continued)

DSM-III	*RDC*	*Feighner*
Anxiety disorders		
Obsessive-compulsive[a]	Obsessive-compulsive disorder	Obsessive-compulsive neurosis[a]
Agoraphobia[a]	Agoraphobia[a]	Phobic Neurosis
Social phobia[a]	Social phobias[a]	
Simple phobia[a]	Simple phobias[a]	
Summary phobia[a]	Mixed phobias[a]	
Panic[a]	Panic disorder[a,b]	Anxiety neurosis
Agoraphobia with panic[a]		
Agoraphobia without panic[a]		
Somatization disorder	Briquet's disorder[a]	Hysteria
Antisocial personality	Antisocial personality[b]	Antisocial personality disorder[b]
Anorexia nervosa		Anorexia nervosa
Disorders not covered in all ECA sites		
Tobacco use disorder		
Psychosexual dysfunction		

TABLE 2 (Continued)

DSM-III	*RDC*	*Feighner*
Transsexualism		Transsexualism[b]
Egodystonic Homosexuality		Homosexuality[a]
Pathological gambling		

[a]With and without exclusion criteria
[b]Probable and definite

TABLE 3
DIS Features.

Economy:

No clinicians needed.

Single interview sufficient.

No external data to gather.

No coders needed—precoded for computer.

No greater length than similar interviews: about 1 hour.

Accuracy:

All questions fully specified.

Probes for positive answers fully specified.

No "cutoffs" or "skipouts" before definite diagnosis.

No "screening" sections requiring reevaluations with another instrument.

Acceptable to the general population.

Flexibility:

Specific symptoms entered into computer so that alternative diagnostic criteria can be applied.

Diagnoses made with and without preemptions by other diagnoses.

"Current" defined 4 ways—last two weeks, month, 6 months, year.

Examples of phobias, hallucinations, delusions recorded to allow review by a clinician if desired.

Drugs and physical illnesses thought to account for symptoms recorded to allow review for plausibility.

Diagnostic comprehensiveness:

Diagnoses in 3 major systems: DSM-III, RDC, Feighner (Renard).

Supplementary information:

Ages of onset and last symptoms for each qualifying diagnosis.

Severity of each diagnosis obtained, as indicated by duration and number of criteria met.

Use of medical services for symptoms of each diagnosis.

Translations:

The interview has been translated into Chinese, Japanese, Spanish, French, Greek, German, Korean, and Portuguese.

relevant areas noticeably absent from earlier surveys because they were thought too "embarrassing."

Diagnostic programs for the DIS can be flexible because the response to each symptom question is entered into the computer, including the reason a symptom is negative. This means that the three sets of diagnostic algorithms provided in computer programs (for DSM-III, RDC, and Feighner) are not the only ones that could be used to assess the psychiatric status of interviewed persons. A variety of algorithms can be devised and compared. These algorithms can vary in which symptoms are used and how they are combined, in whether or not diagnostic hierarchies are used, and in the strictness of the criteria for deciding whether a symptom is positive, by recoding as positive symptoms that are negative for any of three coded reasons—always explained by physical illness or injury, always explained by drugs or alcohol, or not severe. The assessment of whether a disorder is current or past can be made using any of four definitions of current symptoms: present within the last 2 weeks, within the last month, within the last 6 months, or within the last year. These alternative definitions make it possible to compare DIS results with results from studies using varying definitions of "current."

Because analysis of the DIS is flexible in terms of diagnostic systems used, stringency of criteria, and definitions of "current" disorder, the data it provides can be used to evaluate and improve current psychiatric nosology by comparing the success of different ways of defining disorders in predicting outcome, treatment response, and similarly affected family members, all measures of validity that can help to compare the success of diverse diagnostic schemes (Robins & Guze, 1971).

The current programs ascertain diagnosis according to whatever rules for preemptive diagnosis exist in the three systems served, but also provide diagnoses for which criteria would be met if hierarchical rules were set aside. This is particularly useful in searching for risk factors, since it allows separating factors increasing the risk of positive symptoms of a diagnosis from factors protecting against the diagnosis that preempts it.

In addition to diagnoses, for each diagnosis for which criteria were met, the programs provide age of onset, age at which the last symptom was experienced, and whether a physician was consulted. Negative diagnoses are distinguished from diagnoses in which there is insufficient information to decide on the presence of a diagnosis. A count is provided of symptoms positive in each diagnosis. Overall counts are made of total positive symptoms, positive diagnoses, and number of diagnoses for the symptoms on which a physician was consulted.

Conclusion

The DIS has profited from the vast amount of work on survey instruments assessing mental disorder that has gone before it. It has attempted to combine the replicability of the survey with the attention to clinical significance of the clinical interview. We hope that its use will lead to enlarged understanding of both the etiology and course of psychiatric disorders, by providing well-defined, reliable, and valid assessment of specific mental disorders. Looking for the causes of "mental disorder" in general is clearly not useful. The correlates of different diagnoses vary so profoundly that it is hardly possible that they share causes: depression and phobias are common in women, alcoholism in men, drug abuse in young adults, dementia in the elderly. Failure to distinguish among these disorders can only lead to inconclusive results when seeking risk factors for psychiatric disorder.

But the search for disorder-specific causes is not the only value in making specific diagnoses. One of the most important reasons for analysis by specific diagnosis is to improve communication and comparability of data among studies. Specific diagnoses allow comparing results of one study with those of another even if definitions of mental illness are not identical. Consider the problem created by the single figure for "caseness" in the Midtown Manhattan Study (Srole et al., 1962). That study found only 18% of the general population to be currently well and 23% impaired. Many clinicians thought this figure of 82% not psychiatrically well much too high, and they suspected that if psychosomatic illnesses were excluded, a more plausible figure would have been obtained. Unfortunately, since the caseness rating was a global judgment of mental health, there is no way to calculate what the rate of psychiatrically ill would have been had psychosomatic disorders been omitted. Without the use of specific diagnoses, a study's results can be compared only with results from studies that define mental illness in exactly the same way. In contrast, when specific diagnoses are made, comparisons can be made even with studies that have assessed only a single diagnostic entity.

Acknowledgments

This research was supported by the Epidemiologic Catchment Area Program (ECA). The ECA is a series of five epidemiologic research studies performed by independent research teams in collaboration with staff of the Division of Biometry and Epidemiology (DBE) of the National Institute of Mental Health (NIMH). The NIMH Principal Collaborators are Darrel A. Regier, Ben Z. Locke, and William W. Eaton; The NIMH Project Officer is Carl A. Taube. The Principal Investigators and Co-Investigators from the five sites are: Yale University, U01 MH 34224—Jerome K. Myers, Myrna M. Weissman, and Gary Tischler; Johns Hopkins University, U01 MH 33870—Morton Kramer, Ernest Gruenberg, and Sam Shapiro; Washington University, St. Louis, U01 MH 33883—Lee N. Robins and John Helzer; Duke University, U01 MH 35386—Dan Blazer and Linda George; University of California, Los Angeles, U01 MH 33865—Richard Hough, Marvin Karno, Javier Escobar, and Audrey Burnam. This work acknowledges support of this program as well as Research Scientist Award MH-00334, and USPHS Grants DA-00013, AA-03852, and MH-31302.

References

American Psychiatric Association (1980), *Diagnostic and Statistical Manual,* Third Edition. Washington, D.C.: APA.

Blashfield, R. K. (1982), The Feighner et al. paper, invisible colleges and the Matthew effect. *Schizophr Bull* 8:1-12.

Cohen, M. E., Robins, E., Purtell, J., Altmann, M. & Reid, D. (1953), Excessive surgery in hysteria. *JAMA* 151:977-986.

Dohrenwend, B. P. & Dohrenwend, B. S. (1969), *Social Status and Psychological Disorder: A Causal Inquiry.* New York: Wiley-Interscience Division of John Wiley & Sons.

Dohrenwend, B. P. & Shrout, P. E. (1978), Toward the development of a two-stage procedure for case identification and classification in psychiatric epidemiology. In: *Research in Community and Mental Health,* Vol II, ed. Simmons, R. G. Greenwich, CT: JAI Press.

Eaton, W. W., Regier, D. A., Locke, B. Z., Taube, C. A. (1983), The epidemiologic catchment area program. In: *Epidemiologic Community Surveys,* ed. Weissman, M. M., Myers, J. M. & Ross, C. New Brunswick, NJ: Rutgers University Press.

Essen-Moller, E. (1956), Individual traits and morbidity in a Swedish rural population. *Acta Psychiatr Scand* (Suppl 100).

Feighner, J. P., Robins, E., Guze, S. B., Woodruff, R. A., Jr., Winokur, G. & Munoz, R. (1972), Diagnostic criteria for use in psychiatric research. *Arch Gen Psychiatr* 26:57-63.

Folstein, M. F., Folstein, S. E. & McHugh, P. R. (1975), Mini-mental state: A practical method for grading cognitive state of patients for the clinician. *J Psychiatr Res* 12:189-198.

Fremming, K. H. (1951), The expectation of mental infirmity in a sample of the Danish population. *Occasional Papers on Eugenics,* No. 7. London: Cassel.

Gurland, B. J., Sharpe, L., Simon, R.J., Kuriansky, J. & Stiller, P. (1972), On the use of psychiatric diagnosis for comparing psychiatric populations. *Psychiatr Q* 46:461-472.

Hagnell, O. (1966), *A Prospective Study of the Incidence of Mental Disorder.* Stockholm: Scandinavian University Books.

Helgason, T. (1964), Epidemiology of mental disorders in Iceland. *Acta Psychiatr Scand* 40 (Suppl. 173).

Helzer, J. E., Robins, L. N., Croughan, J.L. & Welner, A. (1981), Renard Diagnostic Interview: Its reliability and procedural validity with physicians and lay interviewers. *Arch Gen Psychiatr* 38:393-398.

Hoeper, E. W., Nycz, G. R., Cleary, P.D., Regier, D.A., & Goldberg, I.D. (1979), Estimated prevalence of RDC mental disorder in primary medical care. *Int J Ment Health* 8:6-15.

Klemperer, J. (1933), Zur balastungsstatistik der durchschnittsbevolkerung. Psychosenhaufigkeit unter 1,000 stickprobenmassig ausgelesenen probanden. *Z Ges Neurol Psychiatr* 146:277.

Lapouse, R. (1967), Problems in studying the prevalence of psychiatric disorder. *Am J Public Health* 57:947-954.

Leighton, D. C., Harding, J.S., Macklin, D.B., Macmillan, A.M. & Leighton, A. H. (1963), *The Character of Danger.* New York: Basic Books.

Reich, T., Robins, L., Woodruff, R.A., Taibleson, M., Rich, C. & Cunningham, L. (1975), A computer assisted derivation of a screening interview for alcoholism. *Arch Gen Psychiatr* 32:847-852.

Robins, E., Gentry, K. A., Munoz, R. A. & Marten, S. (1977), A contrast of the three more common illnesses with the ten less common in a study and 18-month follow-up of 314 psychiatric emergency room patients: I. Characteristics of the sample and methods of study; II. Characteristics of patients with the more common illnesses; III. Findings at follow-up. *Arch Gen Psychiatr* 34:259-265, 269-281, 285-291.

Robins, E. & Guze, S. B. (1971), Establishment of diagnostic validity in psychiatric illness: Its application to schizophrenia. In: *The Schizophrenic Syndrome. An Annual Review,* ed. Cancro, R., New York: Brunner/Mazel.

Robins, E., Murphy. G. E., Wilkinson, R. H., Gassner, S. & Kayes, J. (1959), Some clinical considerations in the prevention of suicide based on a study of 134 successful suicides. *Am J Public Health* 49:888-899.

Robins, E. & O'Neal, P. (1953), Clinical features of hysteria in children, with a note on prognosis. *Nervous Child* 10:246-271.

Robins, E., Purtell, J. J. & Cohen, M. E. (1952), "Hysteria" in men: A study of 38 patients so diagnosed and 194 control subjects. *N Engl J Med* 246:677-685.

Robins, E., Schmidt, E. H. & O'Neal, P. (1957), Some interrelations of social factors and clinical diagnosis in attempted suicide: A study of 109 patients. *Am J Psychiatr* 114:221-231.

Robins, L. (1966), *Deviant Children Grown Up: A Socialogical and Psychiatric Study of Sociopathic Personality.* Baltimore: Williams & Wilkins. Reprinted by Robert E. Krieger, Huntington, New York, 1974.

Robins, L. & Braroe, N. (1964), The lay interviewer in psychiatric research. *J Nerv Ment Dis* 138:70-78.

Robins, L., Helzer, J. & Croughan, J. (1978), *Renard Diagnostic Interview.*

Robins, L., Helzer, J., Croughan, J., Williams, J. B. W. & Spitzer, R. (1979), The NIMH Diagnostic Interview Schedule (DIS), Version II. Washington, D.C.: National Institute of Mental Health.

Robins, L. N., Helzer, J. E., Croughan, J. L. & Ratcliff, K.S. (1981), The NIMH Diagnostic Interview Schedule: Its History, Characteristics, and Validity. *Arch Gen Psychiatr* 38:381-389.

Robins, L. N., Helzer, J. H., Ratcliff, K. S. & Seyfried, W. (1982), Validity of the Diagnostic Interview Schedule, Version II: DSM-III Diagnoses. *Psychol Med* 12:855-870.

Spitzer, R. L. & Endicott, J. (1977a), *Schedule for Affective Disorders and Schizophrenia,* New York.

Spitzer, R. L. & Endicott, J. (1977b), *Schedule for Affective Disorders and Schizophrenia—Life-Time Version.*

Spitzer, R. L., Endicott, J. & Robins, E. (1978), Research diagnostic criteria: Rationale and reliability. *Arch Gen Psychiatr* 35:773-782.

Spitzer, R. L., Fleiss, J. L., Endicott, J. & Cohen, J. (1970), The Psychiatric Status Schedule: A technique for evaluating psychopathology and impairment in role functioning. *Arch Gen Psychiatr* 23:41-55.

Spitzer, R. L. & Endicott, J. (1968), DIAGNO: A computer program for psychiatric diagnosis utilizing the differential diagnostic procedure. *Arch Gen Psychiatr* 18:746-756.

Srole, L. (1975), Measurement and classification of sociopsychiatric epidemiology: Midtown Manhattan Study (1954) and Midtown Manhattan Restudy (1974). *J Health Soc Behav* 16:347-364.

Srole, L., Langner, T. S., Michael, S. T., Opler, M. K. & Rennie, T.A.C. (1962), *Mental Health in the Metropolis: The Midtown Manhattan Study, Vol. I.* New York: McGraw Hill.

Stromgren, E. (1950), Statistical and genetical population studies within psychiatry: Methods and principal results. In: *Proceedings of the First International Congress of Psychiatry,* Vol. VI, pp. 115-192. Paris: Herman.

Weissman, M. M. & Myers, J. K. (1978), Psychiatric disorders in a U.S. urban community: The use of research diagnostic criteria in an epidemiological survey. *Arch Gen Psychiatr* 35:1304-1311.

Wheeler, E.O., White, P. D., Reed, E. W. & Cohen, M. E. (1950), Neurocirculatory asthenia (anxiety neurosis, effort syndrome, neurasthenia). A twenty-year follow-up study of 173 patients. *JAMA* 142:878-888.

Wing, J. K., Cooper, J. E. & Sartorius, N. (1974), *Measurement and Classification of Psychiatric Symptoms.* Cambridge: Cambridge University Press.

Wing, J. K., Nixon, J. M., Mann, S. A. & Leff, J. P. (1977), Reliability of the PSE (ninth edition) used in a population study. *Psychol Med* 7:505-516.

Woodruff, R. A., Clayton, P. J. & Guze, S. B. (1969), Hysteria: An evaluation of specific diagnostic criteria by the study of randomly selected psychiatric clinic patients. *Br J Psychiatr* 115:1243-1248.

Woodruff, R. A., Guze, S. B. & Clayton, P. J. (1972), Anxiety neurosis among psychiatric outpatients. *Compr Psychiatr* 13:165-170.

Woodruff, R. A., Robins, L., Taibleson, M., Reich, T., Schwin, R. & Frost, N. (1973), A computer assisted derivation of a screening interview for hysteria. *Arch Gen Psychiatr* 29:450-454.

World Health Organization (1973), *Report of the International Pilot Study of Schizophrenia,* Vol. I Geneva: WHO.

Chapter 19

Describing and Classifying Psychiatric Symptoms: The PSE-CATEGO System

J. K. WING

The purpose of the PSE-CATEGO system is to help standardize the way that psychiatric symptoms are elicited, recorded and classified with a view to making studies of psychiatric disorders more comparable. Its main scientific uses are for epidemiologic case finding; standardizing the description of cases in research projects; providing a comprehensive profile of symptoms, syndromes, and scores useful for measuring changes; and investigating and comparing clinical nosologies. The system includes: a present state examination (PSE), now in its ninth edition, that provides symptom and syndrome profiles and scores; a means of rating syndromes that appeared in previous episodes (Syndrome Check List or SCL); a method of coding etiological factors (Etiology Schedule or ES); a technique for determining threshold points at which sufficient PSE symptoms are present to allow the recognition of a "case" of psychiatric disorder (Index of Definition or ID); and a computer program for analyzing PSE symptom-profiles, together with data from the SCL and ES, to derive, first, a profile of eight categories (each formed from a group of syndromes) and, second, a set of mutually exclusive classes (which can be used as a 50-class or a 10-class set).

Development of the System

The PSE originated in a brief interview designed to elicit and record the severity of four symptoms (flatness of affect, poverty of speech, incoherence of speech, coherently expressed delusions, or hallucinations) in longstay schizophrenic patients and to provide a simple classification. The results correlated well with those of rating scales completed by nurses and the method was found useful in comparing the effects of hospital environments and in measuring change (Wing, 1961; Wing and Brown, 1970).

The interview was expanded to describe acute and chronic neurotic and other psychotic symptoms, and used in a series of surveys and experiments (Wing, 1968). A paper on the reliability of the third to fifth editions and their use in a wide variety of settings was then published (Wing et al., 1967). The seventh edition was used in the first phase of the US-UK Diagnostic Project and the prepilot phase of the International Pilot Study of Schizophrenia (IPSS) as well as in studies by the Social Psychiatry Unit of the British Medical Research Council (MRC). This experience was used to develop an eighth edition, versions of which were used in the second phase of the US-UK project and the main surveys of the IPSS (Cooper et al., 1972; WHO, 1973). The present (ninth) edition, and the classification program and other techniques were then prepared. By this time the PSE had been translated into 15 languages and widely used in research all over the world, together with the classification program. It was thought that sufficient experience had been gained to allow publication of the schedule and glossary and an instruction manual (Wing et al., 1974).

Subsequent developments involved the testing of a short version (the first 40 PSE items) for use in population surveys by nonmedical interviewers and the construction of the Index of Definition as one method of defining a "case." A supplementary instruction manual has now been produced in order to bring the earlier one up-to-date (Wing and Sturt, 1978).

The system has thus evolved over a period of 20 years and the authors have been careful not to publish until they were fairly sure they could describe the main advantages and limitations. The latter have to be taken into account as well as the former. The system is now developing further as means are found to decrease its limitations.

The Techniques

Description and Measurement of Present Clinical State (PSE)

The ninth edition of the PSE consists of an interview schedule that contains probes and more specific questions designed to elicit responses on the basis of which the examiner can rate the absence, or presence in two degrees of severity, of most of the symptoms of the functional psychoses and neuroses (i.e., conditions classified as 295, 296, 297 and 300 in the International Classification of Diseases). In all, 140 items are rated, mostly on the basis of information supplied by the patient about experiences during the previous month. One month appears to be the best time period for general use but shorter periods (e.g., one week) can be used for special purposes, such as when the examination is repeated after this time in order to measure change. There is also a section for symptoms observed during the examination.

The examiner uses the clinical technique of cross-examination and is free to adapt the interview, within limits, in accordance with the condition and replies of the patient. He continues until he is satisfied that he has enough information to rate each item as present or absent or to decide that further questioning will not be productive of useful information. However, it is usually possible to follow fairly precisely the procedure laid down in the schedule. A system of cutoff points allows the interviewer to pass on to another section if there is no evidence from responses to obligatory, above cutoff, questions that further examination in that section will be productive. Data gathered during the whole examination are taken into account and a return can be made to earlier sections if this becomes necessary later in the interview.

This technique of interview places the onus of deciding whether or not a symptom, as defined in the glossary, is present, squarely on the examiner. The most important factor in rating is whether the patient describes experiences that are close to those defined in the glossary (itself based on descriptions by large numbers of patients). The answer "Yes" to any particular question is *not* of great importance except as a cue to ask what the experience was like. This procedure must be clearly distinguished from that of filling in a questionnaire on the basis of the subject's answers. The instruction is to "rate down" rather than up and not to rate a symptom present if there is any doubt. Provision is made for rating "not known" and "not applicable."

The glossary of definitions is of great importance and is based on symptoms commonly observed in hospital practice. Emphasis is placed, where appropriate, on differential definitions; e.g., between delusions of reference and auditory hallucinations; nervous tension and autonomic anxiety; and thought insertion and delusion of being hypnotized.

The definition of common nonspecific symptoms such as worrying, which can occur in any psychiatric disorder, is important because they make up a substantial part of any total symptom score, particularly in population surveys. For worrying to be rated as present, three criteria are necessary: there must be a round of painful thought, which cannot be stopped voluntarily, and is out of proportion to the subject worried about. Severity is judged on the intensity and duration of the symptom during the month. On the other hand, the definitions of highly discriminating but rare symptoms, such as thought insertion or delusions of control, are important because of their key implications for classification.

Most psychiatrists already experienced in clinical phenomenology can use the PSE satisfactorily after a week's training followed by about 20 practice interviews under supervision. Most patients find the interview completely acceptable since it is based firmly on knowledge of the kinds of experiences that they are likely to describe. If a full range of psychotic and neurotic symptoms is present, the interview lasts about three-quarters to one-and-a-quarter hours. If no symptoms are present, it can be completed in 10-15 minutes. The PSE has now been translated into more than 40 languages, including most of the European ones and several belonging to other families, such as Arabic, Chinese, Finnish, Japanese, Luganda, Thai and Yoruba. Most of the problems that, at first sight, seem likely to occur can be overcome by translating the concepts (as defined in the glossary) rather than the words. It has been pointed out, for example, that some languages do not have separate words to describe the moods of depression, irritability, and anxiety (Leff, 1977). However, it proved possible to identify free-floating anxiety in Luganda-speaking subjects by inquiring about palpitations or dizziness associated with fear (for which a word exists) without good reason.

"Depression" could be translated by using the words for grief or sadness or "crying in the heart, without tears" (Orley and Wing, 1979). On the whole, back-translation is satisfactory and fair reliability can be attained by trained and experienced interviewers (WHO, 1973, chapter 6).

A PSE symptom profile gives a very detailed description of present psychiatric state but it is convenient to condense the information in various ways. One of these is to collate symptoms into 38 syndromes which can readily be presented in visual form as profiles; this condensation, in fact, constitutes the first stage of the CATEGO program. In addition, each syndrome has a score consisting of the sum of its constituent symptom ratings. These syndrome scores can be added to provide four subtotal scores (on specific psychotic, nonspecific psychotic, specific neurotic, and nonspecific neurotic symptoms) and a total PSE score. The use of profiles and scores to measure change will be illustrated later in the discussion of the computer classification program.

Short Form of the PSE

The first 40 items of the PSE describe common symptoms such as worrying, muscular tension, depressed mood, and anxiety. Whereas only psychiatrists and clinical psychologists have examined hundreds of patients with delusions or hallucinations, most people have experienced neurotic symptoms for themselves, at least in mild form. It has proved possible to train nonmedical interviewers to use a short form of the PSE reliably and thus to make feasible fairly large-scale surveys of general populations (Sturt et al., 1981; Wing et al., 1977).

Rating Earlier Episodes of Disorder (SCL)

If good clinical records are available, it is possible to rate the presence or absence of syndromes in previous episodes of disorder, or earlier in the present episode, thus supplementing the information available at the PSE interview. The Syndrome Check List (particularly the first 24 syndromes) is a convenient instrument for this purpose. A supplementary schedule is available that lays down questions to be added to the PSE interview in order to date previous episodes. Experience of population surveys has suggested that informants are not very good at dating the onset of a current episode, or the beginning and ending of previous episodes, unless the symptoms were severe and change points clear-cut or there was some anchoring point such as referral to a specialist. Mild disorders are particularly difficult to date. However, if good information is available (and this usually means from case records), it is possible to rate previous episodes on the SCL and the CATEGO program can then be used.

Causes of Disorder (ES)

The Etiology Schedule contains four lists of possible causal factors (organic, psychosocial, personality, mental retardation) likely to be taken into account, as well as present and past symptomatology, by a clinical psychiatrist when making a diagnosis. For example, if a hallucinatory condition with little or no clouding of consciousness is regarded as due mainly to excessive consumption of alcohol, it will be classified as "alcoholic hallucinosis" (291.2 in the ICD) rather than schizophrenia. Similarly, if a neurotic picture is thought to be largely secondary to personality disorder (ICD 301), the latter will be the primary diagnosis rather than the former. The Etiology Schedule requires the psychiatrist to specify such judgments in explicit form and thus eliminates many of the simple coding differences that lead to unreliability in clinical diagnosis. The schedule does not attempt to standardize a procedure for collecting relevant information or rules for applying it, but the requirement that psychiatrists should systematically review the various etiological factors that might be present, and rate the significance of each one for the diagnosis, does reduce considerably the amount of variation found in clinical practice. An Etiology Schedule can be completed for any episode for which a Syndrome Check List or PSE is available (Wing et al., 1977c).

Computer Classification Program (CATEGO)

When a psychiatrist has examined a patient using the PSE and has completed a Syndrome Check List and an Etiology Schedule for relevant previous episodes of disorder, a substantial proportion of the information required to make a diagnosis (at least of acute conditions) is available in numerical form. The CATEGO program, which incorporates a set of rules for classifying this information, is then applied (Wing et al., 1974; Wing and Sturt, 1978). The rules are partly hierarchical and take the form, approximately, of a logical tree. The program is first applied to condense PSE symptoms into syndromes and then, through several further stages, into eight categories (or groups of syndromes) each of which can be present at once. This provides a useful profile summarizing the clinical phenomena. Finally, a classification is made into 50 subclasses, which can be combined into twelve broad classes. The allocation of a case to one of these classes can be regarded as probable (+) or as uncertain (?) depending on the type and number of syndromes present. These classes are mutually exclusive and jointly exhaustive. Syndrome profiles of each of the main CATEGO classes, derived independently from the US-UK project and the IPSS, are given in the instruction manual (Wing, Cooper and Sartorius, 1974, pp. 119-122).

The CATEGO program can be applied to data from case records that have been rated on the Syndrome Check List. Information about causes, coded on the Etiology Schedule, is finally added, if appropriate.

The Concept of a Case in Population Surveys (ID)

The PSE-SCL-ES-CATEGO procedure works quite well when an acute episode of psychiatric disorder is under examination. The symptoms are likely to be sufficiently severe and numerous to allow the application of classifying rules. The problem of the threshold, below which no diagnosis can be made, rarely arises in such cases. This is not true of a population survey, in which most of the subjects examined have only minor symptoms or none at all. The difficulty can be illustrated by asking how a condition should be classified if the only PSE symptoms rated as present are (a) a moderate degree of worrying and (b) moderately depressed mood. How many more symptoms are necessary in order to make the judgment that this is a case of depressive disorder? The answer to such questions must eventually be resolved by the application of external criteria of validity (discussed in a later section), but meanwhile it is essential for the comparability of population surveys that some method be developed to define standard criteria for determining a threshold.

An Index of Definition was therefore constructed, comprising eight degrees of confidence that the PSE symptoms present were sufficient to allow the application of the CATEGO classification program. The first four degrees are at subthreshold level, the fifth constitutes a minimal threshold, and the other three are more definite. The rules for deriving these eight levels are incorporated in a computer program and the CATEGO program is only applied if disorders reach one of the minimal threshold levels (Wing, 1976; Wing and Sturt, 1978).

In a population study in Canberra, a two-stage technique was used. The main clinical instrument was a self-rated questionnaire, the General Health Questionnaire or GHQ (Goldberg, 1972). An extra sample of subjects was the GHQ, and GHQ results used to discriminate cases at ID level 5 or above. The resulting loadings were used to estimate the prevalence of cases in the Canberra population (Henderson et al., 1979).

Reliability

The Full PSE

The reliability of the full PSE, when used to describe acute episodes of disorder in inpatients and outpatients, has been extensively tested in large and detailed international studies (Cooper et al., 1972, chapter 8; Kendell et al., 1968; Luria and McHugh, 1974; Wing et al., 1967; 1974, chapter 5; WHO, 1973, chapter 8). The following general conclusions can be accepted (though with some reservations in the case of the most rare symptoms):

1. Teams of trained psychiatrists working together can achieve a satisfactory overall degree of reliability when simultaneously rating an interview with a patient in an acute episode of disorder or when rating a videotape or audiotape recording of an interview.
2. Reliability is lower when two psychiatrists rate the patient on different occasions, as would be expected because of changes in the patient's condition and because of variation in interviewing technique. When consecutive interviews are close together in time, reliability is still satisfactory for most groups of symptoms.
3. Symptoms rated on the basis of the patient's subjective descriptions tend to have a higher reliability than symptoms rated on the basis of observation of abnormal affect, speech or behavior during the interview. This is probably due to the different time periods covered; in one case up to a month, in the other only about an hour.
4. Groups of items (e.g., syndrome scores) give more reliable scores than individual items.

5. Reliability between psychiatrists using different languages is difficult to test but the evidence suggests that translation problems can be overcome and a reasonable degree of reliability achieved (WHO, 1973, chapter 8; Orley and Wing, 1979).
6. Symptoms that occur rarely in the general population, such as delusions, hallucinations, obsessions, and hypomania, can only be rated reliably by experienced examiners who have seen many such cases.
7. Some psychiatrists are unable to learn the techniques or to achieve a useful degree of reliability. This is particularly true of psychiatrists who can use only nondirective interviewing techniques.
8. When PSE symptoms are rated reliably, all the indices based upon them, such as syndromes, subscores and total score are also reliable. The Index of Definition and the CATEGO program are, of course, absolutely reliable in application.

Shorter Form of PSE

More recently, studies have been made of the reliability of the shorter form of the PSE, used by nonmedical interviewers as well as by psychiatrists (Cooper et al., 1977; Duncan-Jones et al., 1978; Sturt et al., 1981; Wing et al., 1977a,b). The major problem to be overcome by training is to specify the threshold at which a neurotic symptom is recognized to be present by reference to the severity of disorders observed in inpatients and outpatients. Naive interviewers are likely to have a lower threshold than psychiatrists and subjects rating themselves a lower threshold still. We have approached this problem by training nonmedical but experienced interviewers belonging to a social research unit, using videotapes of inpatients with depressive disorders and anxiety states and, when the initial tendency to overrate has been corrected, live interviews with inpatients.

In a pilot population survey in a district of southeast London, nonmedical interviewers trained in this way saw a random sample of women aged 18-65 and, following a present state examination (which was tape-recorded) made a global judgment as to whether a case of disorder was present or not. Psychiatrists then visited (blind) all the cases and a sample of the "noncases." They also rated many of the audiotapes. In general, reliability of symptoms, syndromes and scores was found to be high on audiotapes and when the interview was repeated within a week, although certain symptoms such as anxiety were less reliable than others. Reliability over longer periods of time was low, presumably due to fluctuations in clinical state (Wing et al., 1977b).

More recently, Agency interviewers with no previous experience of psychiatric interviewing were given the same training, and a similar design was followed during a much larger-scale survey. Again, there was a reasonable reliability in general but in these circumstances, there was evidence for persistent overrating by one or two interviewers. Rather more than one week's training is required to achieve a high reliability. There was, however, no evidence of drift away from the standard first achieved although no further training was given during the course of the survey (Sturt et al., 1981).

Agreement with Other Methods of Classification

Global Clinical Judgment in Population Surveys

In several surveys, psychiatrists have made global judgments as to whether the symptoms observed in members of population samples or of series of patients not directly referred to psychiatrists amount to a diagnosable disorder. These judgments can be compared with the above and below threshold distinction made by the application of the ID program to PSE symptom profiles. In five such surveys, the global judgments were made by psychiatrists who administered the PSE before the Index of Definition was designed or who were not aware of its construction. The comparison therefore allows an assessment of the extent to which the rules incorporated in the ID program approximate those used by a variety of clinical psychiatrists familiar with the PSE. It would be surprising if the thresholds of subjective judgment did not vary with the setting in which the judgments were made, e.g., that in a hospital setting the threshold was not set higher than in a population survey. On the other hand, the definitions of PSE symptoms (even of common and nonspecific symptoms such as worrying), which are based on hospital practice and the standard procedure of interviewing, are designed to minimize such influences. The ID level based on PSE symptoms should therefore be more stable than subjective global judgments.

In the pilot sample survey of women in southeast London, the agreement between global psychiatric judgment and discrimination on the basis of ID level was 90% (Wing et al., 1978). In a study of the adult population of two Ugandan villages, the equivalent agreement was 91% (Orley and Wing, 1979). In a sample survey of a Hebridean island, the agreement was 91% (Prudo, unpublished data). There was, however, one less concordant result. It emerged from a survey of a consecutive series of people who had attempted suicide and had been referred to a medical service for treatment. Here, the clinical judgment had a higher threshold which fell roughly between ID levels five and six (Urwin and Gibbons, 1979). In the survey of the Hebridean island, the concordance was increased to 97% by separating a sublevel 5a (PSE score under 15) from sublevel 5b (PSE score 15+).

Private global judgment is likely to be more variable than the more public, specific, and standardized judgments required in symptom rating, to which a set of classifying rules can then be applied with absolute reliability. It is possible that small teams of workers can reach a high degree of reliability among themselves on clinical judgments (as in the diagnostic judgments in the US-UK study) but other teams may reasonably adopt different, though equally reliable, criteria. There can also be an insensible change over time so the basis for agreement is different at the end of a project from that at the beginning. This does not, of course, mean that a case defined at or above the ID threshold level necessarily has clinical validity (any more than a global judgment has).

Using the full PSE rather than the short version in population samples results in the registration of a somewhat higher frequency of cases, since hypomania, delusions, hallucinations, and observed abnormalities are included. These symptoms are uncommon in the general population, however, and the difference is not great.

Analysis of data from the pilot London survey suggests that there is a continuum of severity that can be represented by total PSE score and which may best be designated by a term such as *distress* rather than *illness*. This might include many conditions at the threshold level (ID5) which should not, in that case, be separated into "depressive disorders" and "anxiety states," for example. However, as the total score increases, more key symptoms, such as subjective anergia, pathological guilt, retardation, and depressive delusions begin to appear (Sturt, 1982; Wing et al., 1978). At ID level 6 and above, the CATEGO classes are more securely based on the presence of recognizable syndromes. No studies of validity or long-term course have yet been carried out and it is premature to interpret population data in terms of clinical diagnoses.

In addition, there are of course many other ways of defining a case. For example, someone with a phobia of flying would not reach threshold level on the ID unless there had actually been an episode of anxiety symptoms during the previous month severe enough to be rated on the PSE. Similarly, an investigator who wished to test a method of relieving tension states might adopt a definition of a case that included conditions below the ID threshold. The Index of Definition provides only one approach and all that is claimed for it is that it allows the application of identical rules to PSE profiles thus allowing comparability and replicability in epidemiologic studies. Other techniques will undoubtedly be added as knowledge advances.

Clinical Diagnosis

In several large studies, the clinical diagnoses of acute disorders in inpatients have been compared with the classification produced by applying the CATEGO program to PSE data. In the International Pilot Study of Schizophrenia there was good agreement (82%) on a three-way classification into schizophrenic and paranoid psychoses, manic conditions, and depressive disorders. The major discrepancy was that psychiatrists at centers in Moscow and Washington tended to use a broader definition of schizophrenia than those in the other seven centers, by reference to the CATEGO classification. Even in these centers, however, there was substantial agreement on a large central group of schizophrenic and paranoid disorders. Since the CATEGO program was partially constructed on the basis of IPSS data, this may not seem a surprising result but when applied to independently collected data from the US-UK project, the degree of concordance was equally high (81%). Adding information from the narrative histories of the present episode of disorder, rated on the SCL, improved the concordance with IPSS diagnoses to 87%. It was found that the SCL could be used reliably in this way by two independent raters (Wing et al., 1974, chapter 7).

The value of investigating each individual discrepancy between clinical and reference classifications, by consulting the detailed clinical records for examples of particular symptoms, was clearly demonstrated. Many of the changes in the ninth edition of the PSE and the examples given in the glossary of definitions were based upon this exercise. Since then, other European studies using the ninth edition have confirmed the high agreement between three broad groups of clinical diagnoses (including with the diagnoses made by hospital psychiatrists not connected with the project) and three broad CATEGO classes.

In none of these international studies was there any indication that psychiatrists distinguished between schizophrenic and paranoid psychoses on the basis of rules that could even approximately be matched by a standard procedure. The differentiation between CATEGO classes S and P may nevertheless be of value. It is simple to combine the classes but no test can be made of the distinction if it is not possible also to consider them separately.

The Etiology Schedule has also been used to codify a much wider range of diagnoses, including organic psychoses (ICD 290-294), personality disorders (ICD 301), and addictions (ICD 303 and 304), with a high degree of agreement (Wing et al., 1977c).

Investigation of Taxonomic Systems

A great advantage of a system of clinical classification based on precisely specifiable rules and closely related to a diagnostic system in wide current use is that it offers a means of comparison with other techniques of classification, whether purely clinical as with psychiatric diagnosis or purely mathematical as with various clustering techniques. The difficulty in making comparisons with the statistical taxonomic procedures is that they have usually been used in conjunction with a numeric input that does not allow the representation of symptoms that many clinicians would regard as diagnostically important. Thus Lorr (1965), for example, has derived statistical types, in which anxiety and depression could not be separated from each other; similarly, retarded speech, retarded movement and flat affect were combined together, as were restlessness, agitation, overactivity, and elation. The factor analysis by Spitzer and his colleagues (1967) gave rise to very similar results.

Fleiss et al., (1971), however, using similar statistical techniques based upon an input derived from PSE ratings, found that phobic anxiety could be distinguished from depression, retarded speech from retarded movement and flat affect from both, and restlessness from manic symptoms. These discriminations are important for the differential diagnosis between mania, anxiety states, depression, and subgroups of schizophrenia. The authors conclude, unsurprisingly, that output depends upon input. Clinically rich procedures such as the PSE, quite apart from the advantages derived from standard definitions of symptoms and partial standardization of the interview technique, are likely to give rise to a larger number of factors, clusters or types when subjected to statistical analysis. These clusters are also likely to be closer to the diagnostic categories used by clinical psychiatrists who take diagnosis seriously.

If the principles incorporated in the CATEGO program are indeed similar to those adopted by most diagnosticians in practice, it is evident that there is another very fundamental difference between statistical and clinical methods of allocating cases to categories. This is that clinical diagnosis is partly hierarchical. If organic symptoms such as disorientation or loss of memory or epilepsy are present, other symptoms are regarded as of less diagnostic importance. In fact, practically any other symptom can be present, including first rank symptoms of schizophrenia, elation, depression, obsessions, anxiety, or hysterical conversion symptoms, without being regarded as having diagnostic value in themselves. If there are no organic phenomena, the symptoms (if properly ascertained) with the highest diagnostic significance are usually the first-rank schizophrenic symptoms. Again, any other symptoms lower in the hierarchy may be present, but they can usually only modify the diagnosis (e.g., help in subclassification) rather than determine it. Although the principle becomes less clear in the lower reaches of the diagnostic hierarchy, it can still be discerned and specified. Some clinicians would alter the order, for example, by placing bipolar psychosis above schizophrenia, but they still use the principle.

Nearly all statistical studies ignore the hierarchical principle, since they are built on the premise that every input datum must be given the same weight as every other. From a clinical point of view this assumption is nonsensical, not least because it is evident that many symptoms depend upon the presence of others. For example, in clinical terms, an individual may worry because he has something to worry about, because he is a worrier, because he has phobias, because he has depressive preoccupations, because he has persecutory delusions, because he has first-rank symptoms, or because he has noticed that his memory is failing. To give the symptom "worrying" the same weight diagnostically as any of the others makes no clinical sense at all.

Kendell (1973) has shown that reasonable diagnoses can be made after reading transcripts of 5-minute interviews with acutely ill patients concerning their main symptoms, in response to questions about why they were coming into the hospital, what had been going wrong recently and whether they regarded themselves as ill. If the hierarchical principle is correct, all that need be known in many cases are the highly discriminating symptoms at each level of the diagnostic hierarchy. An example of how this principle applies to mania and severe depressive disorders is given in the Instruction Manual (Wing et al., 1974, p. 104).

The Question of Validity

One of the ways in which psychiatrists and their colleagues try to improve their methods of helping people referred to them is to look for patterns of experience or behavior and for factors that cause, exacerbate, relieve, or prevent them. The more recognizable and communicable the pattern (or syndrome or disorder), and the easier it is to differentiate from other patterns or from none, the more readily can other workers test the validity of claims that are made about it. One of the weaknesses of psychiatric research to date is the relative paucity of replications. Indistinguishable from the question of validity, therefore, is the problem to which the first part of this book is addressed—that of reliable case finding. Discovering workable solutions is not only of fundamental importance to epidemiology but to the whole of psychiatric research and practice. This means attempting to standardize interviewing methods.

The US-UK study illustrates one very simple use of a standardized system in hypothesis-testing, since it was based on the observation that the first admission rates for schizophrenia to U.S. hospitals were much higher than in the United Kingdom and rates for affective disorders much lower. The study showed that when a single set of definitions was used on each side of the Atlantic, there was no difference in rates, although the diagnoses made by local hospital psychiatrists still showed large discrepancies. This study emphasized the need to validate the diagnostic concepts used by the two groups of clinicians and, in particular, to discover whether including "extra" cases under the broad concept could be justified by their having specific causes or pathology or treatment in common with the agreed central group of schizophrenia, in spite of the difference in clinical picture.

Such validation studies are not impossible. For example, it has been demonstrated in controlled trials that Class S conditions (defined by PSE-CATEGO) are less likely to recur if oral or injected phenothiazines are continued after initial recovery (Hirsch et al., 1973; Leff and Wing, 1971). How far is this true of conditions not so defined? To answer this question, and others concerning validation, it will be useful to construct an item-pool containing all the data necessary for the other classifications, e.g., DSM-III or the French nosology, and algorithms for deriving them. If a sufficiently large data base is constructed, several algorithms could be applied and several different classifications tested at once (Wing, 1983).

Another attempt at replication, this time of an experimental study, was made by Hirsch and Leff (1975). The earlier study showed that the parents of people with schizophrenia had far more communication deviances than parents of neurotic patients but the term "schizophrenia" was not clearly defined (Wynne and Singer, 1963). The failure of the second project to find the same clear-cut distinction between groups of parents was probably due to sampling problems, in particular to different definitions of schizophrenia. Such difficulties in replicating studies, on the basis of which important conclusions have been reached, are found just as commonly in genetic, biochemical, therapeutic, and prognostic research. Studies of the validity of diagnostic concepts could progress more rapidly if comparable descriptions were more often used. This is the value of a set of techniques such as PSE and CATEGO. It is not intended to provide a new taxonomy but to be useful in investigating already existing systems (Wing, 1983).

Sample Surveys of General Populations

Five general population surveys in which the ninth edition of the PSE was used have now been completed: two, a pilot and a main survey, in southeast London; one in the Scottish Hebrides; one in Canberra, Australia; one in

Uganda; and one in Edinburgh. The results can be compared across surveys and also with data from a consecutive series of outpatients and another of inpatients from the same London area where, in addition, there is a psychiatric case register (Wing and Hailey, 1972).

The pilot London survey was carried out by four female nonmedical interviewers from the Social Research Unit at Bedford College, London, who were trained by us to use the short version of the PSE. A sample of 290 housing units was drawn at random from the local tax registers of a defined geographic area. A list of women aged 18-65 resident in these households was visited by the four interviewers. Immigrants (except from Eire) were excluded. One woman was selected for interview at random from each household but 52 (17.9%) declined and one interview was incomplete, leaving 237 women in the sample. The interviewers made a global judgment on the basis of each interview, after a team discussion, as to whether there was a definite or a borderline degree of caseness, or whether disorder was absent. All the subjects in the borderline and definite groups and a sample of the rest, 130 women in all, were referred to psychiatrists from the MRC Social Psychiatry Unit who were able to interview 95 of them using the full PSE, on average 3 weeks later, and rate the audiotapes of 28 more. Details of the Social Research Unit's procedure and analysis will be found elsewhere (Brown and Harris, 1978). The Social Psychiatry Unit participated in order to test the instruments and obtain preliminary prevalence data. The data concerning reliability have been summarized earlier (Wing et al., 1977, 1978).

The main London survey was carried out using a similar design, though with tighter sampling, but this time interviewers from a Social Survey Agency, trained on the short version of the PSE, saw a sample of 800 men and women aged 18-65, including immigrants. Information was also collected about experience of loss and separation during childhood. All those with an ID level of 5 or more and a sample of the rest were referred to the Social Psychiatry Unit. There was a loss at this stage of 10%. Two psychiatrists and a psychologist from the Unit examined 310 of the 355 people selected (a loss of 12.7%), nearly all within 4 weeks. Information was collected about the course of symptoms during the previous year, about social performance in a number of key activities (work, household, marriage, children, and personal relationships) and about life events occurring during the year, as well as an occupational history. By checking against the local psychiatric case register, it will be possible to discover which subjects contacted specialist services before and after the survey. There has also been a 6-month followup psychiatric examination of the cases found during the initial survey by Agency interviewers. Finally a series of 74 consecutive outpatients beginning new episodes of contact, and living in the same area, was interviewed by the MRC team in order to collect the same data, and followed up 4 weeks later. The purpose of this series of studies is to test hypotheses concerning the associations between adverse experiences occurring in childhood and more recently and present psychiatric state and use of specialist services (Bebbington et al., 1982).

The Ugandan survey was undertaken in 1972 by Dr. John Orley and a local research assistant using a translation into Luganda of the short form of the ninth edition. Nearly all the adult population of two rural villages, one 48 km and the other 16 km from the capital Kampala were interviewed (Orley and Wing, 1979).

The survey in Canberra (a sample from the electoral roll) was carried out by the Social Psychiatry Research Unit of the Australian National Health and Medical Research Council (Henderson et al., 1979). The London and Canberra surveys yielded remarkably similar rates of disorder: about 10% in women and 7% in men. Depressive disorders account for approximately two-thirds of this morbidity and are twice as common in women as in men. As would be expected, paranoid and hypomanic disorders are relatively rare in the population samples interviewed using the full PSE. The Ugandan rates for depressive disorder are much higher than in London and syndrome profiles show that pathologic guilt, subjective anergia, and hypochondriasis are more frequent (among women: 83%, 89%, and 39% compared with 23%, 32%, and 5%). The differences would probably be greater still if the full PSE had been used.

Considering the very few population samples yet available and the enormous size and diversity of the world's population, only very modest claims can be made. At the least, however, it can be suggested that the techniques show promise and deserve further use.

A comparison of ID levels found in the main London population survey (full PSE) compared with those in the consecutive outpatient series from the same area shows, as expected, that disorders in people referred to specialist services are much more severe. Data from the main London survey are presented in table 1. The more severe depressions in the outpatient series are characterized by symptoms such as delusions, retardation, and guilt

TABLE 1
Levels of Index of Definition in a Population Sample and a Consecutive Outpatient Series From the Same London Area.

ID level	*General population* %	*Outpatient series* %
1	44.8	—
2	30.8	4.1
3	9.1	4.1
4	6.4	4.1
5	5.8	21.6
6	2.3	32.4
7	0.9	28.4
8	—	5.4
	(N800 estimated from N310)	(N74)

which are uncommon in the population sample. Analysis of other data, including the clinical course, allows an estimate of how far severity of disorder can explain which individuals are selected for referral to specialists and whether different symptomatic patterns are related to earlier environmental experiences (Hurry et al., 1980; Tennant et al., 1980; Wing et al., 1981).

Uses and Limitations of the Techniques

The main instruction manual ended with a chapter on the uses and limitations of the PSE and CATEGO system (Wing et al., 1974, chapter 8). Five years later the uses have expanded somewhat and the limitations have expanded with them. Many of the limitations are built into the system, which would be useless without them, but results are liable to misuse if they are not remembered.

Organic, hysterical, and psychosomatic symptoms are not dealt with in any detail in the PSE; other instruments should be added in order to take account of them. The interview covers only the past month; earlier parts of the present episode, and previous episodes, need to be covered by using the Syndrome Check List. The SCL is necessarily less reliable than the PSE in general, although if rated from good clinical records, it can be used reliably and adds important information. Possibly causal factors are codified using the Etiology Schedule but this does not standardize the judgments themselves. No classification of clinical course has yet been tested for reliability.

Ratings based on observations of behavior, speech, and affect during the interview are less reliable than those of subjectively described symptoms, probably because of the fact that the latter cover a month's experience while the interview lasts only an hour or so. This limitation is particularly obvious when patients with chronic disorders (such as schizophrenic impairments) are examined rather than patients in acute episodes of disorder. Other techniques are required to measure such behavioral deficits and change (Wing, 1961; Wing and Brown, 1970) but they cannot, of course, assist in diagnosis of the acute state.

The fact that most symptoms can only be rated as absent, present in moderate degree, or present in severe degree has been regarded by some admirers of analog scales as a disadvantage. It is doubtful, however, whether extra *useful* information is gained by increasing the number of intermediate rating points or by using analog scales.

The differential definitions laid down for symptoms, and the rules adopted to distinguish between absent, moderate, and severe are not, and can never be, precise. A fair degree of reliability can be achieved but even high indices of reproducibility and repeatability may conceal differences in interpretation of particular symptoms. This is particularly crucial in the case of rare symptoms that are highly discriminating diagnostically. Examples of the misrating of first-rank symptoms are given in the first volume of the IPSS report (WHO, 1973, chapter 11). The training of raters is an essential part of the PSE procedure and there is no guarantee that those who use it without training will be able to achieve comparability with the results of users who have been trained.

The final limitation is the most obvious: the system has to be used as it is recommended to be. Comparability cannot be achieved in any other way. A degree of standardization means the introduction of a degree of rigidity. This does not mean, however, that the system does not incorporate flexibility; within limits it does. Nor does it mean that the system cannot be changed. On the contrary, it has changed very substantially and will continue to do so. But changes must be introduced in a controlled way, each one based upon a firm foundation of knowledge derived from earlier studies.

Having described these restrictions on the application of the system, it is fair to point out that there are definite advantages to be gained from operating it within the limits laid down. Its main uses are scientific, educational, and clinical, in that order, and are briefly summarized below:

1. To provide a standard description, in terms of symptoms, syndromes, or classes, of certain psychopathologic characteristics of groups of people during defined periods of time. This allows comparison, within given limits, between samples of referred and nonreferred patients, between samples from general populations that differ in sociocultural characteristics, and between subgroups within any one sample;
2. To allow a degree of comparability between the results of studies carried out by different investigators by providing a standard against which to describe the selection of subjects;
3. To measure change in clinical condition. Symptom and syndrome profiles and scores are the most convenient means of doing this;
4. To help investigate the taxonomy of psychiatric disorders by comparison with other systems of classification;
5. To provide an educational aid to clinical examination. Tapes or live interviews can be compared and any differences discussed in order to illuminate the technical problems of diagnostic interviewing and of differences in defining symptoms;
6. Since the system is simply a standardized clinical approach, many psychiatrists have found that their techniques of interviewing and ability to elicit psychopathology improve after using it. It is emphasized, however, that all clinical decisions must remain the responsibility of the psychiatrist and not of any particular instrument or aid.

Future Development

The development of the DSM-III has shown that it is possible to specify the criteria for using diagnostic categories more precisely, even in a national system, than would have been thought conceivable a generation ago. The idea behind such a system is not principally to ensure that clinical diagnostic practice becomes more uniform, though there might be such an effect. On the contrary, clinicians need not agree with the "standard" diagnosis at all. The idea is to promote comparability in statistical and research studies. The International Classification of Diseases is intended to be used in this way and the next, tenth, revision, is bound to be influenced by the methods of DSM-III.

The next step in the development of systems such as PSE-CATEGO is to construct a data base substantial enough to allow the application of several sets of algorithms, so different systems of classifying rules can be compared. The tenth edition of the PSE and associated techniques, now being tested, are designed to be part of such an international development (Wing, 1983).

Summary

The Present State Examination (PSE) is a structured interview for eliciting and rating 140 symptoms differentially defined in a glossary. It has now reached its ninth edition. An Index of Definition contains criteria for recognizing a threshold level of symptomatology above which a set of classifying rules (the CATEGO program) can be applied. There are accessory instruments for describing previous episodes and codifying etiological factors.

Various components of the system can be used for different purposes. Symptom and syndrome profiles and scores give a description of psychopathology at one moment of time and allow the frequency of cases in population surveys (for which a short version of the PSE is available), and the CATEGO classes make it possible to check the comparability of research studies carried out in different parts of the world as well as to aid the investigation of other taxonomies.

The reliability of the PSE has been tested in small-scale and in large international studies and a good deal is known about the problems of translation since there are versions in over 40 languages. The system has been found useful, within the limitations specified, in a wide range of studies and is being developed further in light of the results.

References

Bebbington, P., Hurry, J., Tennant, C., Sturt, E. & Wing, J. K. (1982), Epidemiology of mental disorders in Camberwell. *Psychol Med* II:561-580.

Brown, G. W. & Harris, T. (1978), *Social Origins of Depression.* London: Tavistock.

Cooper, J. E., Kendell, R. E., Gurland, B. J., Sharpe, L., Copeland, J. R. M. & Simon, R. (1972), *Psychiatric Diagnosis in New York and London.* Maudsley Monograph No. 20, London: Oxford University Press.

Cooper, J. E., Copeland, J. R. M., Brown, G. W., Harris, T. & Gourlay, A. J. (1977), Further studies on interviewer training and inter-rater reliability of the Present State Examination (PSE). *Psychol Med,* 7, 517-524.

Duncan-Jones, P. & Henderson, S. (1978), The use of a two-phase design in a prevalence survey. *Soc Psychiatr* 13, 4, 231-237.

Feighner, J. P., Robins, E., Guze, S. B., Woodruff, R. A., Winokur, G. & Munoz, R. (1972), Diagnostic criteria for use in psychiatric research. *Arch G Psychiatr* 26, 57-63.

Fleiss, J. L., Gurland, B. J. & Cooper, J. E. (1971), Some contributions to the measurement of psychopathology. *Br J Psychiatr* 119, 647-656.

Goldberg, D. P. (1972), *The Detection of Psychiatric Illness by Questionnaire.* London: Oxford University Press.
Henderson, S., Duncan-Jones, P., Byrne, D. G., Scott, R. & Adcock, S. (1979), Psychiatric disorder in Canberra: a standardized study of prevalence. *Acta Psychiatr.* In press.
Hirsch, S. R., Gaind, R., Rohde, P. D., Stevens, B. C. & Wing, J. K. (1973), Outpatient maintenance of chronic schizophrenic patients with long-acting fluphenazine: double-blind placebo trial. *Br Med J* 1:633-637.
Hirsch, S. R. & Leff, J. P. (1975), *Abnormality in Parents of Schizophrenics: A Review of the Literature and an Investigation of Communication Defects and Deviances.* London: Oxford University Press.
Hurry, J., Tennant, C. & Bebbington, P. (1980), Selective factors leading to psychiatric referral. *Acta Psychiatr.*
Kendell, R. E. (1973), Psychiatric diagnoses: a study of how they are made. *Br J Psychiatr* 122, 437-445.
Kendell, R. E., Everitt, B., Cooper, J. E., Sartorius, N. & David, M. E. (1968), Reliability of the Present State Examination. *Soc Psychiatr* 3:123-129.
Knights, A., Hirsch, S. R. & Platt, S. D. (1980), Measurement of clinical change as a function of brief admission to hospital. To be published.
Leff, J. (1977), The cross-cultural study of emotions. *Cult Med Psychiatr* 1:317-350.
Leff, J. P. & Wing, J. K. (1971), Trial of maintenance therapy in schizophrenia. *Br Med J* 3:599-604.
Lorr, M. (1965), A typology for functional psychotics. In: *Classification in Psychiatry and Psychopathology,* eds. Katz, M. M., Cole, J. O. & Barton, W. E. Chevy Chase, MD: National Institute of Mental Health.
Luria, R. E. & McHugh, P. R. (1974), Reliability and clinical utility of the "Wing" Present State Examination. *Arch Gen Psychiatr* 30, 866-871.
Orley, J. & Wing, J. K. (1979), Psychiatric disorders in two African villages. *Arch Gen Psychiatr* 36, 513-520.
Spitzer, R. L., Endicott, J. & Fleiss, J. L. (1967), Instruments and recording forms for evaluating psychiatric status and history. *Compr Psychiatr* 8:321-343.
Sturt, E. (1981), Hierarchical patterns in the distribution of psychiatric symptoms. *Psychol Med* II:783-794.
Sturt, E., Bebbington, P., Hurry, J. & Tennant, C. (1981), The PSE used by interviewers from a survey agency. *Psychol Med* II:185-192.
Tennant, C., Hurry, J. & Bebbington, P. (1980), Parent-child separations during childhood: their reaction to adult morbidity and to psychiatric referral. *Acta Psychiatr* Sup. 285:324-331.
Urwin, P. & Gibbons, J. L. (1979), Psychiatric diagnosis in self-poisoning patients. *Psychol Med* 9:501-507.
Wing, J. K. (1961), A simple and reliable subclassification of chronic schizophrenia. *J Ment Sci* 107:862.
Wing, J. K. (1968), Social treatment of mental illness. In: *Studies in Psychiatry,* eds. Shepherd, M. & Davies, D. L. London: Oxford University Press.

Wing, J. K. (1976), A technique for studying psychiatric morbidity in inpatient and outpatient series and in general population samples. *Psychol Med* 6:665-671.

Wing, J. K., Bebbington, P., Hurry, J. & Tennant, C. (1981), The prevalence in the general population of disorders familiar to psychiatrists in hospital practice. In: *What is a Case? The Problem of Definition in Psychiatric Community Surveys,* eds. Wing, J. K., Bebbington, P. & Robins, L. N. London: Grant McIntyre.

Wing, J. K., Birley, J. L. T., Cooper, J. E., Graham, P. & Isaacs, A. (1967), Reliability of a procedure for measuring and classifying "Present Psychiatric State." *Br J Psychiatr* 113, 499-575.

Wing, J. K. & Brown, G. W. (1970), *Institutionalism and Schizophrenia.* London: Cambridge University Press.

Wing, J. K., Cooper, J. E. & Sartorius, N. (1974), *Description and Classification of Psychiatric Symptoms.* London: Cambridge University Press.

Wing, J. K. & Hailey, A. M. (1972), *Evaluating a Community Psychiatric Service.* London: Oxford University Press.

Wing, J. K., Nixon, J. M., Mann, S. A. & Leff, J. P. (1977a), Reliability of the PSE (ninth edition) used in a population survey. *Psychol Med* 7:505-516.

Wing, J. K., Nixon, J., von Cranach, M. & Strauss, A. (1977b), Further developments of the PSE and CATEGO system. *Arch Psychiatr Nervenkr* 224:151-160.

Wing, J. K., Henderson, A. S. & Winckle, M. (1977c), Brief communication: The rating of symptoms by a psychiatrist and a non-psychiatrist: a study of patients referred from general practice. *Psychol Med* 7:713-715.

Wing, J. K. & Sturt, E. (1978), *The PSE-ID-CATEGO System: A Supplementary Manual.* London: Institute of Psychiatry.

Wing, J. K. (1983), The use and misuse of the PSE. *Br J Psychiatr* 143:111-117.

World Health Organization. (1973), *The International Pilot Study of Schizophrenia,* Vol. 1. Geneva: WHO.

Wynne, L. C. & Singer, M. T. (1963), Thought disorder and family relations of schizophrenics I. A research strategy. *Arch Gen Psychiatr* 9:191.

Afterword

Psychiatric Epidemiology in the 1980s, a WHO Perspective

A. JABLENSKY

Although by the early 1980s the application of the epidemiologic method to the study of mental disorders has a long history, its major contributions to the understanding and control of these disorders probably still lie ahead. Several of the papers in this volume refer, as postscripts or reviews, to milestones of epidemiologic research in psychiatry. Others outline recent methodologic advances and types of studies that hold promises for the future. To a certain extent, therefore, this publication presents a selection of past achievements and gives the reader a few glimpses of developments that might, in the future, take us one step further. Of course, it is not possible to present a panorama of the current state of epidemiologic knowledge about the mental disorders in a single volume, and the choice of themes in this book shows that a comprehensive overview was not the aim. With one exception, significant, or potentially significant, developments in parts of the world other than Europe and North America are not included (let us hope they will be, in a future volume), although at present the generation of innovations and interesting findings in psychiatric epidemiology is not limited to the technologically advanced countries.

Short of epoch-making discoveries, psychiatric epidemiology has reached a stage where advances in knowledge can be cumulative, and studies carried out in different parts of the world point to several areas of consensus regarding the nature, patterns of occurrence, course, and prognosis of mental disorders.

First, epidemiologic research has demonstrated that psychiatric disorders are ubiquitous (no human group, society, or culture has been convincingly shown to be free of mental illness) and rank among the most serious public health problems because of their prevalence, duration, and social consequences (WHO, 1980). Yet, such generalizations should not obscure the complexity of the picture. Mental disorders are not a homogeneous class of phenomena, their rates of incidence and prevalence probably vary across different populations, and epidemiologic correlates found in one setting (e.g., with social class) are not necessarily present in other settings. Even the "hard" data of genetics are not generalizable, and there is a long way to go before the map of descriptive epidemiology of mental disorders will be fully charted.

Second, the search for causes is no longer chained to the metaphysical "nature or nurture" paradigm, even though no new paradigm to replace it has yet emerged. Genetic mechanisms operate through environmentally and culturally determined pathways, and environmental insults and stresses seem to be pathogenic mainly when they fall on intrinsic vulnerabilities. There is evidence suggesting that this may be so in the case of schizophrenia, and many observations point to the validity of this principle in other groups of disorders, including the neuroses. However, a mere recognition of the multifactorial causation of mental disorders is only a way of stating the obvious, and epidemiologic research that does not attempt to elucidate necessary and sufficient causes is unlikely to take us farther afield. Counts of incidence and prevalence are not very informative on their own, unless they serve as tools for disentangling etiologically meaningful connections.

Third, the phenomenology and natural history of the major groups of mental disorders, seen from the epidemiologic perspective, appear to be less uniform than existing classifications and diagnostic concepts based on clinical observations of symptoms, course, and outcome would suggest. This diversity calls for revisions and adjustments of the nosological boundaries.

Fourth, there is, at present, a great variety of treatment and service systems and therapeutic approaches whose impact on the epidemiology of the mental disorders has not been fully evaluated. There is evidence that certain aspects of chronicity in the mental disorders are the result of adverse social reactions to the phenomena of illness, rather than intrinsic characteristics of a morbid process, and there is hope that much of the disability associated with psychiatric morbidity can be contained, reduced, or even prevented.

The tools of psychiatric epidemiology are today considerably more refined and efficient than they were two or three decades ago, and the imputation of a lack of objective measurement in psychiatric research has now less ground than in the past. Among the many areas open for epidemiologic research, there are two approaches that are particularly capable of enhancing the effectiveness of the epidemiologic method.

One is the development of a *comparative* epidemiology of the mental disorders in different populations. This strategy is closely related to the cross-cultural approach but is not identical with it because comparative studies can also be done within the same culture. What needs to be compared is the variation in incidence rates, expectancy of disease, and other epidemiologic indicators, in relation to genetic, ecological, and cultural characteristics of populations selected for their particular suitability to serve as natural laboratories. With a few notable exceptions, which include investigations of genetic isolates and population groups with unusual patterns of occurrence of specific disorders, this approach has not yet been systematically applied. An international register of unusual populations and findings of special epidemiologic interest could be a valuable tool in this respect.

A second type of strategy is the *multidisciplinary* study of the major groups of mental disorders. Few, if any, studies have attempted to test in an epidemiologic context a hypothesis derived from biological investigations. Biological psychiatry has not yet made much use of epidemiologic sampling strategies in the selection of subjects for investigation. The epidemiology of mental disorders has been studied in isolation from the epidemiology of physical disease, although some important etiologic and pathogenetic clues could be found on the interface of the two approaches. In contrast, it can be said that the link between psychiatric epidemiology and the sociological study of mental illness has been a fairly close one. The main bridges that are needed, therefore, appear to be those between psychiatric epidemiology and the biomedical disciplines.

Regarding such developments, the World Health Organization can play a useful role. Since 1959, WHO has made many efforts to promote the epidemiologic approach to the study and control of mental disorders, and in recent years it has initiated and coordinated a great number of multicenter and cross-cultural projects (reviewed by Sartorius, 1980). Several areas of the WHO Mental Health Program deserve special mention in this context.

The standardization of psychiatric diagnosis, classification, and statistics and the development of methods that should lead to a common language in the mental health disciplines, is an important objective of WHO. The collaboration of experts from more than 40 countries in the period 1965-1973 led to a revision of the classification of mental disorders in the International Classification of Diseases (ICD-9) and the development of a glossary that is now an integral part of the classification (WHO, 1978). A multiaxial classification of the mental disorders in childhood, classifications of cerebrovascular disorders, psychiatric impairments and disabilities, alcohol-related problems, a dictionary of epilepsy, and the beginnings of a standard psychiatric nomenclature and terminology are also among the products of this particular program. Since 1979 WHO, in a joint project with the U.S. Alcohol, Drug Abuse, and Mental Health Administration, has initiated a world-wide review of the state of psychiatric diagnosis and classification in the 1970s, with a view to launching a new program of multicenter collaborating studies that should provide a valid empirical base for future revisions and improvements of psychiatric nosology and diagnosis (WHO, 1981).

Another program area in which WHO is playing a unique role is the development of cross-cultural collaborative studies of specific psychiatric disorders or mental health problems. The International Pilot Study of Schizophrenia (1965-1976), the first large-scale collaborative effort of this kind, involved teams of investigators in nine countries and included an initial assessment and a 2-year and a 5-year followup of 1,200 patients (WHO, 1973; WHO, 1979). The project was initially designed as a methodologic and feasibility study aiming to apply standardized assessment techniques to series of patients diagnosed as schizophrenic in different settings and to evaluate the comparability of the concept of schizophrenia across several cultures. A major finding of the study was that schizophrenic patients with similar characteristics could be found in all the cultures in which the investigations took place. In the course of the followup, however, it became clear that in spite of initial clinical similarity, these patients developed different patterns of course and outcome, and that on the whole, their prognosis was more favorable in certain developing countries (e.g., Nigeria and India) than in industrialized societies. Considering the complexity of all the factors involved, it was not possible to give an unequivocal answer to the various questions evoked by such a finding. A new study, on Determinants of Outcome of Severe Mental Disorders, was designed and started in 1977 by 12 centers in 10 countries, to collect data on the incidence of various subtypes of schizophrenic disorders and other functional psychoses in defined catchment areas. The study also aims to test specific hypotheses about factors that may be implicated in the differential prognosis of such conditions in various cultures.

Other collaborative studies, initiated and coordinated by WHO, include a cross-cultural study on depressive disorders, a multicenter study on impairments and disabilities of psychiatric patients, and a case-control prospective evaluation of the psychosomatic sequelae of female sterilization. The first of these, which included the standardized assessment and 5-year followup of about 700 depressive patients contacting treatment agencies in five countries, showed a great similarity in the clinical manifestations of depression in different cultures (Sartorius et al., 1980). An additional investigation, based on monitoring of nonpsychiatric health services, indicated that up to 5%-12% of the caseload of general practitioners and general outpatient departments consist of patients with clinically manifest depressive illnesses. The study on impairments and disabilities of psychiatric patients (focusing mainly on schizophrenia) in six countries is currently collecting prospective data on some 700 patients to test hypotheses about the interrelationships between clinical course and the degree of social disability (Jablensky et al., 1980). The study on psychosomatic sequelae of female sterilization in five countries aims to evaluate certain psychosocial aspects of family planning programs and, in addition, to collect baseline data on the mental state of samples of healthy women in several cultures.

All these studies have contributed to the development of cross-culturally applicable technology for mental health research, and more than 20 different assessment instruments, ranging from the Present State Examination (Wing et al., 1974) in its 25 language versions, to schedules for assessment of depressive disorders (WHO/SADD), disability (DAS), life events (LES) are now available.

Epidemiologic approaches are also used in other WHO-coordinated studies whose primary goal is the development of new methods for mental health service delivery or evaluation of treatment. Thus the study on Strategies for Extending Mental Health Care in developing countries, which tested new techniques for the provision of essential mental health care in the context of primary health care in several countries in Africa, Asia and Latin America, included a survey of the types of psychiatric problems encountered at community health centers in rural areas. It was found that more than 13% of the population receiving services at such centers present manifest psychiatric problems (Harding et al., 1980). Another WHO study is at present testing the dose/response relationship for antidepressants, neuroleptics, and minor tranquilizers in patient series drawn from diverse, including tropical populations (Vartanian, 1980). Yet another study has developed a simplified, reliable technology for carrying out census investigations of psychiatric patients using different kinds of health services.

Within this broad spectrum of WHO work in the field of psychiatric epidemiology, a special place is occupied by training activities and institution-building. The overriding priority in this respect is cooperation with Third

World countries where the development of psychiatric epidemiology is closely linked with the planning of services. The overwhelming size of the problem of mental disorders in such countries, especially when seen in relation to the scarce resources, makes the adoption of ready-made solutions from other parts of the world questionable, to say the least. Epidemiologic thinking and data can stimulate the search for alternative approaches to service development, and encouraging experiments are already taking place.

WHO contributes to such developments not only by providing fellowships to Third World researchers, but also by directly organizing training courses, seminars, and workshops tailored to specific needs. One such activity is the WHO Joint Training Program in Epidemiological and Social Psychiatry which started in 1976 and has by now provided advanced training experience in epidemiologic methods to more than 30 postgraduate students from developing countries. The program consists of a 4-month intensive course during which a group of trainees spend periods of work at leading WHO research centers in Denmark, United Kingdom, Federal Republic of Germany, and Czechoslovakia, and at least a month in a center of excellence in a developing country (India or Columbia). Another form of training is the brief, intensive seminar organized on a country or regional basis, in which local developments in psychiatric epidemiology are reviewed and focused training in new methods and approaches is provided by a faculty of visiting experts.

A mechanism through which WHO implements its activities in the field of psychiatric epidemiology is the network of over 40 collaborating and field research centers in all parts of the world. Some of these centers are designated for a specific research project, while others have broader functions and serve as a resource for training, information, and consultation to public health authorities in the country or region.

This overview of the activities of WHO shows that an infrastructure for the global advancement of epidemiologic research in the mental health field is already in existence. The question of how it could best be used and how the priorities should be selected for future collaborative work now occupies the attention of a broad expert constituency in connection with the preparation of the next medium-term WHO mental health program (1984-1989). Some of the technical options for this period include studies of the variation in the incidence of the major groups of mental disorders and their sociocultural and demographic correlates; family and pedigree studies; search for genetic and disease markers in epidemiologic population samples; assessment of environmental influences on brain development and behavior (e.g., effects of nutrition, environmental pollution, radiation, infectious and parasitic diseases, stress, and psychosocial factors).

The experience accumulated in the mental health program so far suggests that in the 1980s WHO will be in a good position to play a leadership role in the international coordination and promotion of epidemiologic research in the mental health field.

References

Harding, T. W., de Arango, M. V., Baltazar, J. et al. (1980), Mental disorders in primary health care: A study of their frequency and diagnosis in four developing countries. *Psychol Med* 10:231-241.

Jablensky, A., Schwarz, R. & Tomov, T. (1980), WHO collaborative study on impairments and disabilities in schizophrenic patients. *Acta Psychiat Scand* 285:152-159.

Sartorius, N. (1980), The research component of the WHO mental health program. *Psychol Med* 10: 175-185.

Sartorius, N., Jablensky, A., Gulbinat, W. & Ernbert, G. (1980), WHO collaborative study: assessment of depressive disorders. *Psychol Med* 10:743-749.

Vartanian, F. E. (1980), WHO program activities in the area of biological psychiatry. *Zh Nevropatol Psihiatr* 80:123-128.

Wing, J. K., Cooper, J. E. & Sartorius, N. (1974), *Measurement and Classification of Psychiatric Symptoms.* London: Cambridge University Press.

World Health Organization (1973), *Report of the International Pilot Study of Schizophrenia,* Vol. I, Geneva: WHO.

World Health Organization (1978) *Mental Disorders: Glossary and Guide to Their Classification in Accordance with the Ninth Revision of the International Classification of Diseases.* Geneva: WHO.

World Health Organization (1979), *Schizophrenia. An International Follow-up Study.* Chichester: Wiley and Sons.

World Health Organization (1980), *Sixth Report on the World Health Situation,* Part I, Geneva: WHO, pp. 153-163.

World Health Organization (1981), *Current State of Diagnosis and Classification in the Mental Health Field. A Report From the WHO/ADAMHA Joint Project on Diagnosis and Classification of Mental Disorders and Alcohol-and Drug-Related Problems.* Geneva: WHO/MNH/81.11.

About the Contributors

JEROME K. MYERS, Professor and Chairman of the Department of Sociology at Yale University, is co-editor with MYRNA M. WEISSMAN, of Volume 4 of the monograph series in psychosocial epidemiology entitled *Community Surveys*. Born in Lancaster, Pennsylvania, Myers attended Yale University where he received the doctorate in sociology in 1950 and has continued to teach until the present. He has served as a consultant to numerous committees and organizations that interface with medical sociology and psychosocial epidemiology. His current commitments include chairing the Epidemiologic and Services Research Review Committee of NIMH and consulting to the United States Public Health Service, the Connecticut Department of Mental Health, and the American Nurses Foundation. He is the Principal Investigator of the Epidemiologic Catchment Area Research Program funded by NIMH, based in New Haven, Connecticut. It was the first such funded program; subsequently two additional centers have been funded at Washington University in St. Louis and The Johns Hopkins University in Baltimore. Myers has published numerous papers in the areas of his research interest: social psychiatry and medical sociology, psychiatric utilization review, and evaluation in epidemiologic and field studies. Professor Myers' current address is the Department of Sociology, Yale University, 140 Prospect Street, New Haven, Connecticut 06520.

MYRNA M. WEISSMAN, Professor of Psychiatry and Epidemiology at Yale University, was born in Boston, Massachusetts and was educated at the University of Pennsylvania and Yale University, where she received a doctorate in chronic disease epidemiology in 1974. Author of over 200 articles and books including the pioneering treatise, *The Depressed Woman: A Study of Social Relationships* (together with Eugene S. Paykel) as well as *Interpersonal Psychotherapy of Depression* (together with Gerald L. Klerman, Bruce Rounsaville & Eve Chevron), Weissman has distinguished herself as a major figure in the application of epidemiologic techniques to the evaluation of pharmacologic and psychotherapic interventions in the management of affective illness. She was formerly Visiting Senior Scholar at the Institute of Medicine at the National Academy of Sciences (1979-1980), recipient of the Foundations Fund Prize for Research in Psychiatry, and a member of the White House Task Force on Epidemiology of Mental Health of the President's Commission on Mental Health (1977-1978). Included among her current memberships and affiliations are the Collegium Internationale Neuro-Psychopharmacologicum, the American College of Neuropsychopharmacology, the International Epidemiological Association, the Society for Epidemiologic Research, and the Society for Life History Research in Psychopathology. She is an editorial consultant to the *Archives of General Psychiatry*, the *Journal of Nervous and Mental Disease*, and the *Journal of Health and Social Behavior*. Professor Weissman's current address is the Depression Research Unit, Yale University School of Medicine, 904 Howard Avenue, Suite 2A, New Haven, Connecticut 06519.

URI AVIRAM is at the School of Social Work at the University of Tel Aviv, in Israel.

ROGER A. BELL is Associate Professor, Department of Psychiatry and Behavioral Sciences, University of Louisville, School of Medicine, Health Sciences Center, Louisville, Kentucky, 40292.

JOANNE M. BUHL was Research Assistant in the Department of Psychiatry and Behavioral Sciences at the University of Louisville School of Medicine, at Louisville, Kentucky, 40208. She is presently Research Assistant in the Department of Psychiatry, University of Florida, Gainesville, Florida.

BRUCE P. DOHRENWEND is Foundations Fund for Research in Psychiatry Professor at Columbia University and Head of the Social Psychiatry Research Unit. With his wife, Barbara Snell Dohrenwend, Professor Dohrenwend is editor of Volume III of *Monographs in Psychosocial Epidemiology* on the study of stressful life events. His address is the Social Psychiatry Research Unit of Columbia University, College of Physicians and Surgeons, 100 Haven Avenue, Tower 3-19H, New York, New York, 10032.

H. WARREN DUNHAM is Professor Emeritus of Sociology at Wayne State University and Professor of Psychiatry at the State University of New York at Stony Brook. Professor Dunham's address is 15 Stephens Path, Port Jefferson, New York, 11777.

WILLIAM W. EATON is Associate Professor, Department of Mental Hygiene, Johns Hopkins School of Hygiene and Public Health, 615 N. Wolfe Street, Baltimore, Maryland, 21205.

JEAN ENDICOTT is Professor of Clinical Psychology, Department of Psychiatry, Columbia University, and Director, Research Assessment and Training Unit, New York State Psychiatric Institute, 722 W. 168th Street, New York, New York, 10032.

ANITA KASSEN FISCHER is a Research Associate in Psychiatry at the College of Physicians and Surgeons of Columbia University, 722 West 168th Street, New York, New York, 10032.

TÓMAS HELGASON is Professor of Psychiatry at the National University Hospital, 101 Reykjavik, Iceland.

AUGUST B. HOLLINGSHEAD, prior to his death, was William Graham Sumner Professor Emeritus of the Department of Sociology, Yale University.

ASSEN JABLENSKY is Senior Medical Officer in the Division of Mental Health of the World Health Organization, 1211 Geneva 27, Switzerland.

THOMAS S. LANGNER is Professor of Epidemiology in the Division of Epidemiology of the School of Public Health of Columbia University, 600 West 168th Street, New York, New York, 10032.

PAUL V. LEMKAU is Professor of Mental Hygiene at the School of Hygiene and Mental Health of The Johns Hopkins University, 615 North Wolfe Street, Baltimore, Maryland, 21205.

ITZHAK LEVAV is Visiting Associate Professor of Psychiatry at the Social Psychiatry Research Unit of the College of Physicians and Surgeons of Columbia University, 100 Haven Avenue, Tower 3-194, New York, New York, 10032.

BEN Z. LOCKE is Chief of the Center for Epidemiologic Studies, Division of Biometry and Epidemiology, National Institute of Mental Health, 5600 Fishers Lane, Rockville, Maryland, 20857.

JANE M. MURPHY is in the Department of Psychiatry at Harvard Medical School and at the Massachusetts Mental Health Center, 58 Fenwood Road, Boston, Massachusetts, 02115.

LENORE SAWYER RADLOFF is Social Science Statistician at the Center for Epidemiologic Studies of the National Institute of Mental Health, Room 18C-05, 5600 Fishers Lane, Rockville, Maryland, 20857.

DARREL A. REGIER is Director of the Division of Biometry and Epidemiology of the National Institute of Mental Health, 5600 Fishers Lane, Rockville, Maryland, 20857.

LEE N. ROBINS, Professor of Sociology in Psychiatry at Washington University in St. Louis, is the editor of Volume VI of *Monographs in Psychosocial Epidemiology* on drug use studies. Dr. Robins' address is the Department of Psychiatry, Barnes and Renard Hospitals, Washington University, 4940 Audubon Avenue, St. Louis, Missouri, 63110.

CATHERINE E. ROSS is an Associate Professor in the Department of Sociology at the University of Illinois, Urbana, Illinois, 61801.

JOHN J. SCHWAB is Professor of Psychiatry and Chairman of the Department of Psychiatry and Behavioral Sciences of the University of Louisville School of Medicine at Louisville, Kentucky, 40208.

PATRICK E. SHROUT is Assistant Professor of Public Health (Biostatistics) Columbia University, 600 West 168th Street, New York, New York, 10032.

ROBERT L. SPITZER is Professor of Psychiatry at Columbia University's College of Physicians and Surgeons and Chief, Biometric Research Department of the New York Psychiatric Institute. His address is Biometrics Research, 722 West 168th Street, New York, New York, 10032.

LEO SROLE is Professor of Psychiatry at Columbia University's College of Physicians and Surgeons, 722 West 168th Street, New York, New York, 10032. He is also Visiting Professor of Social Science at the New York University Graduate School of Arts and Sciences.

CARL A. TAUBE is Deputy Director, Division of Biometry and Epidemiology, National Institute of Mental Health, Parklawn Building, Room 18C-26, 5600 Fishers Lane, Rockville, Maryland, 20857.

GEORGE WARHEIT is Professor of Psychiatry at the University of Florida and guest editor of the forthcoming volume on needs assessment in *Monographs in Psychosocial Epidemiology*. Dr. Warheits's address is Box J-256 at the University of Florida, Gainsville, Florida, 32610.

JANET B. W. WILLIAMS is Assistant Professor of Clinical Psychiatric Social Work (in Psychiatry) at Columbia University and Research Scientist at New York State Psychiatric Institute. Ms. Williams' address is the Psychiatric Institute, 722 West 168th Street, New York, New York, 10032.

J. K. WING is Professor of Social Psychiatry and Director of the MRC Social Psychiatry Unit of the Institute of Psychiatry, DeCrespigny Park, London SE5 8AF, England.